Advance Praise for *C. Miller Fisher*

Dr. Fisher's sharing his sense of human neurology was the defining experience for me as a neurologist and scientist. Nothing has really come close. Lou Caplan's biography of Dr. Fisher's thinking, and description of his methods of observation and analysis will bring others into his orbit. If not, then I fear science may wait a very long time until another similarly extraordinary person achieves his level of insight into how the human brain works.

—Walter Koroshetz, MD, Director, National Institute of Neurological Disorders and Stroke

Caplan has captured the remarkable life and times of one of the most admired and recognized neurologists of the 20th century. The personal attributes of Dr. Fisher are intertwined with the numerous advances he brought to the clinical and pathological appreciation of many neurological diseases and syndromes, some of which eponymously bear his name—the Miller Fisher variant of Guillain-Barre syndrome for example. This book is a must read for any scholar interested in advances in medicine and how important thoughtful approaches and new organizational thinking move the central tenets of the field. A great contribution.

—Joseph Martin, MD, PhD, Edward R. and Anne G. Lefler Professor Emeritus of Neurobiology and Former Dean of the Faculty of Medicine, Harvard Medical School, Boston, MA

Lou Caplan has written a brilliant and insightful account of the extraordinary life of C. Miller Fisher, the pioneer of modern stroke medicine. He not only recounts his pivotal contributions to both stroke and general neurology, but provides an insight into his unique personality, his humanity, his ability to meticulously study and document a vast range of cerebrovascular and other brain disorders, and his seminal contributions to modern therapeutic strategies in stroke. Caplan chronicles Fisher's wartime experiences through to his formative and then hugely productive years at the Montreal Neurological Institute, the Boston City, and Massachusetts General Hospitals.

This book is a gem and captures the essence of a remarkable neurologist and neuropathologist, with an amazing mind. A riveting read for all interested in the human brain and the compelling story of one of its greatest medical explorers, written by an esteemed stroke neurologist, close colleague, and friend of Miller Fisher.

—Professor Stephen Davis, AM, MD, FRCPE, FRACP, FAHMS,
Director Melbourne Brain Centre, Royal Melbourne Hospital,
Professor of Translational Neuroscience,
University of Melbourne, Parkville,
Victoria, Australia

C. Miller Fisher
Stroke in the 20th Century

Louis R. Caplan, MD
Professor Neurology, Harvard University
Senior Neurologist, Beth Israel Deaconess Medical Center, Boston, MA

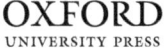

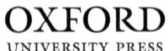

Oxford University Press is a department of the University of Oxford. It furthers the University's objective of excellence in research, scholarship, and education by publishing worldwide. Oxford is a registered trade mark of Oxford University Press in the UK and certain other countries.

Published in the United States of America by Oxford University Press
198 Madison Avenue, New York, NY 10016, United States of America.

© Oxford University Press 2020

All rights reserved. No part of this publication may be reproduced, stored in a retrieval system, or transmitted, in any form or by any means, without the prior permission in writing of Oxford University Press, or as expressly permitted by law, by license, or under terms agreed with the appropriate reproduction rights organization. Inquiries concerning reproduction outside the scope of the above should be sent to the Rights Department, Oxford University Press, at the address above.

You must not circulate this work in any other form
and you must impose this same condition on any acquirer.

Library of Congress Cataloging-in-Publication Data
Names: Caplan, Louis R., author.
Title: C. Miller Fisher : stroke in the 20th century / Louis R. Caplan.
Description: New York, NY : Oxford University Press, [2020] |
Includes bibliographical references and index.
Identifiers: LCCN 2020002323 (print) | LCCN 2020002324 (ebook) |
ISBN 9780190603656 (hardback) | ISBN 9780190603670 (epub) |
ISBN 9780190603687
Subjects: LCSH: Fisher, Charles Miller, 1913–2012. |
Neurologists—Canada—Biography. | Cerebrovascular disease—Treatment.
Classification: LCC R464.F48 C37 2020 (print) | LCC R464.F48 (ebook) |
DDC 616.80092 [B]—dc23
LC record available at https://lccn.loc.gov/2020002323
LC ebook record available at https://lccn.loc.gov/2020002324

This material is not intended to be, and should not be considered, a substitute for medical or other professional advice. Treatment for the conditions described in this material is highly dependent on the individual circumstances. And, while this material is designed to offer accurate information with respect to the subject matter covered and to be current as of the time it was written, research and knowledge about medical and health issues is constantly evolving and dose schedules for medications are being revised continually, with new side effects recognized and accounted for regularly. Readers must therefore always check the product information and clinical procedures with the most up-to-date published product information and data sheets provided by the manufacturers and the most recent codes of conduct and safety regulation. The publisher and the authors make no representations or warranties to readers, express or implied, as to the accuracy or completeness of this material. Without limiting the foregoing, the publisher and the authors make no representations or warranties as to the accuracy or efficacy of the drug dosages mentioned in the material. The authors and the publisher do not accept, and expressly disclaim, any responsibility for any liability, loss, or risk that may be claimed or incurred as a consequence of the use and/or application of any of the contents of this material.

Acquire a teacher and mentor for yourself.
Choose companions and colleagues for learning.
Render everyone the benefit of the doubt.
—Joshua, son of Perichiah (as cited in Berkson, William. *Pirke Avot: Timeless Wisdom for Modern Life*. Philadelphia, PA: Jewish Publication Society, 2010, p. 185)

CONTENTS

Acknowledgments ix
C. Miller Fisher's Life: Timeline xi
Introduction xiii

PART I: Early Years and University and Medical Training

1. Fisher's Early Years   3

2. Toronto University and Medical School and Internship in Detroit   12

PART II: War Experiences

3. World War II and Experience as a British Naval Officer   25

4. Prisoner of War, 1941–1944   39

PART III: Repatriation and Reintroduction to Medicine and Neurology in Montreal

5. Reintroduction to Medicine and Neurology in Montreal   67

PART IV: Neuropathology Fellowship and Experience as a Neurologist Specializing in Stroke

6. Pathology at Boston City Hospital   83

7. Montreal, 1950–1954   106

PART V: Boston and Massachusetts General Hospital: Fisher's Personal Characteristics, Methods, and Major Contributions

8. Boston and Massachusetts General Hospital: Fisher's Activities and Methods   *133*

9. Fisher's Collegiality, Personality Traits and Idiosyncrasies, and "Rules"   *156*

10. Neurological Examination of the Stuporous Patient, Lacunar Infarction, Intracerebral Hemorrhage, and Aneurysmal Subarachnoid Hemorrhage   *170*

11. Carotid Artery and Cerebral Atherosclerosis, Transient Ischemic Attacks, Symptoms and Signs Correlated with Lesions at Various Brain Locations, Cervical and Cranial Arterial Dissections, and Hydrocephalus and Gait Abnormalities   *192*

12. Atrial Fibrillation, Memory, Timing and Quantity of Behavior, Randomized Therapeutic Trials and Anticoagulation of Brain Ischemia Patients, and Headache and Migraine   *213*

13. Eye Signs, Syndromes, and Reviews and Opinions   *232*

PART VI: The Last Decades of Fisher's Life

14. Retirement and Beyond: Fisher's Last Decades   *243*

Name Index   *255*
Subject Index   *259*

ACKNOWLEDGMENTS

This volume would not have been possible without the detailed memoirs that C. Miller Fisher wrote during his life. I have relied on his memory and notes taken during the various events described in this volume. I also relied on Fisher's comments made during an interview that I did with him in 1993. His son, Dr. Hugh Fisher, his daughter Elizabeth Fisher, and his daughter-in-law, Susan Fisher were helpful at all times in obtaining additional information and pictures and reviewing many of the chapters. The remainder of Fisher's family and relatives—Jamie and Sally Patterson and Charles and Elaine Grierson—provided much biographical information about the family and also provided many of the pictures that are included in the volume.

The following libraries were very cooperative and helpful in directing me to historical data: the libraries at Waterloo, the Montreal Neurological Institute, and the Montreal General Hospital, Ontario, Canada; the Countway Library of Medicine at Harvard Medical School and its Center for the History of Medicine, Boston; and the Agoos Medical Library at Beth Israel Deaconess Medical Center (BIDMC), Boston. Especially helpful at these libraries were Nathan Morris, Julia Whelan, Diane Young, and Margo Coletti at BIDMC; and Jessica Murphy, Jack Eckert, and Scott Padulsky at the Countway Library of Medicine. Access to the C. Miller Fisher collection at the Center for the History of Medicine was facilitated by Jack Eckert. Richard Leblanc was very helpful at the Montreal Neurological Institute in supplying photographs and helping me navigate the institute's library.

Many physicians who were colleagues of Dr. Fisher and/or mine were immensely helpful in providing information and reviewing chapters in this volume: Drs. Garth Bray, Joe Martin, Alan Ropper, Martin Samuels, Eva Andermann, Fred Andermann, Robert Ackerman, J. Phillip Kistler, Jay P. Mohr, Ron Kobayashi, Verne Caveness, Merit Cudkowicz, Walter Koroshetz, Ken Tyler, Praful Dalal, Ernie Picard, Jerry Winkler, Robert

Daroff, Steve Cramer, Joe Rizzo, and others. Joe Hanaway was especially helpful in long discussions with me on Fisher's time in Montreal, at McGill University, and at Massachusetts General Hospital before my time there.

A very special thanks to Dr. Robert Hart, Dr. Tom Brott, Dr. Karen Thallinger Brott, Dr. Joe Hanaway, and Charley Radin for reading the entire document and making important suggestions and critiques.

The Oxford University Press staff, especially Craig Panner, Emily Samulski, and William Allen, shepherded the book through its paces in a very professional and collegial manner. Craig read several drafts and made suggestions that helped me submit the final manuscript. My secretaries Ana Tyree and Leslie Magson were very helpful during the long writing and editing process. Leslie was instrumental in helping obtain permission for some of the figures.

Most of all, I thank my wife of more than half a century, Brenda Fields Caplan, for understanding the many hours, days, and weeks away that writing this volume dictated. My time spent on creating this volume also impacted on my children—Laura, Dan, Jonathan, David, Jeremy, and Benjamin—and their spouses and children, and I thank them for their understanding and patience.

C. MILLER FISHER'S LIFE: TIMELINE

December 5, 1913: Birth—Waterloo, Ontario, Canada
1931–1937: University of Toronto College and Medical School, Toronto, Ontario, Canada
1938–1939: Medical internship, Henry Ford Hospital, Detroit, Michigan
Summer 1939: House staff, Royal Victoria Hospital Montreal, Quebec, Canada
November 1939: Married Doris Stiefelmeyer in Montreal
May 1940–1941: Surgeon-Lieutenant, Royal Canadian Navy, Montreal
May 4, 1941: Sunk at sea and captured by the Germans during World War II
1941–November 1944: German prisoner-of-war camp, Sandbostel, Germany
1945–1948: Reintroduction to medicine in Montreal
1949–1950: Neuropathology Fellowship, Boston City Hospital, Boston, Massachusetts
1950–1954: Staff Neurologist and Neuropathologist, Montreal General Hospital, Montreal
1954–2004: Staff Neurologist, Massachusetts General Hospital, Harvard Medical School, Boston, Massachusetts
1980: Official "retirement" from active Massachusetts General Hospital practice
2008: Death of his wife Doris and move to Albany, New York
April 14, 2012: Fisher died in Albany at age 98 years

INTRODUCTION

Views of stroke almost completely flip-flopped during the 20th century. At the midpoint of the century, there was little public or medical interest in stroke. By the end of the century, stroke care and research were among the most intensely active areas within all of medicine. This book is the story of that change and of one physician, Dr. C. Miller Fisher, a main architect and driver of that change.

The word "stroke" indicates being *stricken* with sudden loss of brain function. The term dates back to the 16th century when such events were characterized as a "stroke of God's hand." Attributing the cause to a supernatural force clearly indicates the very limited medical state of knowledge at that time. Scientific knowledge about strokes began to develop in the 19th century when physicians described the appearance after death of stroke-related brain damage.[1,2] Stroke became defined as an injury to the brain caused by abnormalities in the blood vessels that supply and drain blood from the brain. Bleeding into the brain was distinguishable from softening of parts of the brain due to interruption of the blood supply to the brain-damaged regions.[1,2]

Today, stroke is one of the most common and most feared human conditions. The effect of a stroke on an individual and on their family and loved ones is often devastating. What could be worse than the sudden inability to speak, move a limb, stand, walk, see, read, feel, understand spoken language, write, think clearly, or remember? Loss of function is often very sudden and totally unanticipated. The loss can be temporary or permanent, devastating or minor.

Strokes are very common. It is estimated that in the United States at the beginning of the 21st century, nearly three-quarters of a million people had a stroke each year, and 150,000 (90,000 women and 60,000 men) died from stroke annually.[3] At any one time, there were approximately 2 million stroke survivors living in the United States. In China, approximately

1.5 million people died each year because of stroke.[4] In 2015, stroke deaths accounted for 11.8% of total deaths worldwide, making stroke the second leading global cause of death behind heart disease.[3]

In the United States, a stroke occurs every 40 seconds, and someone dies of stroke every 4 minutes.[3] Three times as many women are affected by stroke compared with breast cancer, and yet stroke receives much less public attention and less research funding. For a long time, stroke has been the third leading cause of death in most countries in the world, surpassed as a killer only by heart disease and cancer. Stroke is an even more important cause of prolonged disability. Stroke is the leading cause of serious long-term disability in the United States. Survivors of strokes are often unable to return to work or to assume their previous effectiveness as spouses, parents, friends, and citizens. The economic, social, and psychological costs of stroke are enormous. In the United States, each ischemic stroke costs on average $140,000, and the annual costs related to stroke nationwide are estimated to reach over $183 billion by 2030.

As this book goes to press, stroke is one of the most targeted medical conditions. The public and ambulance personnel are urged to learn about stroke and its warning signs. The news and social media bombard the public with the message that they must get to a hospital very quickly at the earliest signs of stroke in order to maximize chances for effective treatment. In the United States, individuals and families are directed to call 911 at the earliest symptoms that could indicate a stroke. Hospitals are now designated as primary and advanced stroke centers. More neurologists, internists, radiologists, and surgeons are trained each year to specialize in stroke care than ever in the past. More research is performed on the causes, recognition, and treatment of stroke than ever before. Many stroke journals throughout the world publish the latest information about strokes and their treatment and outcomes.

What a change from the mid-20th century, when researching and treating stroke were extremely low on lists of health care priorities. General physicians dreaded having to take care of stroke patients because there was no known or accepted treatment and these patients lingered on the wards for long periods. There were no doctors who viewed stroke as their specialty. There were few neurologists, and internal medicine, not neurology, was considered the medical specialty group that cared for stroke patients. There was little stroke research, and there were no journals dedicated to stroke.

When Charles Miller Fisher was born in 1913, there was very little scientific knowledge about stroke. During the late 19th century and the first quarter of the 20th century, the anatomic details of the arteries that supply the brain were studied carefully and described in London and Paris.[5] During the 1920s, French physicians analyzed the distribution of brain softenings (*ramollissements*) in various arterial brain territories and correlated the anatomy with abnormalities of function found during life.[6] By 1938 when Fisher graduated from the University of Toronto Medical School, physicians were taught how to recognize stroke clinically by taking a history and examining patients. However, there was no way during life to visualize either the brain damage or the disease in the heart or blood vessels that supplied the brain that caused the damage. Strokes, like pneumonia, were thought to be the last pathway toward death. No treatments were known or approved. Therapeutic nihilism about caring for stroke patients was rampant. Stroke patients were often relegated to the back wards of hospitals. Few physicians were interested in caring for those who had what was considered a hopeless condition.

Fisher grew up in a small community in southern Ontario, Canada. Even as a young boy, he was often referred to as "doctor."[7] His interest in the brain and neurology was kindled in Montreal after graduating from medical school. He enlisted as a doctor in the Canadian Navy, but his ship was sunk by the Germans early during World War II. He spent 3½ years in a prisoner-of-war camp in Germany. After the war, he was determined to be productive and not waste further time. His studies and research began by defining changes due to disease in the blood vessels that supply the brain and in the brain itself. These studies and his drive to translate knowledge gained from research into practical ways to help patients led to detailed studies of the manifestations of cerebrovascular disease and strokes in men and women. After moving to Boston in 1954, he devoted his career and the great majority of every waking day to the study of stroke, both in the pathology laboratory and in people. He created the first stroke training program. Fisher's discoveries and contributions and those of the individuals whom he trained changed the knowledge basis of stroke and vascular disease for everyone who practiced medicine and neurology in the latter half of the 20th century and the beginning years of the 21st century. Fisher played a leading role in catapulting stroke into prominence by the end of the 20th century. This book is his story—his life, his method of study and research, and his contributions. Much of the story is told in his own words since in his later years he authored his own memoirs. In the text, I refer to him as Fisher. He disliked the name Charles and never used it. His wife, family, and friends who were contemporaries called him Miller. He often signed his notes and correspondences "CMF."

This book is also in many ways a biography of a disease (stroke) as it evolved during the 20th century. Necessarily included are the disciplines of medicine and neurology that also grew and changed during the lifetime of Fisher. This biography provides a window into Fisher's attributes as a person, physician, researcher, writer, teacher, and colleague. I do this from the point of view of a former trainee and long-term colleague. In 1969–1970, during slightly more than a year as his only stroke fellow, I spent 4–6 hours each day, 6 days a week with him as a private tutorial. I have consulted many of his residents, fellows, and colleagues to be able to attempt to characterize his attributes and accomplishments.

The initial four chapters describe the life and experiences of Fisher before his immersion into research and the care of stroke patients. His war experiences are described in Chapters 3 and 4. Chapters 5–7 describe his re-entry into medicine and his early training and career activities in Boston and Montreal. Chapters 8 and 9 describe his activities, style, and modus operandi during his career at the Massachusetts General Hospital and Harvard Medical School in Boston. Chapters 10–13 summarize his major contributions to stroke and neurology. Finally, Chapter 14 briefly describes Fisher's life and accomplishments after his official retirement.

NOTES

1. Fields WS, Lemak NA. *A History of Stroke: Its Recognition and Treatment.* New York: Oxford University Press, 1989.
2. The following are the primary anatomical studies were made primarily by: Morgagni GB. *The Seats and Causes of Diseases Investigated by Anatomy.* Translated by B. Alexander, Miller and Cadell, London:, Miller & Cadell, 1769;. And by Cheyne J. *Cases of Apoplexy and Lethargy with Observations upon the Comatose Diseases.* J Moyes printer, London: Moyes, 1812.
3. Rosamond W, Flegal K, Friday G, et al. Heart disease and stroke statistics—2018 update: A report from the American Heart Association Statistics Committee and Stroke Statistics Committee. *Circulation* 2018;137(12):e67–e492.
4. Chen ZM, Xu Z, Coillins R, Li WX, Peto R. Blood pressure, blood cholesterol and stroke mortality in a population with low mean cholesterol level. *Cerebrovascular Diseases* 1998;8(Suppl 4):1.
5. Vascular anatomy was clarified mostly by Duret in Paris and Stopford in London: Duret H. Sur la distribution des arteres nouricieres du bulbe rachidien. *Archives Physiologie Normale et Pathologique* 1873;2:97–113; Duret H. Recherches anatomiques sur la circulation de l'encephale. *Archives Physiologie Normale et Pathologique* 1874;3:60–91, 316–353; Stopford JS. The anatomy of the pons and medulla oblongata. *Journal of Anatomy and Physiology* 1928;50:225–280.
6. Charles Foix (1882–1927) could well be considered the first stroke neurologist. He died prematurely of pneumonia at age 45 years: Caplan LR. Charles Foix, the first modern stroke neurologist. *Stroke* 1990;21:348–356; Foix C, Hillemand P. Irrigation de la protuberance. *Comptes Rendus des Seances de la Societe de Biologie (Paris)* 1925;92:35–36; Foix C, Hillemand P. Les arteres de l'axe encephalique

jusqu'au diencephale inclusivement. *Revue Neurologique (Paris)* 1925;41:705–739; Foix C, Masson A. Le syndrome de l'artere cerebrale posterieure. *Presse Medicale* 1923;31:361–365; Foix C. Hillemand P. Les syndromes de l'artere cerebrale anterieure. *Encephale* 1925;20:209–232; Foix C, Levy M. Les Ramollissements Sylviens. *Revue Neurologique (Paris)* 1927;43:1–51.
7. Fisher CM. *Memoirs of a Neurologist*. Vol. 1. Rutland, VT: Sharp, 2006.

PART I
Early Years and University and Medical Training

Miller Fisher was born in a small town in southern Ontario. His mother died when he was 11 years old. Miller and his nine siblings were raised mostly by their father. He received his university and medical education in Toronto. He had praise for his basic science mentors, but clinical work was decidedly non-academic. He was not an exceptional student. He gained valuable clinical experience as an intern at Henry Ford Hospital in Detroit, Michigan.

CHAPTER 1

Fisher's Early Years

WATERLOO–KITCHENER, ONTARIO, CANADA

Charles Miller Fisher was born on December 5, 1913, in Waterloo, Ontario, Canada. Like his older sister Ruth and his older brother Munro and the six other siblings who followed, Fisher was delivered at home. The family, Fisher's parents George Middleton Fisher and Frieda Kaufman Fisher and the children, lived in a simple frame house in Waterloo.

Fisher's early years were spent almost entirely within the area of Kitchener and Waterloo, two separate but connecting townships located approximately 108 km (67 miles) from Toronto in southern Ontario, often referred to as the twin cities. The towns were originally settled during the early years of the 19th century by Mennonite farmers who left Lancaster County, Pennsylvania, to travel in Conestoga wagons to southern Canada. Even into the first quarter of the 20th century, Mennonite farmers driving horses and buggies would bring their produce into markets in Kitchener and Waterloo once or twice a week.

Kitchener

In addition to Mennonites, many German immigrants also settled in this region. Kitchener was originally named Berlin, Ontario, with approximately 15,000 inhabitants. By the 1880s, it was often referred to as Canada's "German Capital."[1,2] The first German settlers were mainly farmers, but their progeny became builders, masons, carpenters, mechanics, and furniture makers. They became pillars of the community.

When Germany became the enemy during World War I, being a namesake of its largest city, Berlin, became problematic. In 1916, during the middle years of the war, the name of the town was changed from Berlin to Kitchener by a vote of 3,057 Berliners. The voters chose the new name from alternatives proffered, ultimately honoring a British military hero, General Lord Horatio Herbert Kitchener, who died in June 1916 when the ship on which he was a passenger struck a German mine.[3] At the time of the official proclamation of the new name, a band played "Die Wacht am Rhein" ("The Watch/Guard on the Rhine," a German patriotic anthem) and "God Save the King." After the vote had been cast, an alderman telephoned King George V of Britain and informed his majesty that Berlin had "cast off forever the name of the Prussian capital."[2]

Waterloo

In 1913, the year of Fisher's birth, the population of Waterloo was approximately 45,000. Waterloo was known as the "furniture capital of Canada" and was also the headquarters of the Mutual Life Insurance Company. In addition, Waterloo was the original home of Seagram's whiskies. At the historic Waterloo Distillery, Joseph E. Seagram asked distiller William Hortop to craft his original product, Seagram's VO (VO stood for "very own"). As in Kitchener, many Mennonite farms were located in the region and sold their goods.

Fisher commented in his memoirs on life in Kitchener–Waterloo in then rural Ontario after World War I:

> The community was deeply religious and the several churches were the center of community life for children and adults. There was neither radio nor television. In the summertime boys were busy with softball, tennis, swimming, and fishing when not engaged in tending their pets, building model airplanes or kites, and hiking in the woods. In the winter, hockey, ice-skating, tobogganing, badminton, and volleyball provided recreation. Ice curling was for the adults. Alley bowling was just being introduced. As the snow melted each spring, the game of marbles held sway for a few weeks. Puppy-love was common at 14 or 15, but usually one did not "invite a girl out" until the age of 17 or 18.
>
> Church societies were probably the most common meeting ground but the last year of high school was also a period of mating. The young people together enjoyed wiener roasts, corn roasts church picnics, band concerts in the park, and sleigh-ride parties and often ice skating. The simple amusements of blind man's bluff, drop the handkerchief, button–button, pinning the donkey, crokinol, and Parcheesi sufficed for

entertainment. Recreational dancing was little engaged in except for square dancing and an occasional waltz night. The use of alcohol or whiskey before the age of 18 must have been a great rarity. High school students do not smoke openly.[4]

FAMILY GENEALOGY

Fisher's grandfather, Mirabeau M. Fisher, was born in 1856 and died in a fire at age 32 years.[5] In 1881, he married Elizabeth England (Fisher's grandmother), who was born in 1857 and died long after her husband, in 1928. George Middleton Fisher (Fisher's father) was born in 1886 in Kincardine, Ontario, before the family moved to Kitchener–Waterloo after Mirabeau's death in 1888. George married Frieda Kaufman (Fisher's mother) in November 1908. Frieda, the daughter of Anna (Mueller) and Adam Kaufman, was 2 years younger than George. The family tree is shown in Figure 1.1. Anna's father, Charles, started the Charles Mueller Cooperage in 1872, a firm that soon became one of the largest producers of barrels and vats, which it sold locally and also exported to the United States and Europe. The cooperage was later sold to Seagram's Distillery.

Fisher commented on his family background:[6]

> *Our family heritage was a mixture of pure English, originally from Huddersfield on one side, and pure German from Alsace on the other. Both sides arrived in Canada in the 1840s via the United States. One great-grandfather owned a foundry; the other great-grandfather was a cooper who supplied barrels to the newly established Seagram*

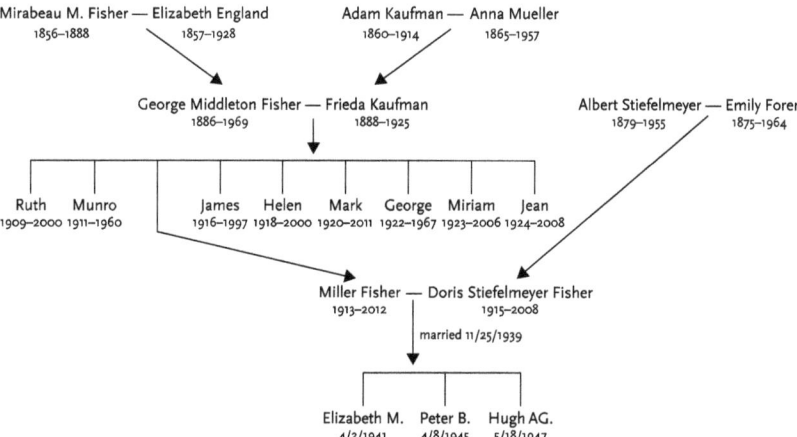

Figure 1.1 Fisher family tree.

Distillery and eventually developed a national enterprise. This man for whom I am named, apparently always had a habit of being busy trying to "figure things out." His wife would upbraid him with "you're no company—do bist ein Rätselkönig (puzzle fanatic)." In his late 80s he still enjoyed making the most attractive wooden pails and tubs as family presents. Our grandmother was a delicate lovely gentle lady who was church organist and choir master. She was widowed tragically and left to raise three children 6, 4 and 2 years of age. Our maternal grandmother was the matriarch and in her 90s welcomed us all with kindness and witticisms.[6]

FISHER'S FATHER, THE PATRIARCH OF THE FAMILY

George Fisher (Figure 1.2) and his wife Frieda lived in a small home on 115 Park Street in Waterloo, where Fisher was born in 1913. George and Frieda had nine children: Fisher was the third oldest; his older siblings were Ruth and Munro. After the next two siblings, James and Helen, were born, the house was too small for the growing family. When Fisher was 7 years old, George and Frieda moved to a larger home on the corner of Erb Street and Tweed Street in Waterloo, where Fisher spent most of his childhood (Figure 1.3).

Fisher's father worked his entire career at the Mutual Life Insurance Company, whose headquarters were based in Waterloo. By all accounts, George was a very hard-working traveling insurance salesman who spent the great majority of his time at the office or on the road. He took many

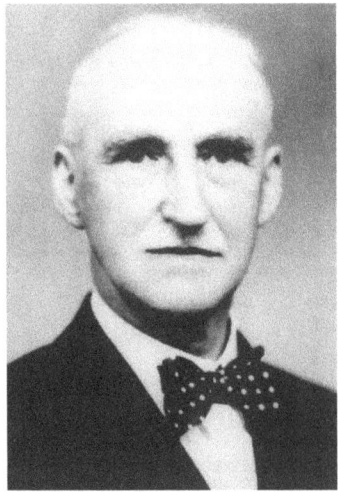

Figure 1.2 George Middleton Fisher.

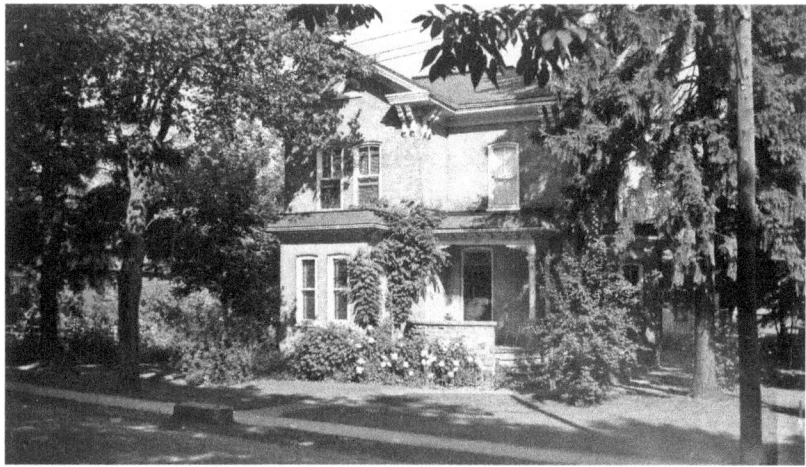

Figure 1.3 78 Erb Street.

courses by mail. He kept physically fit and played ice hockey for much of his life and even coached a hockey team of Mutual Life workers. He was a walker, disciplining himself to spend a good part of each day walking. He also was a disciplined gardener, spending much time treating his flowers and vegetables. Fisher later characterized his father as a "sportsman."

George was formal; he dressed formally, wearing his signature bow tie even when he worked in his garden—his major recreational outlet. He was a strict disciplinarian and quite compulsive in his record-keeping. He had a reputation for being very penurious. For many years, he kept meticulous records in a log book concerning each penny spent on groceries and garden and household expenses. He followed a strict routine of reading the newspaper each morning and then going to work quite early. He returned punctually each late afternoon and insisted that dinner be served at 6 p.m. The children were to be seated by then. He enforced the rule that each child must finish their plate and eat each pea and morsel before being excused from the table. He was religious and regularly attended the First United Church of Waterloo.

George retired in 1953 at age 67 years. During his retirement years, he paid loving attention to his garden. Although George was strict, Fisher had fond memories of his father, whom he respected for his diligence and self-discipline. Fisher retained great admiration for the milieu that his father demanded in his home and in his life. Fisher thought of his father and the home model of his youth when he raised his own family. Hard work, education, and physical conditioning were important and keys to success.

Cursing, drinking alcohol, and gossip were prohibited. Emphasis was on a moral life of serving others. George died in 1969 at age 83 years.

Fisher later reflected on his father and his methods:

> *The upbringing was strict with emphasis on honesty, piety, and civility. Never did I hear my father say an unkind word about another person no matter the provocation. His advise to us children was brief "Avoid bad company." As a family we were abstemious. Children were not permitted to have tea or coffee in the home. There was great emphasis on the development of vocabulary and the use of correct words. When he was on his deathbed at the age of 84, confused with an intravenous running into one arm, my father struggled with a crossword puzzle and asked me for a six letter word for a mountain climber's tool. That night he slipt away.*[7]

FISHER'S MOTHER, THE MATRIARCH OF THE FAMILY, AND HER SUCCESSORS

Fisher's mother, Frieda, died while giving birth to her 10th child, who also died. Fisher was 11 years old at the time of his mother's death and later had only very faint memories of her. Fisher and his siblings (shown in Figure 1.4)

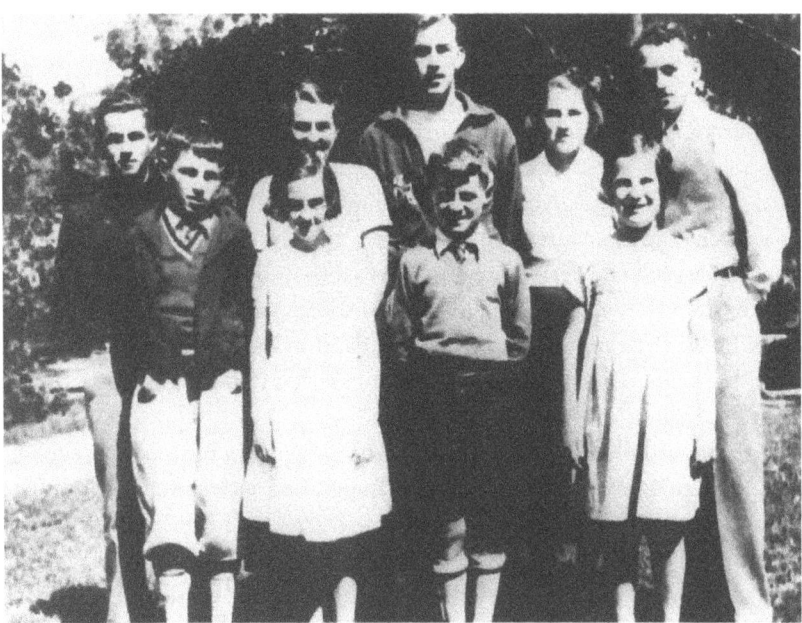

Figure 1.4 Fisher and his siblings. Fisher is the tall one in the middle of the back row.

[8] *Early Years and University and Medical Training*

were mostly raised by two Mennonite sisters who were housemaids and lived with the family at the Erb Street domicile. Fisher and his siblings had pet names for the women—"horse and cow" and "Chasta and Canasta."

After Frieda's death in 1925, George married Ella Knechtel in 1928. Ella was 27 years old at the time, and she became the matron of nine children ranging from Ruth, who was 17 years old, to Jean, who was 3 years old. Ella died in 1964, after which George married her sister, Margaret Knechtel, in 1965.

FISHER'S EARLY YEARS

Fisher must have spent considerable time in various stores and emporiums in his hometown.[8] More than a half century later, in his memoirs he included a note titled "Memories of Waterloo Ontario Circa 1928." This note also serves as a testimony to his prodigious memory for details and as a glimpse into small-town Canada during that time period:

> My memories of Waterloo especially King St., the main St. are still fairly vivid. King St. runs North–South. On the east side of King St. proceeding North from William St. there was first Rollie Plantz' ice cream and sandwich parlor occupying the first floor of the Alexandra Hotel, a handsome structure of four stories. Proceeding North there were a Red and White grocery store, a shoe repair shop, Shinn's store combining picture framing and funeral supplies, then McPhail's bicycle shop, Dobbins motor car repair shop, a flower shop, Rahn's shoe store, Wettlauffer's department store. Next was one of the last private dwellings on King St, Cressman's realty office was next, followed by Adam Kaufman's residence, a former mayor of the town and a paternal uncle of my mother. Then came a blacksmith shop, Pinto's fruit store, a store selling electric fixtures, Bruegemann's tailor shop, and the City Hotel, a two story building, and a favorite watering spa on Saturday afternoons. A street, Herbert Street branched off of King at this point. On the other side of Herbert Street there was a dry goods store, then a Chinese Café, Longo's Fruit store, Sturm's Tobacco Shop, a photographic studio, the Hub cigar store, Urstadt's candy store, Doersam's Stationary Store, Lippert's Furniture Store, Detenbeck's Haberdashery, A. B. Learn's Drug Store, Weichel's Hardware Store. Lippet's Hardware Store, Frank's Jewelry Store, Frowde's Investment, Haehnel's Drug Store, and Klopp's Store for women and children.[9]

The memoir went on to detail the makeup of the other stores on King and Erb streets.

Fisher attended the public school system in Waterloo through high school. By age 11 years, he was known as the "doctor" in the family. He was uncertain as to how that name came about: Doctors were held in very high esteem in town at that time, but Fisher did not cite any particular physician as a role model. He was always very active in sports. He loved the water, most often preferring distance swimming, 1- and 2-mile races. He was a lifeguard at the swimming pool and played water polo. He fished with his father and siblings, played football and hockey, and often played golf on a nearby nine-hole golf course. He built model airplanes and kites, and by his

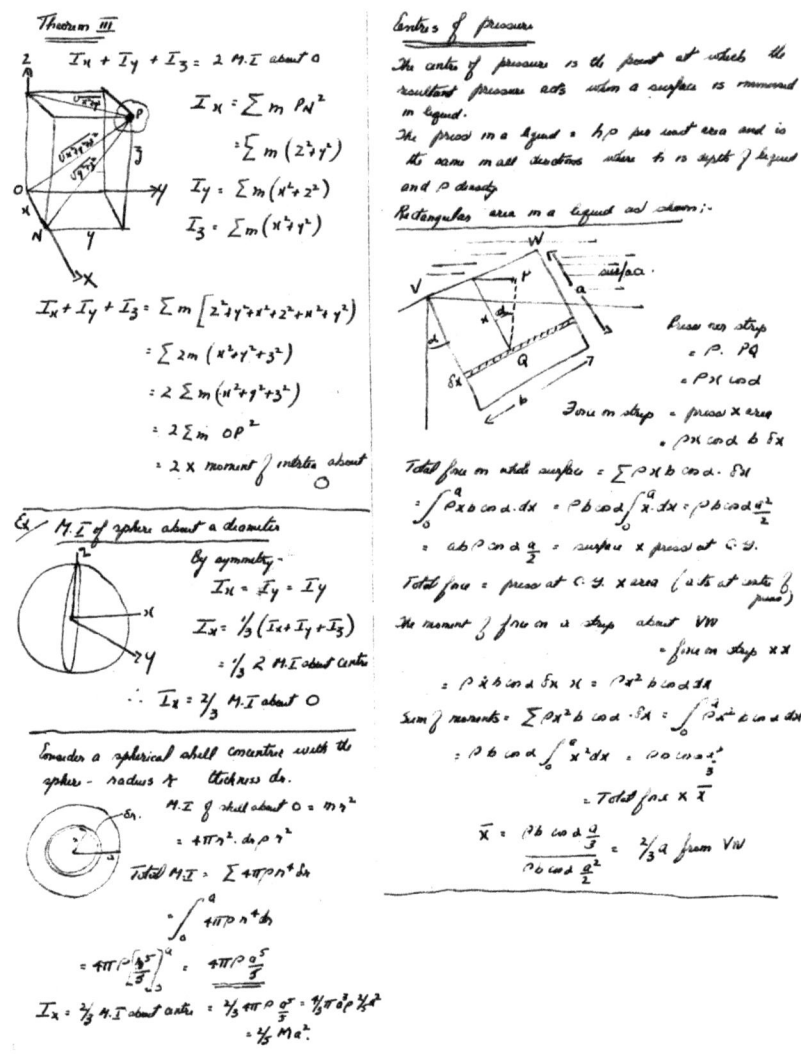

Figure 1.5 Calculus homework during high school.

own admission he spent little serious time as a student and did little homework until age 15 or 16 years.

Somehow during his last 2 years in high school, Fisher "turned up the burners" and began to study more assiduously. One of the reports that he submitted had been criticized by a respected teacher who emphasized that he could do much better. This admonishment stimulated him to work harder at school. His reports and notes from the last two high school years showed features that were predictive of his later modus operandi: He kept copious, well-organized notes and read avidly. Figure 1.5 is a page from his calculus course notebook that illustrates his attention to detail. By graduation, he was recognized as "the scholar in the class." He was awarded a scholarship to the University of Toronto in recognition of his academic performance during high school. Only a small minority of students from his high school went on to college.

NOTES

1. Moyer B. *Kitchener. Yesterday Revisited: An Illustrated History*. Burlington, Ontario, Canada: Windsor, 1979.
2. English J, McLaughlin K. *Kitchener: An Illustrated History*. Waterloo, Ontario, Canada: Wilfred Laurier University Press, 1945.
3. Kitchener's career is detailed in Pollock J. *Kitchener: Architect of Victory, Artisan of Peace*. New York: Carroll & Graf, 2001.
4. Fisher CM. *Memoirs of a Neurologist*. Rutland, VT: Academy Books, 1992, Vol. 1, p. 1.
5. Many details about the Fisher family were provided by Fisher's cousins, Jamie Paterson and Charles Grierson, who kept family histories and memorabilia.
6. Fisher CM. *Memoirs of a Neurologist*. Rutland, VT: Academy Books, 1992, Vol. 1, pp. 4–5.
7. Fisher CM. *Memoirs of a Neurologist*. Rutland, VT: Academy Books, 1992, Vol. 1, p. 5.
8. Some recollections of his early life came during an interview of Fisher for the American Association of Neurological Surgeons in 1984 (available on YouTube).
9. Fisher CM. Memories of Waterloo Ontario Circa 1928. In *Memoirs of a Neurologist*. Rutland, VT: Academy Books, 1992, Vol. 5, pp. 89–90.

CHAPTER 2

Toronto University and Medical School and Internship in Detroit

TORONTO MEDICINE BEFORE FISHER'S MATRICULATION

For 21st-century readers, medical education and medicine in general at the time of Fisher's matriculation seems quite primitive and undisciplined. A very brief review of the history of medicine and medical education up to that time[1,2,3] places the situation during the 1930s when Fisher matriculated in perspective. If a prospective student from the Canadian province of Ontario wanted to learn medicine in the 1830s, he could attend one of three proprietary medical schools in Toronto that were sometimes affiliated with Trinity College, the University of Toronto, or the Methodist' Victoria University.[1] These "medical schools" would in no way be recognized as such today. None of the schools had libraries, laboratories, or pathology facilities. Lecture halls were rented. Some had dissecting rooms in the basement. Students paid for their courses directly to the professors, attended a few short courses that they chose, did some dissections, and saw some patients at the Toronto General Hospital. The Toronto Medical School was owned and run by a group of physicians, and courses were taught in a building rented from the University of Toronto. Teachers were paid from students' fees. Graduation led to qualification as a physician and surgeon. Biology, anatomy, pathology, and materia medica (the substance of various drugs) were the major courses taught. A former student reflecting on his time as a medical student made the following comments about education offered at the Toronto Medical School:[4]

The teachers in their professorial chairs rayed out from these high and sunless peaks mere cold and darkness, without enthusiasm, humour, and human geniality. Their lectures were given without cases or specimens and were a compound of textbook material and quotations from authorities, the whole being flung at us pellmell without word of guidance, and leaving us standing helpless, bewildered, and starved in the midst of what seemed a superabundance of wealth. . . . Scholarship students found they could learn faster from books at home and only appeared for the compulsory number of lectures.[4]

When the Toronto General Hospital opened in 1868, the hospital cared for only 25 indigent patients at any one time and medical students were only permitted to see their own professor's patients.[5] The education received depended almost entirely on the diligence of the student. It was not until the last half of the 19th century that the practice of medicine in Canada became more scientific[1,2] while medical schools and medical education remained rather primitive. Anatomy and pathology were taught in laboratories, but clinical training was often not systematic and was performed mostly by volunteer physicians. Sir William Osler, often considered the most important figure in the history of modern clinical medicine, began his study of medicine at the Toronto Medical School in 1868 and remained there until 1870.[6]

FISHER'S COLLEGE AND MEDICAL SCHOOL TEACHING IN TORONTO

In 1931, Fisher journeyed to Toronto, where he was determined to learn to become a physician. The Toronto Medical School and McGill University in Montreal were the foremost respected training institutions for future physicians in Canada. The educational facilities and the reputation of the Toronto Medical School had greatly improved since Osler's time. Frederick Banting and Charles Best isolated insulin while working in the Physiology Department at the Toronto Medical School. This discovery and their award of the Nobel Prize in Physiology or Medicine in 1923 had catapulted the school into the limelight and resulted in an international reputation. The university had been able to attract many faculty members who became well known for their discoveries and productivity.

Students who matriculated at the Toronto Medical School in 1931 had a choice of entering one of two different academic pathways to a medical degree. The main track, which most students chose, was titled Straight Medicine. This curriculum took 6 years and was divided into 3 years of preclinical study (predominantly anatomy, histology, pathology, physiology, and biochemistry) and 3 years of clinical medicine and surgery. The other track was titled Biology and Medicine (B&M). Students who elected the B&M pathway matriculated during their first 4 years at one of the arts colleges affiliated with the University of Toronto (Victoria, Trinity, University, and St. Michael's Colleges). These students were exposed to religion, philosophy, English literature, French or German, psychology, and mathematics. Physics and repetition of key physics experiments were an important feature of the arts and sciences teaching at that time. The arts and science courses were intermingled with the standard preclinical medical classes in anatomy, pathology, and physiology (taken along with the students who had chosen the Straight Medicine track). At the end of 4 years, the B&M students were awarded a Bachelor of Arts degree and then became full-time students at the medical school for the next 4 years. Fisher, along with 25 other men, chose the B&M pathway. On the other hand, the Straight Medicine pathway attracted 120 men and 20 women students.

Fisher wrote enthusiastically about his course in physics:

In our laboratory periods in physics we were privileged to repeat many of the classical experiments that underlie the major discoveries concerning the structure of matter—Becquerel's decay of radium and pitchblend, JJ Thomson's cathode ray tube, Crooke's phenomenon, Wilson's cloud chamber etc. Radio tubes and photoelectric cells were the objects of experiments. On one occasion primitive television was demonstrated. . . . The first electron microscope on the continent had been installed and was demonstrated to the students. Buttressing the entire exposition was the introduction to statistics by the exciting Dr. John Satterly who made the Fundamentals of Scientific Measurement an almost enjoyable exercise.[7]

Later, during his medical career, Fisher maintained a strong commitment to accurate measurement and quantification of physical signs and observations, a discipline he first learned in Toronto as a student.

Concerning the B&M course that combined medicine and arts, Fisher commented,

In retrospect the method of presenting them simultaneously rather than consecutively was perhaps conducive to a more harmonious blend. . . . I have always thought that the B&M course prepared me superbly for the practice of medicine providing me with the fundamentals of the scientific method while at the same time broadening my perspectives on what are called the Arts.[8]

The preclinical curriculum included a full year in Anatomy—12 hours a week of lectures and dissections with four to six students dissecting each cadaver. The practical examination in Anatomy consisted of each student advancing along tables on which 100 human specimens were displayed, with each student having a minute to answer a question posed about each specimen. Fisher's histology course was taught by Dr. Arthur Ham, a leader in the field, and physiology was taught by Dr. Charles Best (one of the discoverers of insulin). His lectures on the function of each organ system became the foundation of the book, *Best and Taylor's Textbook of Physiology*. Biochemistry and pharmacology, on the other hand, were rather rudimentary at that time. Fisher commented on the preclinical curriculum and teaching: "In retrospect how thrilling all this was. Yet most of us were only 18 or 19 years of age when served this fascinating feast. Were we too young?"[9]

Teaching during the clinical years focused on bacteriology and pathology. During the laboratory experience in bacteriology, students learned to perform their own complete systematic bacterial analyses.

During Fisher's entire active medical career, he emphasized the importance of pathology and neuropathology in clarifying the cause and extent of neurological conditions, especially stroke. Fisher's lifelong emphasis on pathology must have begun during the medical school years:

> *Pathology under the direction of Professor Oscar Klotz was the cornerstone of teaching in clinical medicine. The bedside discussion of symptoms and signs was always in terms of pathological anatomy. ... Klotz insisted on clear thinking and precise exposition ... the main emphasis was on the recognition and meticulous description of microscopic structures. Attendance at autopsies was obligatory.*[10]

Clinical teaching in both medicine and surgery occurred mostly during bedside clinics held for groups of 10–12 students. Each student was regularly assigned one patient to examine and write up in detail. Teaching emphasized the history and physical examination. At that time, X-rays and laboratory analyses were very rudimentary. Diagnosis was almost entirely clinical, with little help from investigations. Fisher noted, "Didactic lectures in Medicine, Surgery, and Therapeutics were usually conducted by personable, able and even somewhat flamboyant senior staff members who were assured an attentive audience."[11] At that time, the pharmaceutical agents available for treatment were very limited—insulin, thyroid extract, laxatives, antacids, liver extract, aspirin barbiturates, atropine, vitamins, digitalis, and colchicine. In 1937, one of the first sulfonamides was introduced to treat gonorrhea. There were no other antibiotics and no available antihypertensives, antidepressants, anticoagulants, or anticonvulsants. The wards were mostly occupied by patients with infectious diseases—pneumonia, gonorrhea, syphilis, tuberculosis, diphtheria, and poliomyelitis.

In his memoirs, Fisher reflected rather critically on his clinical years in medical school:

> *It probably was not a very disciplined period of apprenticeship. . . . No student was particularly well known, if at all, to any staff member. Full time hospital-based staff physicians literally did not exist. A philosophic view of the students was that if you did not learn a particular thing today, you would learn it tomorrow. Attending medical school was a stimulating experience in a relaxed atmosphere. . . . Special effort was not always encouraged or welcomed. For example, I once went along to practice examination, particularly auscultation of the heart and lungs. When the Chief inquired what I was up to, he said "You should be out throwing the ball around on such a nice day." And I went. Instructors were more authoritative at that time and discussion was not easily entered into.*[12]

FISHER'S EXPERIENCES, ACTIVITIES, AND INTERESTS WHILE IN TORONTO LEARNING MEDICINE

During his college and medical school years, Fisher was interested in general biology, interior decorating, and music, as well as medicine, as cited in the inscription under his picture in the 1935 yearbook (Figure 2.1).[13]

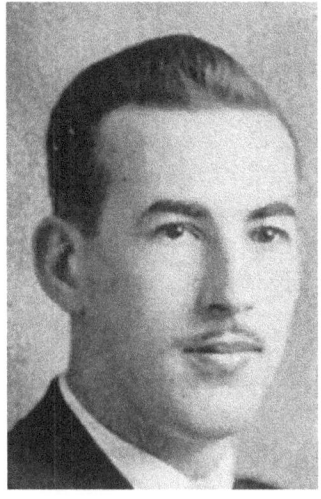

Figure 2.1 Fisher's 1935 yearbook photograph.

While matriculating in Toronto, Fisher spent most of his time within the confines of the university. He waxed eloquent about the facilities available to him: Recall that he was from a small town and this was his first exposure to a very large metropolitan area and a major university. He lived in "the distinctive ivy-covered Burwash Residence"[14]—a long line of adjoining buildings, each of which housed approximately 30 male students. Rooms were predominantly single, measured approximately 11 × 8 feet, and many contained fireplaces. Housemen made the beds and tidied the rooms for the students so that when Fisher returned from a full day, he was welcomed by "a cozy room and a fire in the grate."[15] There was always abundant heat, even on the coldest days in winter. Meals were served in Burwash Hall, "a magnificent Great hall traditional in English Universities."[16] The windowed walls rose three or four stories, and the hall was crowned with a high arched ceiling. Large polished oaken tables were surrounded by long benches that seated 8 students on each bench. Food was served by uniformed waitresses. Fisher commented that "unfailingly the meals were unbelievably abundant, tasty, and nourishing."[17] Alcohol was not allowed in Burwash Hall, and cigarette smoking was not common among students. Fisher noted that "the vast majority of our Victoria University class came to Toronto with a background of religious upbringing, faithfulness to the Church, and ingrained Christian ethical behavior."[18]

Sports were an integral part of university life. A full-sized football field, hockey and skating rink, tennis courts, an indoor gymnasium, and handball courts were available for student use and for organized team activities. Fisher was very active in athletics and was one of the stars of the water polo team (Figure 2.2).

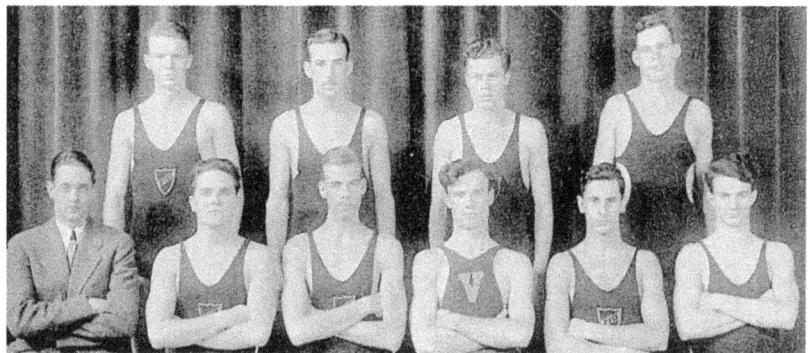

Figure 2.2 The water polo team. Fisher is second from the left in the upper row.

When reflecting back on his years at the university, Fisher lauded

> the grandeur that was the University of Toronto, the magnificence of Hart House, Burwash Hall, Trinity College, Knox College, the beauty of the campus, the throng of robed Scholars dedicated to baptizing us in the swelling tide of Man's achievements since the beginning of time.[19]

Figure 2.3 is a graduation picture of Fisher.

MEDICAL INTERNSHIP IN DETROIT

Fisher took a competitive written examination for an internship at Henry Ford Hospital in Detroit, Michigan. Detroit was only a short distance across the border into the United States, and Henry Ford Hospital had an impressive reputation.[20] A few days after sitting for the examination, he received a letter informing him that he was accepted for this prized

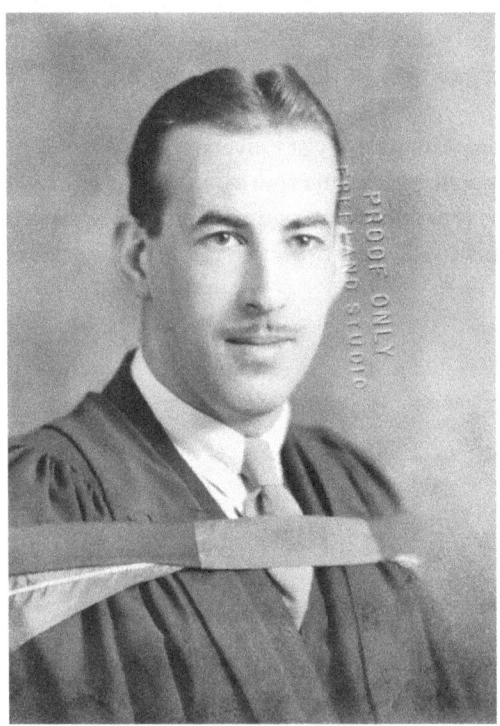

Figure 2.3 Fisher's medical school graduation photograph.

internship. He began his internship on July 1, 1938. When he arrived in Detroit, he learned that he had to arrange his own housing because none was available for hospital house officers at that time. Along with nine other house staff, he found lodging at a large private home only two houses from the hospital.

During the second day on duty, July 4, he heard noises and assumed they were youngsters firing off firecrackers. He soon found out that the sounds were from exchanges of gunfire between a carload of fleeing bank robbers and two police officers who chased them on motorcycles. This procession circled the hospital, even going through the circular drive located just in front of the hospital. Fisher commented, "This was strong medicine for a country boy". Fisher proceeded to spend the vast majority of his internship year within the confines of the hospital and his lodging several houses nearby. He had virtually no time for social activities or exploring Detroit or nearby regions.

At Henry Ford Hospital, one of his colleagues was William S. Fields, who became a lifelong colleague.[21] Each focused their careers on stroke. Fisher lauded his training in general medicine during his internship: "In every specialty the physicians and surgeons of Henry Ford Hospital were superb and effective clinicians. It was medicine at its best."[22] Because Fisher was a Canadian citizen, his stay in Detroit at Henry Ford Hospital was limited by statute to 1 year. After his internship in Detroit, he returned to his native Canada.

During his time in Toronto and later in Detroit, he continued intermittently to communicate with and woo his girlfriend and future wife Doris Stiefelmeyer, whom he met during high school and who still lived in Kitchener. He married Doris in Montreal on November 25, 1939. At the time of the marriage, according to Doris, married women in Canada were not allowed to work. For financial reasons, she returned to her job in Kitchener and continued to live with her parents, keeping their marriage a secret. Doris did not wear her wedding ring to work. Doris later told Elizabeth, her daughter, that one day she wore the ring by mistake and was fired from her job.[23]

NOTES

1. An account of medicine in Toronto and in general is included in Bliss M. *William Osler: A Life in Medicine*. New York: Oxford University Press, 1999, pp. 54–56.
2. McHenry L. *Garrison's History of Neurology. Revised and Enlarged with a Bibliography of Classical, Original, and Standard Works in Neurology*. Springfield, IL: Charles C Thomas, 1969.

3. An account of medical teaching during the 19th and early 20th centuries is contained in the Flexner report: Flexner A. *Medical Education in the United States and Canada: A Report to the Carnegie Foundation for the Advancement of Teaching*. New York: Carnegie Foundation, 1910.
4. Crozier JB. *My Inner Life: Being a Chapter in Personal Evaluation and Autobiography*. London: Longmans, 1898, pp. 225, 227. These comments are quoted in Bliss M. *William Osler: A Life in Medicine*. New York: Oxford University Press, 1999, p. 54.
5. Cosbie WG. *The Toronto General Hospital 1819–1965*. Toronto: Macmillan, 1975, pp. 71–81.
6. Sir William Osler was the first Professor of Medicine at Johns Hopkins Hospital. He later became the Regius Professor of Medicine at Oxford. Many volumes of his textbook, *The Practice of Medicine*, became the bible for medical students throughout the world. Osler spent much of his time at the Toronto Medical School studying botany and general biology. He spent very little time in Toronto studying human disease or human pathology. When his mentor, Dr. James Bovell, left, Osler moved to Montreal and McGill University, where hospital advantages were considered superior to those offered in Toronto. Osler set up a laboratory for human pathology in Montreal. Fisher later occupied the same laboratory that Osler had used. Osler's time in Toronto and Montreal is described in Bliss M. *William Osler: A Life in Medicine*. New York: Oxford University Press, 1999; and in Cushing H. *The Life of Sir William Osler*. Oxford, UK: Oxford University Press, 1925.
7. Fisher CM. *Memoirs of a Neurologist*. Rutland, VT: Academy Books, 1992, Vol. 1, pp. 13–14.
8. Fisher CM. *Memoirs of a Neurologist*. Rutland, VT: Academy Books, 1992, Vol. 1, pp. 23–25.
9. Fisher CM. *Memoirs of a Neurologist*. Rutland, VT: Academy Books, 1992, Vol. 1, p. 14.
10. Fisher CM. *Memoirs of a Neurologist*. Rutland, VT: Academy Books, 1992, Vol. 1, pp. 16–17.
11. Fisher CM. *Memoirs of a Neurologist*. Rutland, VT: Academy Books, 1992, Vol. 1, p. 18.
12. Fisher CM. *Memoirs of a Neurologist*. Rutland, VT: Academy Books, 1992, Vol. 1, pp. 19–20.
13. *Torontonensis*, the yearbook of the University of Toronto, 1935.
14. Fisher CM. *Memoirs of a Neurologist*. Rutland, VT: Academy Books, 1992, Vol. 1, p. 26.
15. Fisher CM. *Memoirs of a Neurologist*. Rutland, VT: Academy Books, 1992, Vol. 1, p. 26.
16. Fisher CM. *Memoirs of a Neurologist*. Rutland, VT: Academy Books, 1992, Vol. 1, p. 26.
17. Fisher CM. *Memoirs of a Neurologist*. Rutland, VT: Academy Books, 1992, Vol. 1, p. 26.
18. Fisher CM. *Memoirs of a Neurologist*. Rutland, VT: Academy Books, 1992, Vol. 1, p. 30.
19. Fisher CM. *Memoirs of a Neurologist*. Rutland, VT: Academy Books, 1992, Vol. 1, p. 30.

20. A history of the Henry Ford Hospital is included in Rodengen J. *Henry Ford Health System: A 100 Year Legacy*. Fort Lauderdale, FL: Write Stuff Enterprises, 2014.
21. William (Bill) Fields was one of the first full-time academic neurologists interested in stroke. He spent his entire career in Houston, Texas. Fields edited many volumes concerning the diagnosis, evaluation, and treatment of stroke patients. He was one of the first neurologists active in stroke randomized therapeutic trials.
22. Fisher CM. *Memoirs of a Neurologist*. Rutland, VT: Academy Books, 1992, Vol. 1, p. 33.
23. Recollections of Elizabeth Fisher.

PART II
War Experiences

After brief internal medicine training in Montreal, Fisher enlisted in the Canadian Navy in 1940. In April 1941, the ship on which he served was sunk by the Germans. After floating in the ocean for some time, he was captured by the Germans and taken to a prisoner-of-war camp in Sandbostel, Germany. He spent 3 years as a medical officer in the camp and finally returned to Canada at the end of 1944.

CHAPTER 3

World War II and Experience as a British Naval Officer

The winds of war hovered over Europe and North America during the mid-1930s. Hitler had taken control of Germany in 1933, and in 1938, while Fisher was an intern in Detroit, Hitler annexed Austria and added a portion of Czechoslovakia to Nazi Germany's Third Reich. On September 3, 1939, soon after Hitler's army invaded Poland, Canada officially entered World War II, joining the United Kingdom on the side of the Allies.

WAITING TO ENTER MILITARY SERVICE: MONTREAL

Fisher returned to Canada from Detroit in the summer of 1939. He volunteered to become a member of the Canadian reserve militia soon after Canada entered the war. He was a very loyal Canadian and believed it was his duty to serve his country.

In 1939, the future in Canada was quite uncertain. While Fisher awaited mobilization, he sought a medical position that would further his training. He recognized that he could not make a long-term commitment because he could be called to active service at any time. Dr. Jonathan Meakins invited him to become a member of the Medical House staff at the Royal Victoria Hospital in Montreal, with the fledgling Montreal Neurological Institute across the street. His time was divided between the general medicine and diabetic wards at the Royal Vic; the Alexandria Hospital for Infectious Diseases, where diphtheria was a major problem; and a 200-bed tuberculosis sanitarium. Fisher had considerable exposure to rheumatic conditions, infections, and diabetes. The diabetic service emphasized careful measurements of blood sugars, food intake, and insulin requirements. House staff received no stipend but were given room and board. They were on call 24 hours a day. They were allowed an occasional night and every other weekend off provided that all of their work was up to date. The house staff also served on ambulance duty, traveling to accidents and other urgencies at high speed.

In his memoirs, Fisher rendered very high praise for one mentor encountered during this period of his training: Dr. Kenneth Evelyn. Evelyn was a biophysicist who worked with Meakins, Fisher's sponsor, on studies of lung physiology and was an acknowledged expert in biochemistry. As a basic scientist, while working in the pulmonary physiology laboratory, Evelyn discovered a way to measure the concentration of various substances in body fluids using a photoelectrometer. Stimulated by his contact with patients, Evelyn went to medical school and became a house officer at the Royal Vic at the same time as Fisher. The much older and more experienced Evelyn became a mentor for Fisher. Evelyn roamed the wards and was available to consult on all types of biochemical and metabolic issues. The experience with Evelyn and his time on the diabetic ward became important influences on Fisher, so much so, in fact, that Fisher thought at the time that he would specialize in metabolic conditions when he returned from military service. The emphasis on metrics—carefully studying and quantifying variables—appealed to him and later became an important component of his entire neurological career.

EARLY EXPERIENCE IN THE CANADIAN NAVY

In April 1940, Fisher enlisted in the Canadian Navy. He had been in the reserve militia, a branch of the Canadian Army. He characterized his switch to the Navy as an odd twist of fate. Dr. Donald Webster, a Professor of Surgery at McGill University in Montreal, was one of the principal medical officers of the Royal Canadian Navy. When war was declared, Webster considered that his surgical skills would not be utilized as effectively in the Navy as in the Army. He would be of much more use performing needed surgery if he could transfer to the Royal Canadian Army Medical Corps. He requested a transfer, which he was told would be granted if he could find someone to take over his Navy duties. At that time, Webster was examining Naval recruits on a ship docked in Montreal. Webster sought potential volunteers who might switch services with him, and Fisher made a preliminary inquiry. Soon thereafter, Webster sought out Fisher and said, "Fisher, how about it, will you do it?" Pressured by a much senior officer, Fisher quickly, without much reflection, replied that he would. Fisher agreed to take over Webster's duties and to enlist in the Royal Canadian Navy. On May 4, 1940, Fisher was commissioned as a Surgeon Lieutenant in the Royal Canadian Naval Volunteer Reserve in Montreal and assigned to *His Majesty's Ship (HMS) Donnaconda*. (Figure 3.1 is a photograph of Fisher as a young Surgeon Lieutenant.)

Fisher's duty was to examine all naval recruits. Veterans from World War I and others, often in their late 40s or 50s, tried to enlist and were among those to be examined. Fisher soon became bored with the monotony of examining the recruits. Presaging his later career, he gave himself a project that would render the time more profitable: He began to assess and characterize cardiac murmurs found among the recruits.

Meanwhile, the early portion of World War II was not going well for the Allies. France fell, and the British had to retreat from the Battle of Dunkirk. Hitler commented that there remained only one adversary, England. The Royal Canadian Navy received a request to send 12 Surgeon Lieutenants

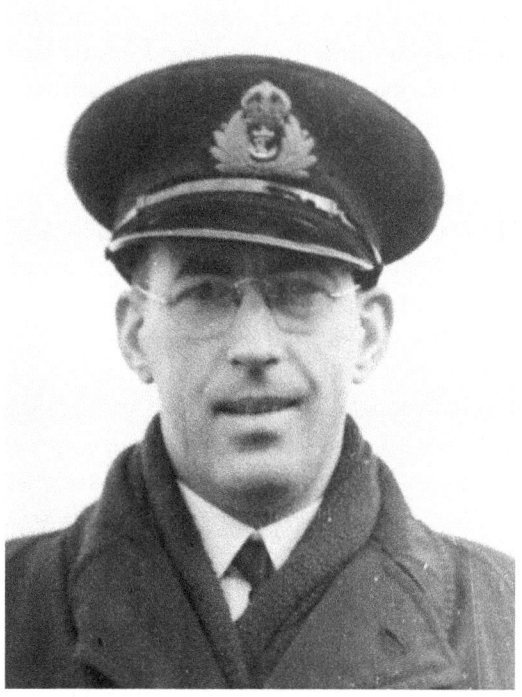

Figure 3.1 Fisher as a young Surgeon Lieutenant.

on loan to the British Royal Navy. Fisher and 11 others who hailed from cities and towns throughout Canada were chosen and were ordered to be sent urgently to the United Kingdom. Nonetheless, Fisher was allowed a short leave to spend with Doris, his bride of 6 months, before being shipped across the ocean. Fisher's leave was interrupted by orders detailing his transfer to the British Navy. He was directed to return immediately to Montreal and to proceed from there to Halifax, Nova Scotia, Canada. At that time, Trans Canada Airlines did not fly to the east coast of Canada, so Fisher rode in a Canadian Pacific Railway Pullman car for the long overnight journey to Halifax.

Fisher was quartered in Halifax at an Admiralty House while awaiting further orders. He was warned not to send laundry out because he would not be staying very long—his departure was supposed to be imminent. This was Fisher's first exposure to regular naval officers and the "spit and polish" of the routine, and he became quite impressed with the disciplinary aspects of the system. After several days of waiting, only 2 of the 12 medical Surgeon Lieutenants had arrived in Halifax, so Fisher telephoned Doris to come meet him. He reserved a room at the plush Lord Nelson Hotel, where he described the service as impeccable.

While awaiting departure, Fisher and the other early arrivals examined naval recruits and manned sick call held at the Halifax shipyards. He also participated in marching drills and evening retreats, during which the manpower at the base marched along with spirits stirred by music from the large naval band.

At that time, Halifax Harbour was the main naval communication pathway between Canada and England. Hundreds of freighters of various sizes came and went each day, traversing a channel in the harbor 5 miles long and a half mile wide that extended from the sea into the land-locked Bedford Basin, which encompassed several miles.

Fisher described the scene as follows:

> *Ship after ship outward bound traversed the channel, silently in single file all day long headed for the open sea to be picked up by their escorting war ships, destroyers, cruisers, minelayers and coastal vessels, moving at a painful 8 to 10 knots, constantly sitting targets for Nazi submarines lurking along the 14 day route to England.*[1]

On September 22, 1940, the 12 navy doctors, who had finally assembled, boarded a gray troop carrier on their way overseas (Figure 3.2 shows the 12 young Surgeon Lieutenants). The *Leopoldville* was a Belgian liner that was approximately half the size of the *Queen Mary* and the *Queen Elizabeth*. It could go as fast as 16 knots. In peaceful times, it had carried passengers

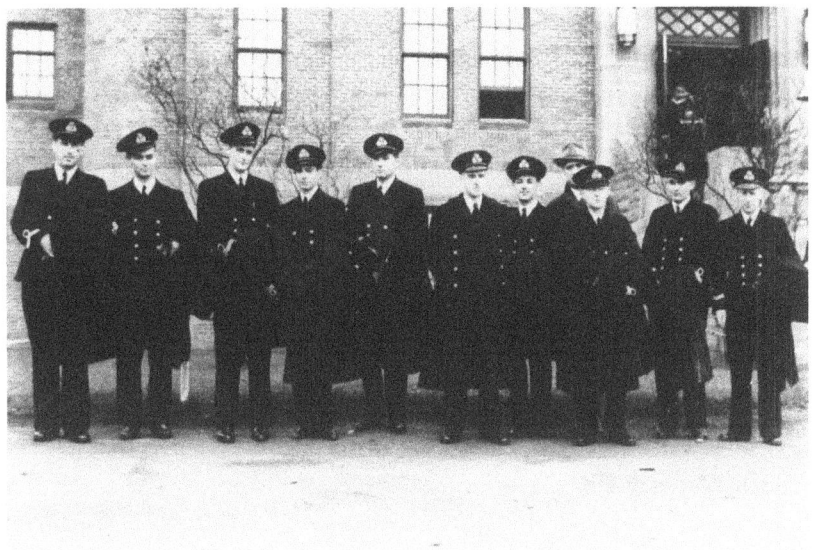

Figure 3.2 The 12 Surgeon Lieutenants.

and freight between Antwerp and the Belgian Congo. But when Belgium came under Nazi control, the *Leopoldville* could not return to Belgium. The ship first came to Canada, where it was painted gray so that it would be difficult to spot by submarines in ocean waters as it transported soldiers to the United Kingdom. Large guns were placed at the front and back decks of the ship to fire at attacking ships and submarines, and machine guns were located on the upper decks to target airplanes.

Fisher boarded the *Leopoldville* in the morning, and at dusk the ship's engines throbbed, lines were cast off, and within 10 minutes the *Leopoldville* was in open sea. In addition to the 12 naval physicians, there were approximately 500 troops, mainly from the army, aboard the ship. Fisher was appointed the senior officer in one small group. The senior army officer was a colonel who confessed to hating the sea. He was the captain of the ship's first trip in these ocean waters, and he appeared very nervous to Fisher and the other passengers. Communication between those guiding the ship and the passengers was limited, and rumors circulated that a warship was supposed to be joining the trip, but none ever appeared. The *Leopoldville* was unaccompanied while traversing dangerous waters. Navy orders at that time dictated that ships that were capable of traveling at 15 knots or faster always traveled alone because of their ability to outrun German submarines. Joining a convoy moving at 10 knots and spread over miles of sea would greatly increase the danger of being sunk. As the *Leopoldville* sailed toward England during a 14-day journey, torpedoed ships could be seen sinking or limping while on fire. For miles, the ocean was strewn with debris from sunken ships, empty lifeboats, and oil slicks from tankers. This time period was later described as the worst week of the war on the seas. German submarines were vigorously attacking the waters around the United Kingdom with the goal of forcing an early surrender. Bombs were also falling on English cities. One day, a long-range Caledonian reconnaissance flying boat passed near the *Leopoldville* and flashed a signal that land was approaching. The next day, the tip of Northern Ireland became visible; the ship entered the Irish Sea and dropped anchor in Liverpool's harbor.

The German air bombings were aimed mostly at the docks several miles from where the *Leopoldville* first anchored. The next day, Fisher and the other Surgeon Lieutenants were transported to Liverpool's grand hotel, the Adelphi. After one-night stays, the Surgeon Lieutenants were taken to a railway station for an overnight train journey to London, which was under siege with nightly bombings and fire bombings.

Fisher described the trip and the landing in London as follows:

> *Our train was blacked out and the trip was a series of stutters, dashes, and pauses, dictated by damaged rail yards and enemy aircraft in the vicinity. It was dawn as we crept into Euston Station. A smoky haze hung over the scene. Bombed-out and burnt-out shells of buildings could be seen for 3 or 4 streets. Firemen, fire wardens, and fire trucks were everywhere. A section of the station roof was missing. The islands were piled high with goods of all kinds awaiting delivery. . . . Women, children, and elderly men were emerging from the underground stations carrying their bed clothing and belongings. The night had been another nightmare of danger. Now a calm, determined business was evident. The apparent disorder was orderly.*[2]

The young naval officers carried medium-sized blue duffel bags because it was thought beneath the dignity of a naval officer to carry a suitcase or a parcel. They made their way to the entrance of the station, trying hard not to be appalled by the scenes they encountered. Within minutes, one London Cab appeared and the officers divided into groups of four and awaited the appearance of more cabs. Fisher was impressed by his London cab driver's coolness and demeanor of civilian courage. Fisher and the other passengers asked the taxi driver about how the previous night had gone. The driver replied in a cheery cockney accent: "Oh 'e buzzed around and around and dropped one now and then, but 'e aint done a wonderful lot o' damage."[3] The driver showed no signs of being disheartened even after the brutal assaults that had Britain virtually on its knees.

The naval doctors reported as directed to the Admiralty office in London. They were greeted by a young lieutenant, who consulted a more senior officer who quickly disappeared into an inner office. Fisher and colleagues could readily hear the conversation that ensued because the door was left ajar. It became obvious that the doctors' arrival was completely unexpected and the main question was what to do with them. They were then ushered into the office of the admiral, who referred to them as "momentarily expected medical reinforcements for the Royal Navy."[4] Rooms were arranged at the Cumberland Hotel very near Marble Arch, where Fisher and colleagues quartered for 3 days.

Fisher observed that London business went on almost normally during the day. Occasionally, air-raid sirens whined as enemy planes neared, but the massive daylight raids on London had almost ceased. When dusk approached, storefronts were boarded up, the city became dark, and people rushed to air-raid shelters located within the underground stations. Because it was considered beneath the dignity of naval officers to go to air-raid shelters, the young navy doctors remained in their beds. At approximately 7:30 p.m., air-raid sirens warned that German planes approached. During the night, the roar of planes was mixed with the high-pitched whine of falling bombs, explosions, and barrages of fire from anti-aircraft weapons stationed in Hyde Park, near the hotel where Fisher was quartered. At approximately 2 a.m., an all-clear signal sounded, quiet returned, and sleep became possible. The doctors hoped that they were as safe in the hotel as in any other place.

Fisher commented:

> *The spirit that is the camaraderie of war is difficult to convey. . . . The fellowship of union in a common perilous and desperate cause created a oneness in which each became significant and essential. . . . Everyone expected to see it through. Pride in sacrifice was the bond.*[5]

While at the hotel, the naval doctors received further orders: 4 were to proceed to Chatham, 4 to Portsmouth, and 4 to Plymouth. Fisher was among those ordered to proceed to Portsmouth on the south coast of the island. Portsmouth was the principal naval base and was an approximately 2-hour train ride from London, during which Fisher observed groups of 8–12 camouflaged planes of the Royal Air Force. These planes, called hurricanes and spitfires, were relatively small and were strategically positioned in order to try to drive off the hordes of German bombers that had been attacking London each day and night.

Portsmouth was a very large naval base, home of *HMS Victory* (Admiral Horatio Nelson's ship). When Fisher arrived, nearly all the ships had been removed to ports that were further distant from Nazi bombers, whose bases were only 75 miles away, directly across the English Channel. Portsmouth was one of the major training areas for the Royal Navy. Fisher's indoctrination into the Royal Navy was characterized as a pleasant experience. His main instructor was a surgeon commander who had served in World War I. Most of Fisher's time was spent in morning lectures, which were delivered with a heavy dose of anecdotes and humor; receiving instructions on how to fill out sick bay reports as well as drill instructions; and joining other recruits in basic training sessions. Fisher was only 29 years old, and all these experiences were very new for him.

Naval officers took turns manning potential casualty stations every few nights. This was accomplished by driving around blacked-out Portsmouth in military vehicles with hooded headlights. Driving was difficult for Fisher, who was accustomed to driving in Canada rather than on the "wrong side of the road." One evening, Fisher was dropped off several blocks from his hotel. The blackness was so complete that he became disoriented. He turned his ankle on a curbstone that he could not see. He could hear and feel his ligaments tearing. Half lost and limping badly, he passed individuals who seemingly were dark adapted. He heard a young lad exclaim, "Look at that drunken sailor."[6]

In early November 1942, Fisher received orders to report to No. 742 at the Admiralty in London. The train journey to London took a few hours, and he arrived at the Admiralty at approximately noon. A senior clerk greeted him and gave him travel vouchers to report immediately to No. 292 at naval headquarters in Glasgow, Scotland. After taking an overnight train to Glasgow, Fisher arrived the next morning at 10 a.m. A senior clerk at naval headquarters informed him that his assigned ship was scheduled to depart from Greenock and the Clyde at noon that day. A driver took him to the railway station, and Fisher took the Greenock train to Gourock, arriving at noon. A small naval boat was waiting for him. The boat sped across the Firth of Clyde, which was filled with hundreds of seagoing craft, and came alongside a huge vessel, the *HMS Letitia*. A ladder was thrown down and Fisher ascended gingerly to the ship's rail, where he was pulled aboard. He saluted the Officer of the Day and was quickly greeted by the ship's senior surgeon, Surgeon Lieutenant Commander Dr. Harvey Hebb, a Canadian-born surgeon with the Royal Navy. The vessel had been waiting for Fisher, and seconds after his arrival the ship began its journey.

Hebb and Fisher were the only Canadians on board. Fisher found Hebb to be very congenial. After being shown around the ship, Fisher was introduced to the sick bay where he would be working during the voyage. Within a few hours, the ship entered the rather turbulent waters in the Minches on the west coast of Scotland. Fisher became quite seasick and commented that this experience allowed him to identify with sufferers of mal de mer.

The *Letitia* was a 15,000-ton British liner that during peacetime sailed mostly to the Far East. It had been painted gray (like the *Leopoldville*) and converted to an armed merchant cruiser that carried numerous machine guns, an anti-aircraft battery, and a full complement of depth charges. The crew engaged in different practice exercises, preparing for action during a real attack. Fisher found that life on board was rather dull for the medical personnel. One task was censoring outgoing mail, especially information concerning Army personnel. Presaging his lifelong need to gain information and to be involved in active learning, Fisher described how he spent his time aboard ship:

> To keep busy, I undertook a study of navigation and spherical trigonometry, tried my hand at repairing watches, and with a machinist's mate tried to understand the practical aspects of motors and generators. Finally, I understood a little about navigation and could use a sextant to a degree. A few amateurish experiments on exposure to cold seawater were carried out.[7]

The main naval task of the *Letitia* was to patrol the North Atlantic entrance to the channel between Iceland and Greenland, the Denmark Strait. The ship could intercept Nazi ships that attempted to enter the Atlantic Ocean from occupied ports in Norway. A rapid cruising speed and a zigzag course among drifting ice packs made the *Letitia* a difficult target for German submarines. For the first months that Fisher was aboard, it was Arctic night and the only daylight was a faint lightening of the sky at approximately 2 p.m. The roll and hum of the engines in the dark became quite monotonous and mind dulling when there was no naval action for long stretches of time. After 3 months at sea, when food supplies were getting exhausted, the ship was ordered to return to Halifax, Canada, for rest and recuperation.

The docking at Halifax was fraught with problems. Halifax was blacked out. The ship was ordered to approach at full speed. The *Letitia* stopped suddenly with a crash when it ran aground approximately 100 yards offshore. The crew and passengers were taken to shore by harbor tugs. An investigation into the cause of the grounding uncovered that the only deck officer familiar with Halifax's harbor was in his cabin too drunk to assume his duties. As a result of the investigation, the captain of the ship, a very

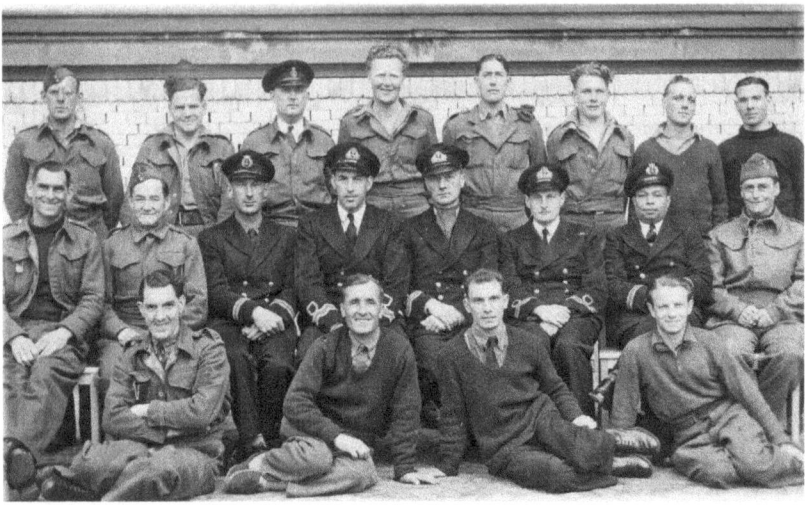

Figure 3.3 Fisher (second row, fourth from the left) and colleagues aboard the *Voltaire*.

promising young naval officer, was relieved of his command and never went to sea again.

Fisher requested and received permission for home leave. His appearance was a surprise to his wife Doris, who was very pregnant with their first child. After a few happy reunion days at home, the leave was cut short by a signal to report to the Halifax shipyard immediately. After a 1,200-mile train trip to Halifax, Fisher was dispatched to Saint John, New Brunswick, for service on the *HMS Voltaire*. The ship was originally a passenger ship out of Liverpool, England, but the British Admiralty had requisitioned it in October 1939 and began converting it into an armed merchant cruiser. The conversion was completed in January 1940, but the ship remained in dry dock undergoing a refitting, which was nearly complete. Fisher was introduced to the other officers and became acquainted with the sick bay and its staff (Figure 3.3). A few days later, the ship was afloat. Fisher was the only Canadian aboard.

DISASTER IN THE SOUTH ATLANTIC OCEAN: SUNK AT SEA

The captain of the *Voltaire* was secretive, and neither Fisher nor the crew knew the destination or the plan. The ship was heading south. Two days after leaving Saint John, a severe storm shook the ship, and it stopped in Hamilton, Bermuda. The *Voltaire* had been on convoy duty. Now in a tropical climate, the entire ship's company had to be issued new gear suitable to the expected very hot weather. Tropical gear had been secretly stashed aboard. Getting it to fit well was another matter.

Fisher described the comic scene in detail in his memoirs:

> Officers' epaulets had to be switched from winter gear to summer. Getting white stockings to stay up was a problem. And, of course everyone had black shoes. Sunday church parade the next morning presented the most hilarious assortment of naval dress the world could ever have witnessed. Short sailors had white shorts that were too long, reaching half-way between the knee and the ankle. Thin sailors had shorts that might have held two of them. Sleeves seemed either to hide hands or expose the forearm. Short black stockings were the rule and added not one whit to the attractiveness of shorts that were much too long. Black shoes did not go well with white tropical gear. Furthermore, the men on parade seemed to have made little or no effort to cover up the discrepancies, but on the other hand used every occasion to highlight their ridiculous garb. The officers on parade viewing the scene lost their composure . . . and laughed their way through the hymn Rock of Ages.[8]

The *Voltaire* spent 4 days in the Caribbean at Port of Spain, Trinidad. Fisher spent time in the hospital library boning up on tropical medicine, a subject in which he had had no prior training. The crew learned that the destination of the ship was Freetown, Sierra Leone, from which they were to lead a convoy of freighters to England.

On the third day out of Trinidad—April 4, 1941—disaster struck: The ship was sunk by the German ship *Thor*, a 400-foot-long, 9,200-ton ship armed with 12 naval guns and four torpedo tubes, with 349 officers and crew aboard.[9] The *Voltaire* was larger than the *Thor*. The *Voltaire* weighed 13,458 tons and had 10 naval guns and at least one anti-aircraft mount, with 269 officers and crew. The *Thor* was returning to Germany when it found the *Voltaire* heading toward Freetown approximately 900 miles southwest of the Cape Verdi islands. Accounts of the battle became available from documents released after the war.[10] The war marine (Kriegsmarine) auxiliary cruiser *Thor* was patrolling the mid-Atlantic Ocean during the spring of 1941 on its way back to Germany when it came upon the *Voltaire*. The German ship had previously engaged two British armed merchant cruisers, the *HMS Alcantara* and the *HMS Carnavon Castle*, in preliminary surface battles, but the skirmishes had ended indecisively. The British referred to the *Thor* and similar ships as "raiders" in reference to their activities in the open waters. When the *Thor* encountered the *Voltaire*, its crew had been battle-tested and was itching to finally sink an enemy combatant.

Crew members of the *Thor* spotted smoke on the horizon at approximately 6:15 a.m. on April 4, 1941. The German captain thought that the vessel was a coal-burning ship, so he headed the ship in the direction of the smoke. When the Germans made visual contact with the *Voltaire*, they suspected that it was a neutral ocean liner because it did not attempt to escape. The British, under Captain J. A. Blackburn, sighted the approaching ship and fired a burst of anti-aircraft fire as a signal for identification. The *Thor* did not return the signal. The British discovered the identity of the approaching ship at approximately 6:45 a.m. when the ship replaced the flag of Greece with a German naval insignia and fired a shot across the *Voltaire*'s bow. The British responded by manning their guns and firing a broadside. After only 4 minutes of dueling at a distance of approximately 9,800 yards, the Germans began striking the *Voltaire* with their larger guns. The first shots entered the radio room and the generator room of the *Voltaire*, heavily damaging the vessel and knocking out communications and steering gear. Heavy fires broke out and nearly covered the entire deck of the British ship. The gunners aboard the *Voltaire* continued fighting for nearly an hour despite the fires aboard the ship. For the next several minutes, the two sides fired, but only one British shot managed to hit the *Thor*, and it caused no casualties. The shot tore off some radio equipment attached to the main mast. By 7:15 a.m., only two of the largest British guns were in action. The *Thor* circled around the *Voltaire*, firing rapidly. At 8:00 a.m., just as the *Thor* was prepared to launch a torpedo, a white flag was observed aboard the *Voltaire* and so the firing stopped. Having lost 72 men killed in action, Captain Blackburn gave the order to abandon ship. During the next 5 hours, the Germans rescued 197 survivors, approximately half of whom were injured and 2 of whom died later. The remainder of the survivors, including Fisher, became prisoners of war.

In his memoirs, Fisher provides a personal account of the battle:

> On the third day out of Trinidad and just about on the equator, at 0600 the alarm was sounded. . . . I could see a large ship three or four miles away, obviously a freighter we had chanced upon. Signals were flashed back and forth between the ships. She had a difficult to identify profile. . . . Suddenly guns flashed and the Voltaire received a full broadside at point-blank range. The bridge was put out of action, the forward signal station received a direct hit, the main mast went down, and at least two of our guns were knocked out. From the beginning, we were paralyzed, coordinated firing was impossible and guns had to be trained and fired individually. . . . My sick bay warrant officer was struck and killed by a shell fragment. It was impossible to move about. Two of our guns fired from time to time and the German raiders kept blasting until these guns were silent. The Voltaire was on fire and a gunnery officer shouted that a

magazine was on fire and ship was to be abandoned. The fear of being sucked down by a sinking ship is deeply ingrained in sailors. The Voltaire was going to turn over and we survivors slid or jumped into the ocean.[11]

A few rafts were floated, and Fisher inflated his and paddled around in the warm water. Others were hanging onto planks or other debris from the ship. Fisher had difficulty seeing far because of ocean swells. From time to time, a higher swell lifted him so that he could see the *Voltaire* lying on its side and finally disappearing. When a rope ladder from the sunken ship came within his reach, he fastened one end to his waist and let the other end dangle off of his feet. He wrote,

One's memories of such a time may be real or fanciful. I recall that when we went into action stations my thoughts were of my dear wife, who on that very day, April 4 was expecting our first child. . . . Once in the water my thoughts were of the possibility that at that moment she might be in labor and I thought only of her welfare. I recall that after a period in the water I thought that if I had to swim it made no difference if I swam back to South America or forward to Africa, the distance was about the same. I conserved my strength by floating idly. I don't recall alarm. After 5 or 6 hours in the water, a wave lifted me and I could see a ship in the distance. It might be a sign of hope. Another view later showed the ship closer and I could hear the crackle of machine gunfire. . . . A few more hours passed and I was by no means exhausted. . . . There came into view a small boat fishing a man out of the water. Now I began to swim and wave and shout. . . . Fortunately in the next minutes I heard a motor and a launch came along the wave trough I was in and spotted me. I was lifted into the boat by two sailors in the uniform of the German Navy and I realized I had been rescued by the enemy.[12]

Two hours or so were spent searching for other survivors, and then Fisher and others were taken back to the raider *Thor*. The *Voltaire* had been unable to transmit signals before going down. The *Thor* had left the scene until the *Voltaire* had completely sunk, and then it returned for the rescue operation. Approximately 200 of the crew of the *Voltaire* lost their lives. Among the 97 survivors, many had shattered limbs, gaping shrapnel wounds, or were weak from blood loss. Two German surgeons took charge of treating the wounded, and Fisher administered the anesthesia when needed. Fisher commented that he received the special treatment accorded medical personnel. He was placed in a specially guarded cabin with some officers from a Swedish freighter that had also been sunk by the *Thor* 2 weeks previously off the coast of Cape Town, South Africa.

Fisher reflected in retrospect on the battle. Although the officers of the *Voltaire* had spotted the raider, apparently the raider had not seen the

Voltaire until the last moment. The silhouette of the *Thor* did not match that of any Allied or friendly ship on the available charts, but in many ways it resembled that of a German raider drawn by Allied naval officers from the *Carnarvon Castle* and the *Alcantara*, which had engaged the raider in battle. Captain Blackburn had been told in Trinidad that a raider was operating in the region through which the *Voltaire* was planning to pass. The captain was apprehensive but failed to tell other officers of the bridge about a potential engagement with one or more raiders during their travel. If the ship's crew had been aware and had reviewed the drawings of potential ship sightings, perhaps the sinking of the ship might have not occurred. The *Voltaire* could have begun the attack and gained an advantage.

April 4, 1941, Fisher was very much under the control of the German enemy to do with what it pleased.

NOTES

1. Fisher CM. *Memoirs of a Neurologist*. Rutland, VT: Academy Books, 1992, Vol. 1, p. 66.
2. Fisher CM. *Memoirs of a Neurologist*. Rutland, VT: Academy Books, 1992, Vol. 1, p. 69.
3. Fisher CM. *Memoirs of a Neurologist*. Rutland, VT: Academy Books, 1992, Vol. 1, p. 69.
4. Fisher CM. *Memoirs of a Neurologist*. Rutland, VT: Academy Books, 1992, Vol. 1, p. 70.
5. Fisher CM. *Memoirs of a Neurologist*. Rutland, VT: Academy Books, 1992, Vol. 1, p. 71.
6. Fisher CM. *Memoirs of a Neurologist*. Rutland, VT: Academy Books, 1992, Vol. 1, p. 74.
7. Fisher CM. *Memoirs of a Neurologist*. Rutland, VT: Academy Books, 1992, Vol. 1, p. 77.
8. Fisher CM. *Memoirs of a Neurologist*. Rutland, VT: Academy Books, 1992, Vol. 1, pp. 8s0–81.
9. Asmussen J. Hilfskreuzer (auxiliary cruiser/raider)—*Thor*. http://Bismarck-class.dk. Retrieved June 21, 2014.
10. Wikipedia: Action of 4 April 1941.
11. Fisher CM. *Memoirs of a Neurologist*. Rutland, VT: Academy Books, 1992, Vol. 1, pp. 81–82.
12. Fisher CM. *Memoirs of a Neurologist*. Rutland, VT: Academy Books, 1992, Vol. 1, p. 83.

CHAPTER 4

Prisoner of War, 1941–1944

THE TRIP TO THE PRISONER-OF-WAR CAMP

Fisher was clearly under the complete control of German officers as a prisoner of war (POW). He and his fellow prisoners spent 10 days aboard the German raider *Thor*. He described it as a trim ship that flew a Spanish flag and was equipped with well-camouflaged, 5.9-inch guns that were accurate at approximately 10 miles. The Nazis who were aboard the ship were convinced that the war would soon end, and the German surgeons took his name and address and promised to visit him in Ontario when the "Teutonic conquest was complete."[1]

On Easter Sunday, after 10 days on the *Thor*, prisoners with minor or no injuries were transferred to an old Dutch prison tanker ship. Fisher accompanied them as a medical officer and as the British Officer in Charge. The prisoners were jammed into the after-hold of the ship, which consisted of three decks built on planks arranged one above the other. A steel drum on each deck represented the common outhouse facility. Prisoners were allowed only a few minutes on the open deck each day and were battened down in a very crowded, very hot, and malodorous hold at night. After a few days, Fisher, as a medical officer, was allowed to be quartered with the Swedish officers aboard. Because the Swedes were not officially classified as prisoners of war, they were allowed some of the amenities that they saved from their ship before it sunk, such as Aquavit, a distilled spirit that was produced in Scandinavia. Drinking lightened a bit the rest of the time on the ship.

The prison tanker arrived on the 10th day at the port city of La Rochelle on the French coast just north of Bordeaux. After disembarking, the prisoners lined up on the dock under the watch of a large contingent of the German infantry. They then marched through the streets to a deserted French cavalry barracks singing one British marching song after another. Somehow spirits remained high among the prisoners. After spending the night lying on straw in a very cold horse barrack, the prisoners were taken to a huge pile of used clothing presumably taken from other prisoners, and they were urged to grab what fit. They then traveled in a train to St. Medard, a town nearer to Bordeaux. The trip, which ordinarily took 2 hours, took 2 days because the train was often halted. At St. Medard, the prisoners were placed in a tiny prison camp, with 70 prisoners sleeping on the floors of large huts. Their diet consisted of a weak flour soup with a trace of vegetables. Merchant marine officers and seamen from British and Allied ships sunk by German raiders kept arriving in the camp. The Germans waited for a count of 400 persons, a trainload, to begin the transfer to Germany.

Once 400 prisoners were captured, they were herded into cattle cars, 40 to a car. A steel drum for sanitary disposal sat in the center of each railroad car and was emptied every 48 hours. On the way, 2 prisoners escaped and others attempted to exit the cars but were intercepted by German guards, who rushed into the cars and began punching, slapping with the flat part of bayonets, and kicking prisoners. Because Fisher was the senior officer, he vigorously protested the guards' actions, with all attention almost immediately centered on him. He commented,

> I was dressed in rags and wore a scraggly thirty-day beard. A huge fat-faced, beady-eyed, brush-cut Prussian madman began to threaten me with his riding crop, bringing it down time and time again within a hairsbreadth of the skull. The guards were evidently under the influence of schnapps, and I thought the sand in my time-glass had run out. Suddenly the train started up again, the guards jumped out and the door slid shut.[2]

At that time, trains moved mostly at night through the blackout. The prisoners' journey took approximately 5 days as the train passed through Bordeaux, Nantes, Paris, Maastricht, Dusseldorf, Hanover, and Bremen. The destination was prison camp Stalag XB.

STALAG XB, SANDBOSTEL

The Stalag XB camp was located in Sandbostel, Germany, 43 km northeast of Bremen. This facility opened in 1932 within the Province of Hanover during the great economic depression. Here, out-of-work singles could congregate for roadwork jobs and jobs involving upgrading other public works. In 1933, the Reich Labour Service took over the camp and later used it as a Nazi internment camp for undesirables. Beginning in 1939 and throughout World War II, the camp served as a POW camp. The camp was expanded when Polish POWs were brought to it.[3] Initially, huts for approximately 10,000 prisoners were built. Figure 4.1 shows photographs of Stalag XB.

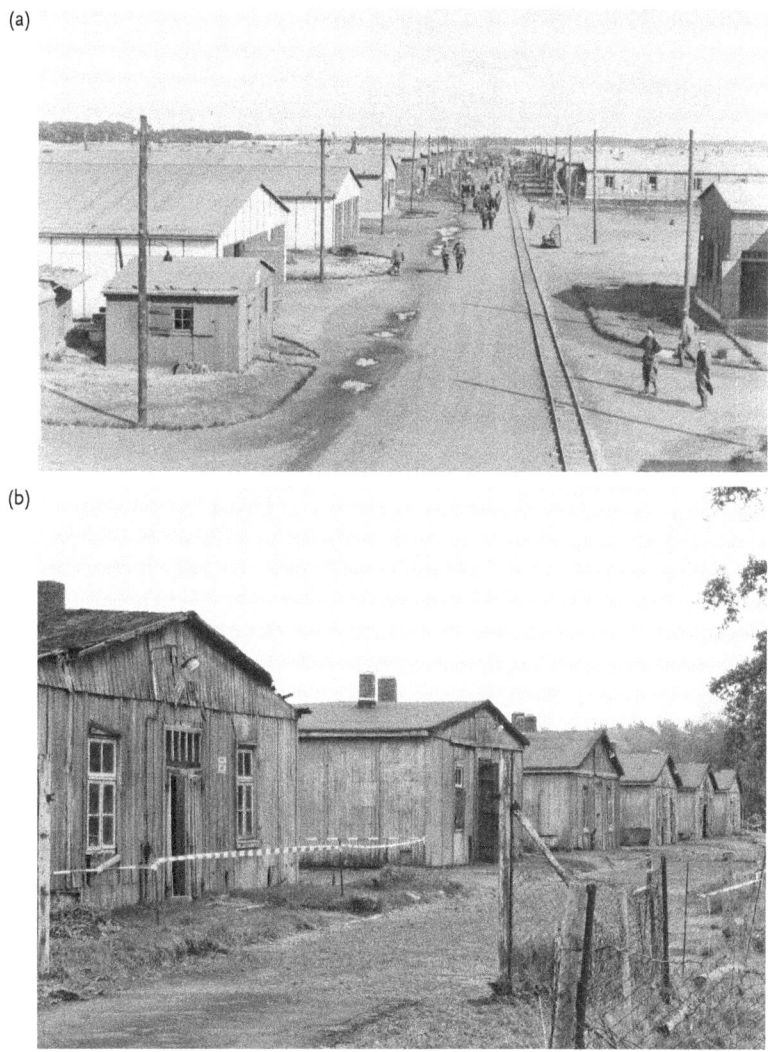

Figure 4.1 (A) Photograph of Stalag XB, Sandbostel, Germany, taken during the 1940s. (B) Recent photograph of barracks at Stalag XB.
Sources: A, provided courtesy of Ronald Sperling and the Memorial Place Sandbostel, with permission; B, reproduced with permission, © Peter Hohenhaus, http://www.dark-tourism.com.

The camp was divided into several smaller camps: a stalag holding enlisted men from occupied countries (Poland, Belgium, the Netherlands, France, southeastern Europe, and Italy after the armistice) and a camp for officers (oflags) from occupied countries. In 1941, this part of the camp was merged with oflags elsewhere—a Marinelager (Marlag), controlled by the Kriegsmarine, holding British sailors, marines, and officers including Fisher. In the fall of 1941, this part of the camp was moved to Westertimke. An Internierungslager (Ilag), or internment camp for civilian citizens of enemy nations, including members of the British merchant marines, was also moved to Westertimke in 1941.

Fisher described the Stalag XB camp as follows:

> *A huge facility situated on the flat barren sand dunes of northern Germany. Throughout the entire camp, not a blade of grass nor a tree could be seen, nor could a tree be seen in the surrounding countryside. Nothing except sand. . . . The whole camp measured 200 yards by 400 yards. It was surrounded by huge double barbed wire fences about 4 feet apart, in between which were bales of more barbed wire. At 100-yard intervals stood guard towers, 15 feet high armed with machine guns and spotlights. In addition to the guards in the towers, guards patrolled the perimeter often with "dogs" more like ponies on leash.*[4]

Figure 4.2 shows photographs of the Marlag camp.

Soon after Fisher arrived, the Germans excavated a large moat around the perimeter of the camp and sunk listening devices into the ground, allowing them to detect any tunneling activity.

Even while floating in the water after the *Voltaire* sunk, Fisher's mind was preoccupied with his Canadian family and the imminent birth of his first child. Before sailing from Saint John, Fisher sent his wife the name of the ship to which he had been assigned. Doris Fisher gave birth to a daughter, Elizabeth, on April 2, 1941. On April 7, Doris' father read in the newspaper of the sinking of the *Voltaire*, the ship name Fisher had sent. On April 14, a Canadian government official called the family to report that the *Voltaire* had been sunk by the German Kriegsmarine, and a week later an official naval telegram arrived stating that Doris' husband was missing in action (Figure 4.3A). During the next 2 months, additional telegrams arrived informing Doris of Fisher's whereabouts, so by the end of June 1941, Doris and her family knew of his confinement at Stalag XB (Figures 4.3B and 4.3C).

Meanwhile, Fisher and the other prisoners were settling into the POW camp. His memoirs contain details of life in the camp; they spell out well the very negative but also some positive experiences. Wartime imprisonment

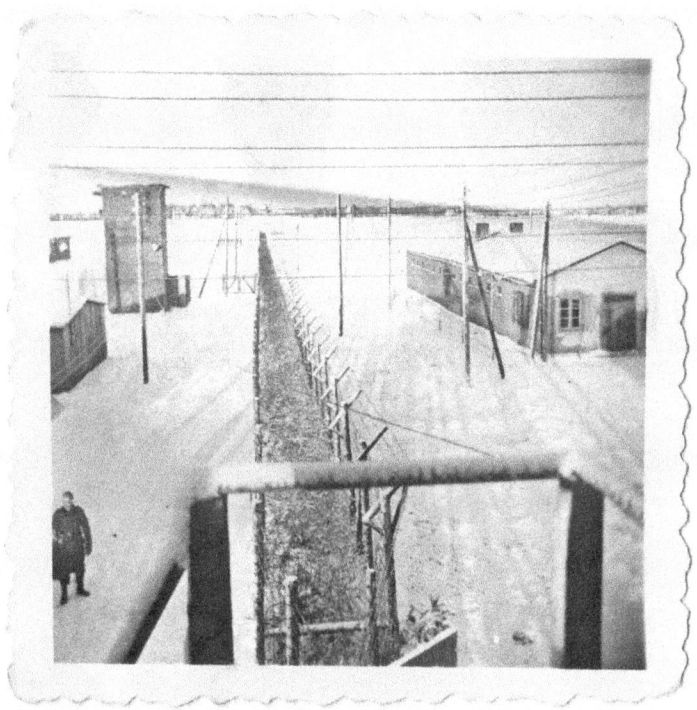

Figure 4.2 Photograph of the Marlag prisoner-of-war camp during the 1940s. The photograph was taken from the main road of the camp from a tower.
Source: Provided courtesy of Ronald Sperling and the Memorial Place Sandbostel, with permission.

is mostly portrayed in literature and motion pictures as a totally negative phenomenon. But there was some humane behavior.

During early spring of 1942, Red Cross parcels began to arrive at the camp. These provided tangible evidence to the prisoners that they were not forgotten. The parcels were packed tightly in 16 × 10 × 8-inch parcels in England or Canada and sent under the auspices of the International Red Cross headquarters in Geneva, Switzerland. Inside the parcels were small cans of meat and vegetable soup, meat paste, margarine, kippers, sardines, plum pudding, ham, marmite, dried milk, mixed fruit, coffee, and tea. Sometimes a chocolate bar and shortbreads were included. Three parcels for each prisoner were delivered during some months, whereas in other months, no parcels were delivered. The Red Cross deliveries fostered solidarity and communication between the officers. The officers of the Royal Navy decided to organize a common mess where parcels were stored centrally; each officer received content suited for individual use, and more stable goods were prepared in a communal kitchen and served in a common

(a)

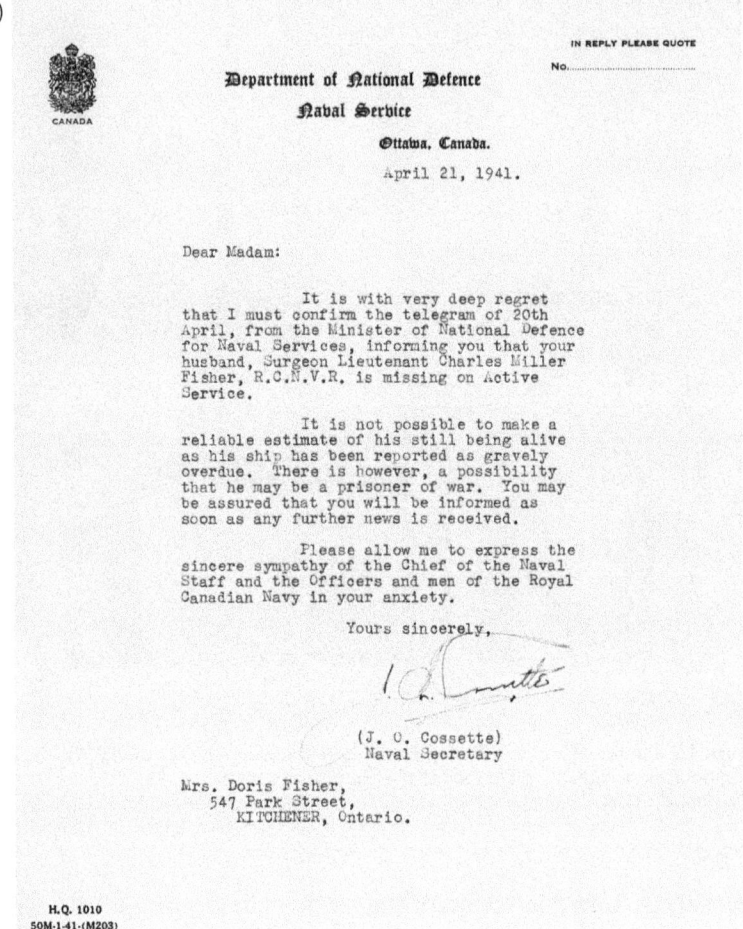

Figure 4.3 Continued

dining barrack. This plan facilitated officers mingling together three times a day at the common barrack site.

There were two British compounds in Stalag XB, each approximately 100 yards square. Each compound had 10 long, low barracks buildings; each barrack was divided into 10 square rooms arranged 5 on each side of a central corridor. Initially, each room slept 20–27 prisoners in three-tier bunks. Mattresses were filled with wood straw. A potbellied stove in the center of each room was the only heating source. The fuel was peat moss and occasional briquettes of coal. The German food ration provided approximately 1400 calories daily, composed mostly of potatoes, sauerkraut, turnips, gherkins, black bread, and fish soup in which whole fish were chopped up.

(b)

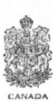

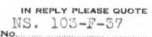

Department of National Defence
Naval Service

Ottawa, Canada.

IN REPLY PLEASE QUOTE
NS. 103-F-37
No.

4th May, 1941.

Dear Madam:

Further to my letter of the 21st April, 1941, I am directed to inform you that your husband, Surgeon Lieutenant Charles Miller Fisher, R.C.N.V.R. (Temp.) was serving in H.M.S. "VOLTAIRE". The Admiralty have announced that this ship is overdue and must be presumed lost.

Unfortunately it is impossible to give you any more news of your husband and until some more definite news is received he will continue to be listed as missing on Active Service.

Please again accept the sincere sympathy of the Chief of the Naval Staff and Officers and men of the Royal Canadian Navy in your great anxiety.

Yours sincerely,

(J.O. Cossette),
NAVAL SECRETARY.

Mrs. Doris Fisher,
547 Park Street,
KITCHENER, Ontario.

Figure 4.3 Continued

The bread was Kommisbrot, a solid, heavy dark brown loaf that hefted like a rock. When cut with a bread knife, the crumbs looked like sawdust. Horse meat filled with maggots was occasionally supplied as well.

There were various ways of getting and trading goods, variously referred to as the camp market, black market, and schwarz market. Fresh eggs, bread, sausage, whiskey, and wine were somehow available in the camp. Prisoners often traded coffee or tea for fresh items such as eggs or white bread. Fisher noted that the market values of items fluctuated from day to day depending on the supply and demand. Two ounces of coffee was variably worth two eggs one day and three the next. Cartons of cigarettes were sent from the Red Cross and could also be sent privately from home.

(c)

Department of National Defence
Naval Service
Ottawa, Canada.

28th June, 1941.

Dear Madam:

    It is with much pleasure that I confirm the telegram of the 28th June from the Minister of National Defence for Naval Services informing you that your husband, Acting Surgeon Lieutenant-Commander Charles Miller Fisher, R.C.N.V.R., previously listed as missing, has now been reported a Prisoner of War in Camp Stalag, X.B., GERMANY. At the present time, no information is available as to his condition, but it may be assumed that he is fit and well.

    Instructions for addressing correspondence to Prisoners of War in Germany can be found in any local Post Office.

    All allotments made by your husband will be continued, and you will receive your monthly cheque as usual.

    You may be assured that all members of the Canadian Naval Forces share with you the good news that your husband is alive.

Yours very truly,

(J. O. Cossette),
NAVAL SECRETARY.

Mrs. Doris Fisher,
  547 Park Street,
    KITCHENER, Ont.

Figure 4.3 (A and B) Letters to Doris Fisher regarding her husband's "missing on active service" status. (C) Letter to Doris Fisher informing her that her husband was found but was in a prisoner-of-war camp in Germany.
Source: Reproduced from a collection of war memorabilia by Dr. Hugh and Susan Fisher.

Cigarettes made excellent currency to trade for goods. When cigarettes were in short supply, high prices were often demanded for them.

Fisher became well aware of the activities and behavior of the guards. To challenge or displease them was potentially very dangerous:

> *The temperament of the guards was mercurial. At times they were friendly but discreet, at other times irritable, volatile, dangerous and impulsive. Then we were still all schweinhunds. Guards would shoot at the slightest pretext. Rescuing a football that had rolled past the guard wire was risky. At night sending a bullet through the corridor of a barrack just in case someone was out of his room constituted amusement.*[5]

Sanitary facilities consisted of an open room with a cement floor. Porcelain toilets were fitted into holes cut through the floor. There was a large septic tank below the floor. The contents of the septic tank were pumped out and used as fertilizer at nearby German farms. The contents were transported in tanks that rested on four-wheel carts that were hauled by prisoners.

The medical facilities consisted of 12 beds. Medical supplies were nearly non-existent. In the room in which the sick bay was held were paper bandages, licorice tablets for gargling, and a one-piece scalpel that was corroded with a quarter of the tip missing. There were also unmarked cough tablets. Sulfa drugs (the only known useful antibiotic at that time) were not routinely provided.[6] The medical facilities were periodically visited by American visitors who were supposed to oversee the care. One of the visitors broke into tears when he saw the virtual non-existence of medicines, supplies, and implements. These visits were likely pro forma and little was ever done to improve the capabilities. Fisher commented that there was little to do medically. Most of the patients who came to the sick bay were there because of injuries. Most of the beds were almost always empty. The lack of effective remedies for those who were ill led to Fisher becoming interested in and much more aware of the placebo response.

Some rooms in the compound had giant maps of the eastern front that showed all Russian towns and villages as they fell to the Germans. Fisher and others could watch at night as British night bombers (the Wellingtons) flew toward the German cities of Hamburg, Kiel, Berlin, and Hanover. These nocturnal scenes must have been very discouraging to view by Fisher and colleagues. Fisher commented,

> Night after night formations of a few "Wimpies" heavily weighted down with bomb loads slowly droned overhead. They faced almost hopeless odds. Countless moving searchlights stabbed the night sky attempting to catch a plane in their beams. German night fighters cruised back and forth until suddenly . . . a point of brilliance appeared in a beam. Immediately the night fighters opened their throttles and sped towards the lumbering victim. The "Wimpie" dove and wove wildly, desperately trying to escape from the pursuing light. The rattle of the night fighters' guns were all too liable to send the bomber down in flames. Some German areas were protected by strong antiaircraft batteries, and when the bombers escaped the night fighters and searchlights, they faced tremendous firepower from the ground as they approached their targets.[7]

There was abundant time to think and to try to distract one's mind away from the carnage of the camp and the war. It is apparent from Fisher's comments in his memoirs that in Stalag XB he became interested in how people thought, how they predicted future happenings, and how they subsequently recalled their own predictions. These analytic techniques were a very important part of his modus operandi later in his medical career. They indicated his tendency to be a keen student of human behavior and thought.

One of his analyses involved the behavior of Germans who often visited the camp barracks. Gestapos and other propagandists frequently came by and were ostensibly interested in the views of the war of the physicians who technically were noncombatants. The visitors were intelligent college graduates. When the topic of Russia arose, the propagandists quickly explained that Hitler and Stalin were very good friends. They had signed a non-aggression pact. Then 1 day later, German guards excitedly ran into the barracks and announced that Hitler had attacked Russia and that panzers had already advanced hundreds of miles into Russia. A week or so after that, the same propagandists who had spoken of Russian and German friendship returned to the camp praising the German coup. Fisher reminded them that they had sung a very different story weeks before. The propagandists retorted that Hitler said that Stalin was about to stab Germany in the back and so pre-empted him and attacked Russia.

Fisher commented, "Herein lies the danger of the totalitarian state with its secrecy, controlled information, and official indoctrination. Dictatorial regimes are aggressive either by arms or by lies and deceit. Devotees (or victims) reverse themselves 180 degrees without protest. Democracy beware."[8]

Fisher joined a poker club of eight members. After cards, the members would discuss the war and other topics and often would make predictions. Fisher noted that they tended to only recall the predictions that came true. After poker on December 7, 1941, the senior British camp commandant of the merchant marines predicted firmly, "I can assure you that Japan will never enter the war on the side of Germany." This prediction was based on the fact that most of his military career had been spent traveling to the Far East. Of course, that very same day, Japan bombed Pearl Harbor. When Fisher became aware of the vagaries of subsequent recall of predictions, he urged his colleagues to write down their predictions for subsequent review.

During Fisher's stay in Stalag XB, there was an attempt at escape by building a tunnel. In his memoirs, Fisher begins the story of the tunnel by declaring "a young naval officer and I began to plan our escape by a tunnel."[9] Others became heavily involved. A senior British officer pointed out to Fisher that according to the Geneva Convention, medical personnel were forbidden from participating in any nefarious activity whatsoever. Fisher then dropped out of active participation in building the tunnel but became an observer. The tunnel was a major accomplishment that was constructed during a 4-month period. One entered the tunnel by lifting a well-camouflaged trapdoor in the floor beneath one of the barracks. When completed, the tunnel was approximately 2 feet square and lay at a depth of 5–9 feet; it was approximately 100 yards long. It extended 20 yards to near the gate, 15 yards under the gate, and 65 yards out into the peat bogs that surrounded the camp. The overhead and walls were shored up with ¾-inch wooden slats taken from the bunks of cooperating colleagues.

The prisoners needed to make inquiries to try to obtain civilian clothing, German money, identification papers, and maps. Word of the tunnel spread widely, not only in the British compound but also among other nationalities—French, Polish, Serb, Belgian, etc. Despite the fact that all prisoners seemed aware of the tunnel, evidently the Germans were unaware that it existed.

Fisher noted that even the most menial and poorly educated men in the camp kept the secret and even under severe duress would not buckle down to German pressures. He cited the example of Chinese crewmen who were ordered to proceed to Hamburg to work in laundries. They refused. Rifles were pointed at their heads. They still refused. "You shoot but still no workee."[10]

The prisoners arranged for a "variety night," during which noise and singing were planned to direct attention away from the escape. Fourteen officers escaped through the tunnel. One of the marine escapees reached a point 125 miles south of the camp but was captured by a German policeman on a motorcycle and the Gestapo was alerted. Unfortunately, the 16 escapees (2 escaped at a later time) were captured and sent to a different punishment high-security camp and likely killed.

Fisher commented,

> Is there a lesson in all of this? I see in it evidence that in every man a nobleness of spirit resides, can we but summon it forth. Silently a common bond united us. We were fighting for right against a ruthless subhuman enemy plain to see. Churchill and the British people set the example.[11]

MARLAG (MILAG NORD), WESTERTIMKE

In the summer of 1942, Fisher was transferred to Marlag (Milag Nord) in Westertimke, 15 miles northeast of Bremen and 7 miles from the Weser

River, into a compound that was solely for naval prisoners. Fisher noted that the new camp was a definite improvement. The barracks were in better condition and were less crowded. The camp was divided into three compounds. Two compounds—a 100-yard square area for the

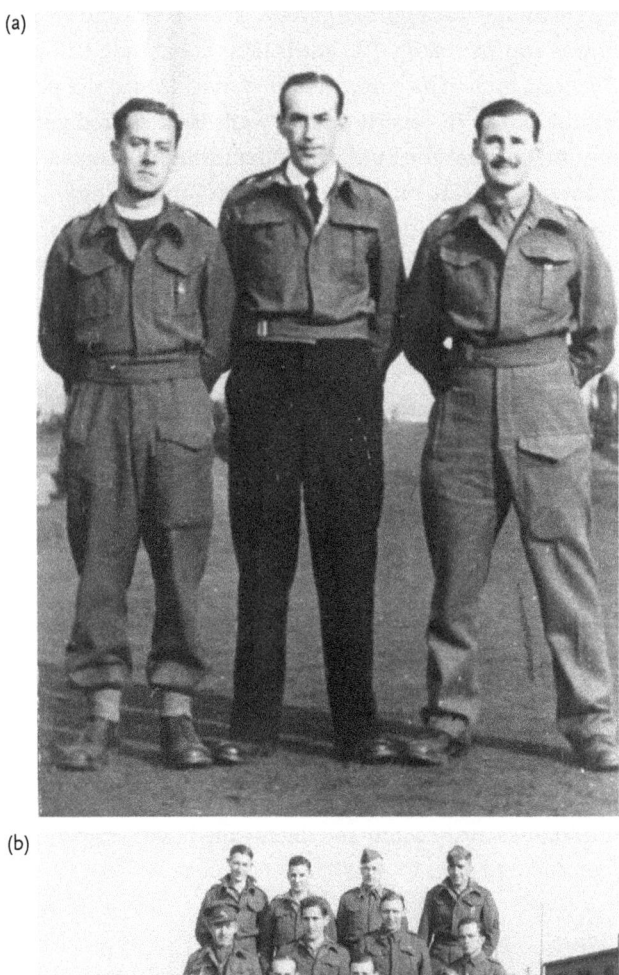

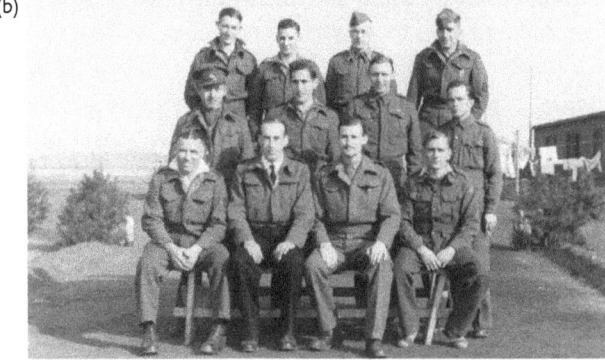

Figure 4.4 (A) Fisher (middle) with two colleagues in the prisoner-of-war camp. (B) Fisher (first row, second from the left) and colleagues in the camp.

150 officers of the Royal Navy and a second region approximately twice as large as the first for the approximately 300 other navy personnel—were called Marlag (Marine Lager). A much larger compound was located a half-mile away for the approximately 2,400 officers and men of the merchant marines. This marine compound was called Milag (Marine International Lager). There was no communication between the compounds except by medical officers from Marlag who rotated to the Milag to assist in caring for the sick bay.

MEDICINE AT MARLAG

The medical facilities and medical care at Marlag were better organized than at Stalag XB. Fisher joined Dr. Gavin Knight working in the sick bay, sharing responsibilities for the sick, sanitation, food, and preventive health measures. Medical equipment and pharmaceuticals were more abundant than at Stalag XB. A sterilizer, a few needles, and suture material were available at the new camp. Medicines such as sulfapyridine, calcium, antacids, aspirin, and cough tablets were all provided. Each sick bay had an adequate number of hospital beds for the population of the camp. The sick bay to which Fisher was assigned had 12 beds, but usually only 6 were filled. The wounded patients continued to stay in the barracks while being treated. An excellent dentist from New Zealand was available. Fisher commented that dental care was probably better in the camp than prisoners had known at home.[12]

During Fisher's time in the camp, there were no major infectious disease epidemics. Lice, fleas, scabies, and bedbugs were minor inconveniences endured by the prisoners. Tuberculosis of the lungs was diagnosed six times. Stomach ulcers were common. Surprisingly, mental illness was rare; only a few patients had schizophrenia or major depression. Fisher noted that although uncommon, both acute and chronic anxiety states responded well to encouragement and time. Homosexual activity, rarely obvious, was abhorred by the other prisoners. The only attempted homicide involved a jilted gay partner. Tobacco addiction was very prevalent, and advice to stop smoking simply because of the unavailability of cigarettes proved unsuccessful. Prisoners somehow were able to get hold of cigarettes by bartering. Fisher stated, "The officers were remarkably resolute, buoyant, resourceful, and resilient, thereby setting a superb example that lifted the entire company. . . . Young healthy males require little medical attention. Insomnia was nonexistent and constipation was hardly spoken of."[13]

According to the Geneva Convention (some aspects of which it seems were grossly adhered to), medical personnel were allowed to go on walks outside of the camp, under guard. Fisher went only twice. The walks made him more aware of his incarceration. He thought it unwise to claim a privilege not available to other prisoners.

Prisoners were sent out of Marlag to work on the surrounding farms. Fisher noted that the prisoners stole many goods, which they kept hidden under their coats. When returning to Marlag, they marched along a road adjacent to the camp, throwing their loot over the wooden fence and the barbed-wire enclosure that surrounded the camp, before the daily searches by guards. Fisher commented,

> Soon it would rain everything a prison camp might desire: bread, a plucked chicken. Coal, a bottle of schnapps, a bicycle wheel, radio tubes, a saw, apples, fresh vegetables, butter, bologna, sausage etc. Inside the camp everything was scooped up quickly.[14]

AWARENESS ABOUT THE TREATMENT OF JEWS AND OTHER PRISONERS

Fisher was able to see and watch guards and prisoners adjacent to his compound, and his medical duties often involved traveling to and through other compounds. He commented,

> Russian prisoners began to arrive in the compounds next to ours. . . . The Russian prisoners were virtually skeletons and obviously dying of starvation. They were dressed in ragged garments that encircled the body rather than hanging normally. Typhus was rampant and bodies were hauled away by the cartload almost every day. To throw them food invited a rifle bullet from a guard. My window was no more than 30 feet from these events.[15]

Fisher tried to maintain an upbeat approach to imprisonment. The pervasive spirit among many officers was "You can't do anything about it, so let's at least be cheerful."[16] Fisher's duties were to look after the wounded and help two doctors care for the daily sick call. Prisoners who had a major illness or needed surgery were transferred to a prison, Lazarett, 3 miles away, where a Yugoslavian surgeon reportedly provided excellent care. One of the sick call physicians was Dr. Mihil Sperber, a Czech surgeon who had escaped to Great Britain but was captured when the merchant marine freighter on which he was traveling was sunk. One morning, Sperber was summoned to the commandant's office and never returned. Fisher knew that Sperber was Jewish. Fisher related in his memoirs that two Jewish officers, a surgeon who worked in the daily sick call and an army dentist who was available on call, were summoned to the commandant's office and disappeared thereafter. It is unclear in his memoirs how much he knew or suspected about the German handling of Jews and other sects and about Nazi atrocities both inside and outside the camp.

RECEIVING INFORMATION ABOUT WAR EVENTS OUTSIDE THE CAMP

Fisher and others in the compound were able to stay informed about wartime events by way of a hidden radio. Swedish officers who were captured when their boat was sunk had been allowed to keep personal belongings because they were not at war with Germany. One Swedish officer had taken his new Phillips radio with him and kept it in a steamer trunk. When the Swedes were repatriated, the Germans transferred all Swedish belongings into a locked hut. The Swedes had given Navy prisoners a key to the trunk that contained the radio. One evening when Fisher was doing sick bay in the Milag compound, a colleague invited him to look under his bunk, where the radio had been stowed. The radio was later moved to a different hiding place.

Use of the radio was strictly regulated by a special news committee of the prisoners. This is another example of the tightly knit cooperation within the compound. Once or twice each day, while lookouts ensured that Germans were not nearby, the British Broadcasting Corporation news was obtained through headphones. The person who obtained the news told it to other men who were responsible for ensuring that everybody interested was informed. Individuals responsible for disseminating the news wrote it on fine paper that could be rolled into a cigarette and so passed on. Some wrote the news on paper that they kept hidden in their socks. Only a few individuals in the camp knew the source of the news.

Fisher and many of the other prisoners were able to follow the war news through the secret radio and the camp correspondents. In addition, the German camp commandant would announce news when it was favorable to Germany. When there was a British naval disaster, the commandant announced, "I hope none of you has relatives on the H.M.S. that was sunk." But the prisoners knew more than their captors. They were aware that the German navy had had even greater losses that were not mentioned. The German guards became aware that many of the prisoners were well informed and often knew of bad news regarding Germany before the guards.

The Gestapo was never able to detect the source of the news. As the collapse of Germany approached, the German guards would ask the British prisoners, "Was ist Neues?" ("What's new?"). Some German guards indicated by their behavior that they were not particularly sympathetic with Hitler and his gang and hoped that the war would end soon.

Fisher could listen to American broadcasts to troops in England, including the big bands of the time—those of Glen Miller, Benny Goodman, and Vaughan Monroe. The radio conveyed news of the war in Russia and the war in the Pacific. The British football scores were received promptly each Saturday evening, allowing many fans to follow their home team and often to bet on the outcome of matches. The presence of the radio and access to the outside world helped buoy the spirits of the prisoners, as did the regular arrival of Red Cross parcels.

CAMP ACTIVITIES

In order to avoid boredom, the prisoners organized many activities. Apparently, the officers and merchant marines were allowed much leeway and were not overly disciplined as long as they did not try to escape or become insubordinate in other ways. Participation in sport events organized by the prisoners was one of the most important outlets. Soccer was the most common sport. Cricket, field hockey, rugger football in which touch supplanted tackling, softball, and basketball were also popular. The weather was rarely cold enough for hockey; however, when it was sufficiently cold, the prisoners demonstrated their ingenuity by constructing makeshift skates. Ship engineers were able to fashion skate blades using door and window hinges; these were fastened upright between two pieces of 1-inch wood and then attached to the bottom of a shoe with straps or rope. Fisher commented that it was truly remarkable that reasonable hockey games could be played on those improvised replicas. Ice hockey was the most popular sport in Canada, and undoubtedly the Canadian prisoners' spirits were buoyed by being able to play even rarely.

A rather colorful story that conveyed the underworkings of POW camps was uncovered after the war ended.[17] Fisher became familiar with a prisoner in the Stalag XB camp, Harry Vosic, who would heckle while Fisher played second base for the Canadian team during camp baseball games. The heckler had a very loud booming voice that would emanate from a window near which he lay on a stretcher. The heckler's real name was Reuben Rabinovitch. He was a Canadian doctor who was training in neurosurgery with Clovis Vincent, a prominent French neurosurgeon. Rabinovitch was also active in the French Underground aiding American airmen who had been shot down over France. He was arrested by the Nazis and identified himself to them as Harry Vosic, a gunnery sergeant. He gave them a factitious serial number that he had memorized for such an eventuality.

Soon after his arrest, Vosic came to the aid of a boy who was writhing on a cement floor clutching his abdomen in pain. After Vosic examined the lad, he spoke to an attendant in French and spoke German to an officer who was summoned to help. Vosic told them that the boy had appendicitis and needed urgent surgery. When questioned about how a gunnery sergeant knew about medicine, Vosic made up a story about how a failed love affair had derailed his medical training and so he had joined the military. In Stalag XB, the Germans put him in charge of an infirmary of sorts in a filthy louse-infested barrack that formerly housed Russian prisoners. Vosic was assigned POWs as aides who had no medical knowledge. When Vosic found white spots in the throat of a prisoner, he trained his makeshift medical corps to identify diphtheria lesions. He urged German officials to provide serum to thwart an epidemic that could spread to the Germans in the camp. Vosic's aides examined the throat of every prisoner in camp and saved many prisoners by administering serum provided by the German officials.

Vosic used every strategy that he could to get as many men as possible out of the camp. He faked X-rays; mixed up case histories; and, using medical double-talk, bamboozled German medical officers into approving the release of many prisoners, some of whose scars and injuries had occurred during football games and accidents on farms before the war. Soon after arriving at Stalag XB, Vosic developed severe back pain, and he often needed a cane for support to make his rounds. The Germans eventually began to suspect Vosic's activities, at which point Vosic converted his back pain into paraplegia. During the remaining years in camp, Vosic pretended to be paraplegic, fooling even Fisher, who did not suspect that he was malingering.[17]

Theater activity was also very popular; various groups worked to present a new play or musical every 2 or 3 weeks. Half of a barrack was transformed into a stage, and approximately 100 POWs could be seated in front of it. Several camp prisoners had been professional actors before the war, and others had experience in amateur theater presentations. Most presentations involved light comedy or whodunits. Gilbert and Sullivan musicals were among the favorites. Ingenuity was clearly critical in creating theatrical props from odds and ends. Of course, the men played female roles, as was the case in early Elizabethan stage productions, but the prisoners soon became accustomed to this necessity. Fisher commented that costumes and sets were often imposing and beautiful. He noted that "only plays of some merit were presented for most prisoners came to dislike any display that was cheap or below the belt". The theater activities kept large numbers of prisoners usefully occupied.

A camp orchestra was organized under the direction of a prisoner who was in peacetime a London Orchestra leader. Some members had been professional musicians, and approximately half of the players learned to play an instrument while in the camp. Instruments were sometimes sent to the prisoners by the Red Cross. The orchestra conducted variety nights, during which old-time vaudeville skits were the major entertainment.

Most important for Fisher was the development of schoolroom-type classes in the camp. Languages were the most popular subject. German, French, Spanish, Swedish, and Russian tutelage was available. Some prisoners studied multiple languages. Fisher took the opportunity to educate himself during his imprisonment in the camp.[18] In addition to German, he also studied Italian and Spanish. He became sufficiently proficient in Spanish that he was able to complete all the lessons in a Spanish learning textbook and to read a Spanish-language newspaper. During the 3½ years that he was confined to the camp, he read widely in history and English literature. The German learned in camp was very useful to Fisher later in his medical studies when he was able to read "Virchows Archiv" which was written in German and was not translated into English.[19] Other subjects taught included engineering, navigation, mathematics, radio, electricity, law, agriculture, botany, economics, history, and English literature. Classes were held from early in the morning until lights out at night. Fisher attended courses on mechanics and calculus taught by a young university professor. A forum was planned each week at which current topics were discussed. Lectures on unusual subjects were presented by prisoners who had special interests and expertise. Self-study was available through books. Prisoners could have the Red Cross or families send books of interest, which were subsequently placed in the central library of the camp available to all prisoners. Fisher commented that many POWs qualified for university examinations when they returned home. Fisher later commented to me "I went to graduate school in the camp." Having explored history, physics, calculus, and the arts, he was ready and anxious to focus on medicine when he was liberated.

According to Fisher, the Red Cross played a major role in helping the POWs keep busy and educated. Items sent included parcels of food, clothing, some medical supplies, instructions on how to read Braille, university courses and examinations, games, sports equipment, books of every kind, art supplies, music, musical instruments, and phonographs and phonograph records. The prisoners were also able to receive gifts.

Fisher commented that family, friends, and medical and naval colleagues sent clothes, novels, medical books, and music. He was particularly grateful to receive *Fowler's Oxford English Dictionary*—gold-limned, leather-bound, and printed on the finest paper.[20] He cherished this book and referred to it often.

Fisher wrote,

> What a privilege to pore over the classics at the age of thirty rather than eighteen, unhurried with no serious distractions. I studied navigation, mathematics, and the theory of music. It seems that young physicians may finish their demanding studies and plunge into practice with a feeling that an important segment of intellectual grandeur has escaped them. After time with the wonders of Shakespeare and Dickens and Macaulay and the others, I was ready to return to medicine. I had at least glimpsed the other realm.[21]

When Fisher later immersed himself in academic medicine in Boston, he wrote often and elegantly. His reports and manuscripts were characteristically long and scholarly. He did not favor others (including myself and his fellows, colleagues, and journal editors) tampering with his descriptions and text. His writings were rich in vocabulary, metaphors, and in references to classic literature of all kinds. He strongly believed in providing detailed, quantitative descriptions of medical phenomena written in clear English. I believe that the self-education and courses taken during the camp years were instrumental in his later being able to write so copiously and so colorfully. He had an individual style of writing that may be evident in the quotes that I have sprinkled herein from his memoirs, which were written long after the camp imprisonment.

WAR EVENTS AND REPATRIATION

On Christmas Eve 1942, a plane dove out of the cloud cover and a hand waved to the prisoners who stood in the camp on parade. The plane quickly disappeared, and a few minutes later the prisoners heard three bomb explosions and hoped that the bombs had landed on target. The plane was recognizable as one of the new British light bombers, the Mosquito. The main turning point in the war came in 1943, when American four-engine bombers carried out the first major daylight air strike by the Allies. The target was Wilhelmshaven, a principal naval base that was evacuated a few days later, at which time the prisoners could see trucks and cars driving by with Germans who appeared gray and quiet. Five days later, the quiet of the

Marlag camp was interrupted by the earthshaking sound of anti-aircraft defenses located along the Weser River, quite near the camp.

Fisher commented,

> Our camp had a front seat at the unbelievable sight of group after group of American fortresses at a great height gleaming in the sunlight, slowly wheeling in perfect formation as they headed back out to sea. Once clear of antiaircraft fire, the bombers were attacked by German fighter aircraft, and for several minutes the sky was crisscrossed by vapor trails and dotted with falling aircraft on fire. One hundred and fifty American fortresses had attacked Bremen in broad daylight. This was war and realistic Germans realized that for them the picnic was over.[22]

Soon after this attack, between 250 and 700 American planes took part in each raid. During the autumn of 1943, the bombers were followed by their own fighter plane escorts. The Marlag camp often lay in the path of the incoming aircraft. During 1944, hundreds of American bombers flew inland over the camp. Britain's Royal Air Force also dramatically increased the frequency of its night bombing. During a heavy attack on Hamburg, 1,000 night bombers passed over the region near the camp. The noise of the night bombers, the roar of night fighters, and the blast of anti-aircraft guns produced a din that created an unforgettable memory for Fisher and the other prisoners. The prisoners hoped and knew that "it wouldn't be long now."

Most German guards behaved in a very authoritarian manner, but a few were anti-Nazi. One example cited by Fisher was a German guard who had been in Hamburg during a night air attack by British bombers. The next day, he returned to the camp obviously shaken and announced to the prisoners, "That was a good raid, but for God's sake send more planes". He shook his fist in frustration. Another guard rounded up propaganda leaflets dropped by British planes. The German guard asked the prisoners to give him all the leaflets. He said, "They are doing no good here, give them to me and they'll be working in Berlin tomorrow."[23] Another guard brought bread taken from German navy mess tables to sick bay patients. Many of the guards participated in the black market, trading eggs, bread, schnapps, cigarettes, and meat for tea, coffee, and chocolates that had been sent to the prisoners.

News of allied gains and Nazi losses continued to be communicated during the fall and winter months of 1943. On June 6, 1944, also known as D-Day, approximately 156,000 American, British, and Canadian forces landed on five beaches along a 50-mile stretch of the heavily fortified coast of France's Normandy region. The attack was code named Operation

Overlord. The invasion was one of the largest amphibious military assaults in history and required extensive planning. Prior to D-Day, the Allies conducted a large-scale deception campaign designed to mislead the Germans about the intended invasion target.

On June 20, 1944, Fisher received a message from a medical colleague at Marlag, Dr. Peter Brownlees, informing Fisher that based on Brownlees' length of time in captivity, he had been designated as one of the medical officers who would accompany the first group of wounded and sick who were to be repatriated to England. Brownlees stated that because he was single and Fisher was married and had a daughter who had never seen her father, he was withdrawing his name and allowing Fisher's name, the next on the list of amount of time imprisoned, to stand in his stead.

Two days later, the repatriates of the camp started the journey home accompanied by Fisher and another medical officer. They traveled by train from Bremen to Annaburg, passing through many towns that were devastated by bombings. In Annaburg, they were housed in an old castle. Repatriates from other camps arrived. After 1,200 men were assembled, plans for the journey to Sweden were announced. While in Annaburg, Fisher and the others witnessed the full might of the American Air Force. Thousands of American planes flew unchallenged in perfect formation hundreds of miles deep into Germany on their way to bomb further key targets.

Fisher anxiously awaited orders that would send him home. On June 23, a list of individuals scheduled to depart the next morning was posted, but Fisher's name, as well as those of four other medical officers, was not on the list.

Fisher commented about his time in Annaburg:

Once out of Marlag and Milag Nord the psychological trappings of captivity fell away and soon one realized what mental blinders one wore without being aware of it. The nightmare was over as relief and thanks and joy welled up. Now in a stroke we were back in captivity. That was cruel. That was bitter. The rest moved off and we were left behind in an otherwise empty old castle.[24]

The remaining prisoners kept active by engaging in sports and games. Games of "rounders" were played with prisoners from Canada pitted against those from the rest of the Commonwealth and also the United Kingdom. Rounders was a popular game that involved hitting a small, hard, leather-cased ball with a rounded-end bat. Players scored by running around four bases marked off on a field. Amputees, patients with cancer and infectious illnesses, and sick bay personnel all participated. Prisoners who were confined to bed were pushed to windows to watch and cheer.

After approximately 1 month, new loads of wounded and sick prisoners began to arrive at Annaburg. The medical officers now had duties to perform. Fisher now thought that the chances were very good that he would be one of the medical officers chosen to accompany these patients. Spirits were high because the news was good. The Allies were advancing in France, Germany had retreated from Russia, Italy's forces had collapsed, and a group of German soldiers led by General von Stauffenberg had tried to assassinate Hitler. The war against Germany was effectively over. By late August 1944, all of northern France had been liberated, and by the following spring the Allies had defeated the Germans.

Finally, orders came to move on, and Fisher's name was on the list. A few days were spent certifying the mode of transport for each prisoner. Fisher and the prisoners then boarded a special Red Cross train for the journey to Sweden. Fisher commented that on the train, he had a seat to himself, on which he stretched out and savored those first precious hours of freedom.

The train went to Sassnitz, a coastal city on the Baltic Sea, after which Fisher and the soldiers boarded a ferry headed to Trelleborg in southern Sweden and then to Göteborg. There, they boarded a Swedish Red Cross ship, the *Gripsholm*, for the trip to England. The ship carried ample food and delicacies, a real treat for prisoners who had been deprived for years. Because Germany had not officially surrendered, there was concern about traveling along the Norwegian coast, which was still occupied by Germany. The *Gripsholm* safely navigated to the north of Scotland and then on to Liverpool, where it docked. That same day, the city's blackout was lifted. The British wounded and sick went ashore in Liverpool, and 36 hours later the *Gripsholm* sailed for New York with the American and Canadian contingents. Fisher and colleagues are shown aboard the ship in Figure 4.5.

The ship docked in New York City 5 days later. Fisher then boarded a Canadian Pacific train to Toronto, where he was met by naval personnel, taken to naval headquarters, and debriefed. His wife and young daughter had traveled to Toronto and were staying at the Royal York Hotel, where a blissful family reunion took place. Fisher was given 1 month's leave.

Fisher commented in his memoirs which were written many years later that the Marlag prisoners of war met annually in London every year after 1946:

> *Virtually all returned to civilian life without incident and succeeded and prospered. Wartime experience teaches one to do with less, to be satisfied with fewer material goods and that may be a good thing. It leaves one envious of no man.*[25]

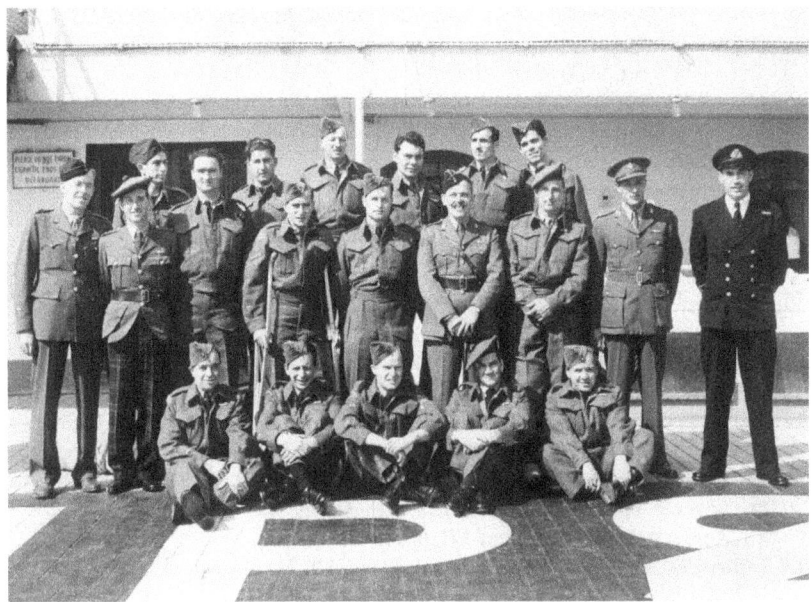

Figure 4.5 Fisher (standing on the far right in a dark uniform) aboard the *Gripsholm* with fellow prisoners of war.

Undoubtedly, Fisher's wartime experiences had a profound effect on his later life and career. He did not pay much attention to material goods, money, or finances. He told me that he believed so much time in his life had been wasted as a prisoner that he was determined to make each subsequent day meaningful.[26] With regard to his career, he was determined to contribute to knowledge and to dedicate himself to the optimum care of patients. He also developed a wide interest in people and human nature, probably at least kindled by the variety of individuals he came in contact with during the war years.

NOTES

1. Fisher CM. *Memoirs of a Neurologist*. Rutland, VT: Academy Books, 1992, Vol. 1, p. 85.
2. Fisher CM. *Memoirs of a Neurologist*. Rutland, VT: Academy Books, 1992, Vol. 1, pp. 89–90.
3. An account of the POW camp Stalag XB is available at https://en.wikipedia.org/wiki/Stalag_X-B.
4. Fisher CM. *Memoirs of a Neurologist*. Rutland, VT: Academy Books, 1992, Vol. 1, pp. 90–91.

5. Fisher CM. *Memoirs of a Neurologist*. Rutland, VT: Academy Books, 1992, Vol. 1, p. 100.
6. The medical supplies were commented on by Fisher in his *Memoirs of a Neurologist*. Rutland, VT: Academy Books, 1992, Vol. 1, pp. 96–97.
7. Fisher CM. *Memoirs of a Neurologist*. Rutland, VT: Academy Books, 1992, Vol. 1, pp. 97–98.
8. Fisher CM. *Memoirs of a Neurologist*. Rutland, VT: Academy Books, 1992, Vol. 1, p. 95.
9. Fisher CM. *Memoirs of a Neurologist*. Rutland, VT: Academy Books, 1992, Vol. 1, p. 101.
10. The story of the attempted escape by tunnel is detailed in Fisher CM. *Memoirs of a Neurologist*. Rutland, VT: Academy Books, 1992, Vol. 1, pp. 101–105.
11. Fisher CM. *Memoirs of a Neurologist*. Rutland, VT: Academy Books, 1992, Vol. 1, p. 105.
12. Fisher described medical facilities and care during his wartime experience in a letter to the Canadian Medical Authorities prepared and sent in December 1944 titled "Marlag 1941–44 by Surgeon Lt-Commander CM Fisher RCNVR." The letter is reproduced in Fisher CM. *Memoirs of a Neurologist*. Rutland, VT: Academy Books, 1992, Vol. VII, pp. 68–71.
13. Fisher CM. *Memoirs of a Neurologist*. Rutland, VT: Academy Books, 1992, Vol. 1, p. 121.
14. Fisher CM. *Memoirs of a Neurologist*. Rutland, VT: Academy Books, 1992, Vol. 1, p. 124.
15. Fisher CM. *Memoirs of a Neurologist*. Rutland, VT: Academy Books, 1992, Vol. 1, p. 96.
16. Fisher CM. *Memoirs of a Neurologist*. Rutland, VT: Academy Books, 1992, Vol. 1, p. 94.
17. The story of Rabinovitch (also known as Vosic) is contained in Feindel W, Leblanc R. *The Wounded Brain Healed: The Golden Age of the Montreal Neurological Institute 1934–1984*. Montreal, Quebec, Canada: McGill-Queen's University Press, 2016.
18. The educational activities described by Fisher that took place at Marlag are similar to Nelson Mandela's experiences during his Robben Island imprisonment in South Africa, which are described in detail in Mandela N, *Long Walk to Freedom: The Autobiography of Nelson Mandela*. New York: Back Bay Books, 1994.
19. After the war, antipathy between the British and French toward Germany led to the rarity of English translations of classical German medical literature. Germany had a very rich tradition of scholarship and clinical studies. Before World War II, many American, Canadian, and British physician trainees received postgraduate training in German medical centers. During his later time at the Massachusetts General Hospital, Fisher could often be found at Boston's Countway Medical Library studying older German texts, particularly those of Rudolph Virchow, an eminent German pathologist who made many observations relevant to the field of cerebrovascular disease. *Virchows Archiv* was written in German and was not translated into English.
20. Fowler's Dictionary was sent to him by the Surgeon Commander Richard Lane. See Fisher CM. *Memoirs of a Neurologist*. Rutland, VT: Academy Books, 1992, Vol. 1, p. 113.

21. Fisher CM. *Memoirs of a Neurologist*. Rutland, VT: Academy Books, 1992, Vol. 1, p. 113.
22. Fisher CM. *Memoirs of a Neurologist*. Rutland, VT: Academy Books, 1992, Vol. 1, p. 118.
23. These two quotes are cited in Fisher CM. *Memoirs of a Neurologist*. Rutland, VT: Academy Books, 1992, Vol. 1, p. 117.
24. Fisher CM. *Memoirs of a Neurologist*. Rutland, VT: Academy Books, 1992, Vol. 1, pp. 125–126.
25. Fisher CM. *Memoirs of a Neurologist*. Rutland, VT: Academy Books, 1992, Vol. 1, p. 129.
26. This and other comments are available in an interview with Fisher by Louis R. Caplan. The interview can be accessed on YouTube ("C. Miller Fisher, MD Interviewed by Louis R. Caplan MD," October 7, 2016).

PART III
Repatriation and Reintroduction to Medicine and Neurology in Montreal

Having been away from medical practice for nearly 5 years, Fisher began retraining in medicine in Montreal. Encounters at the Montreal Neurological Institute stimulated an interest in neurology. He began to gain experience with neurological conditions and developed an interest in headache and hypertension. He found the academic environment in Montreal to be very stimulating.

CHAPTER 5

Reintroduction to Medicine and Neurology in Montreal

After liberation from the prisoner-of-war (POW) camp, Fisher was transported to Toronto during September 1944 and was officially debriefed. His wife Doris and his young daughter Elizabeth had preceded his arrival in Toronto and had a room at the Royal Victoria Hotel. He had been separated from his family for 3½ years, so he was granted a 1-month leave to attempt to reintroduce himself into civilian and family life. In November 1944, he was posted to HMCS Stadaconna, the Canadian East Coast Naval Hospital in Halifax, which reintroduced him to medicine as it was then practiced: Fisher had very limited treatments available to him in the POW camp, and major changes had occurred since the beginning of World War II.

The Surgeon Commander of the Naval Hospital, Wendell MacLeod, was particularly kind to Fisher and his wife. Fisher believed that the hospital's professional staff "represented the very best in medicine and surgery."[1] He considered that the three major changes in medicine that he encountered during his stay in Halifax were the introduction of penicillin to treat infections, albeit it was available only in small amounts; a new emphasis on "psychosomatic" causes of symptoms; and an emphasis on cervical and lumbar disc disease as a cause of back and limb complaints.

Although Fisher heavily praised his stay at the Naval Hospital, he recognized that the practice of medicine there was not really the same as that in the community and nonmilitary settings. At that time, it was the custom of the Canadian Naval Service to grant each medical naval officer who had served 2 or 3 years of service a 6-month refresher course in the subject of his choice at any institution where suitable arrangements could be made. The two Canadian cities that had the most prominent medical reputations were Toronto and Montreal. Fisher had been critical of his medical education in Toronto, where he noted that there were few full-time teachers, academic pursuits were discouraged, and training was suboptimal. More important, before his enlistment in the Canadian Navy, he had had very good medical experiences in Montreal, where he had been appointed a house officer at the Royal Victoria Hospital and he had had some experience at an infectious disease hospital and tuberculosis sanitarium. The choice was clear: He would spend the 6-month grant time in Montreal.

Academic medicine and research were well established in Montreal by the mid-20th century. The two fields and disciplines that were to be the cornerstone of Fisher's later career, pathology and neurology, were among the centerpieces of medicine in Montreal at the time Fisher began his retraining in 1945. It was during these early post-war years in Montreal that Fisher was introduced to and charmed by neurology. Because Montreal, the Royal Victoria Hospital, the Montreal General Hospital (MGH), and the Montreal Neurological Institute (MNI) and its founder and leader, Dr. Wilder Penfield, played such crucial and important roles in Fisher's career, I devote much of this chapter to characterizing them as Fisher found them during the mid-20th century.

MONTREAL MEDICINE, 1945

In the mid-20th century, Montreal was widely acknowledged as the academic medical leader in Canada. By the time Fisher began retraining in 1944, the MGH, the Royal Victoria Hospital, McGill University, and the MNI had all established leadership roles in academic medicine, neurology, and neurosurgery.

In 1811, James McGill, a very successful businessman, bequeathed his 46-acre estate, Burnside, for endowment of a university that would bear his name. Copying the model of Edinburgh, courses in medicine were offered; the medical school contained the first faculty at McGill University. At that time, the MGH was the only hospital that was open to students who matriculated at McGill Medical School. MGH has remained a principal teaching site for McGill students.

The cornerstone of MGH was placed in 1821. Sir William Osler, the most famous Canadian-born physician, had served as the first pathologist at MGH beginning in 1877. Osler served for 10 years, during which time he performed 800 autopsies and published more than 400 academic papers.[2] Osler left Montreal to become Professor of Medicine at the University of Pennsylvania. Later, he became the first Professor of Medicine at Johns Hopkins University. He finished his career as Regius Professor of Medicine at Oxford. The pathology laboratory during Osler's time in Montreal was in the basement of MGH, but in 1895 the laboratory moved to a new building on hospital grounds. By 1911, a new pathology building had been erected, and Dr. Horst Oertel was recruited from Guy's Hospital in London to become the Strathcona Professor of Pathology at McGill in 1914, where he served in that capacity until 1938. During the 19th century and approximately the first 75 years of the 20th century, diagnosis and research on diseases depended very heavily on pathology—viewing tissues taken by biopsy or at necropsy. Bacteriology and culturing of tissues were also important. Bacteriology was often headquartered and housed together with pathology as essential diagnostic and research services.

Two prominent Canadians, Sir George Stephen and Sir Donald Smith, pledged money to be used for the construction of a hospital in Montreal to be named the Royal Victoria Hospital, after the long-reigning Queen Victoria of Britain.[3,4] The Queen granted permission to use her name, and construction of the new hospital was completed in 1893. The Royal Vic, as it was called, opened with 265 beds and eight appointed house surgeons: four in medicine, three in surgery, and one in obstetrics. In time, the MGH and Royal Vic became the major teaching hospitals of McGill University. As in many US and Canadian cities, the teaching hospitals were not located at or near the medical school of the university.

THE MONTREAL NEUROLOGICAL INSTITUTE AND DR. WILDER PENFIELD

During the late 19th century and early years of the 20th century, scientists and doctors began to concentrate on the brain and its functions and malfunctions. Stimulated by activity in Europe—mainly Paris, London, Spain, Germany, and Austria—physicians and surgeons began to specialize in brain and nervous system diseases.[5] Physicians who specialized in medical care of these patients were called neurologists, and surgeons who mainly operated on the brain and spinal cord and its coverings were called neurosurgeons. Understandably, these specialists sought to develop workplaces where patients with nervous system disease could be studied and treated. In this milieu, an institution (the MNI) was developed adjacent and connected to the Royal Vic Hospital,

The recruitment of Dr. Wilder Penfield to Montreal in 1928 and the opening of the MNI (affectionately known as the Neuro) in 1934 positioned Montreal as one of the world leaders in research on the nervous system and care of patients with neurological conditions. Penfield and the Neuro were to play major roles in Fisher's early career.

Penfield was born in Spokane, Washington, on January 26, 1891. His father and grandfather were physicians. Penfield was thoroughly educated in physiology, medicine, neurology, and neurosurgery.[6]

In 1921, Penfield was recruited to New York to the College of Physicians and Surgeons of Columbia University, where he had begun his medical training years earlier. Columbia University and the Presbyterian Hospital had been given generous grants by the Rockefeller Foundation to reorganize their medical and surgical departments into a full-time system. Dr. Allen Whipple was the chief of surgery. He turned over to Penfield the task of developing a neurosurgical service. After all, Penfield's training had been impeccable: He had been exposed to and tutored by the world leaders in basic neuroscience and in clinical medicine neurology and neurosurgery.[6] The "full-time" arrangement at the hospital entailed 9 months of clinical hospital activities, 1 month of vacation, 1 month of travel, and 1 month for working on a scientific project.

In 1924, Penfield became interested in studying the process of healing in the brain. With the approval and support of Whipple, he traveled to Madrid, Spain, and studied in the laboratories of Drs. Santiago Ramon y Cajal and Pio del Rio-Hortega. He learned to use impregnation techniques for viewing nervous system components. He planned to apply the anatomical skills and pathology techniques he had learned in Madrid to launch a fundamental scientific approach to nervous system conditions. On returning to New York, he established a laboratory of neurocytology and recruited Dr. William Cone to work in the laboratory with him. The laboratory was supported by the Rockefeller Foundation. Early publications from the laboratory concerned scarring in the brain, reactions of microglia, and cytology and morphology of encapsulated nervous system tumors. Even before formation of the MNI, Penfield and Cone had joined with Dr. Colin Russel, a neurologist who had worked with Sir Victor Horsley in London, to form a combined Department of Neurology and Neurosurgery at McGill. The department was supported fully by the dean and the Professor of Medicine.

The beginnings of a neurological institute in Montreal can be traced back to a neurosurgical procedure in which Penfield operated on a boy whose epileptic seizures were uncontrolled. Penfield had told the boy's parents before the surgery that he had only previously performed this procedure in monkeys. The boy was greatly improved after the operation.[6] The patient's father was a member of the board of trustees of the Rockefeller Foundation. After his son's surgery, the father discussed Penfield and his work with the newly appointed director of the Rockefeller Foundation's Division of Medical Education, Alan Gregg. Penfield met Gregg in his office in New York in 1931, and the two had long discussions about neurology, neurosurgery, and research in Europe and North America. This visit was followed by prolonged discussions and visits during which the building of a neurological institute in Montreal was discussed. Other potential sites, including the University of Pennsylvania in Philadelphia, were also considered. Finally, with a $1.2 million grant from the Rockefeller Foundation of New York and the support of the government of the province of Quebec, the city of Montreal, and private donors, the MNI was conceived and built. The maple leaf of Canada and the crest of McGill University are found on one side of the bridge that connects the MNI with the Royal Victoria Hospital, and the crest of the Royal Victoria is on the other side of the bridge.[3]

The Neuro (Figure 5.1) was only the second institute/hospital in North America dedicated solely to care for patients with diseases of the nervous

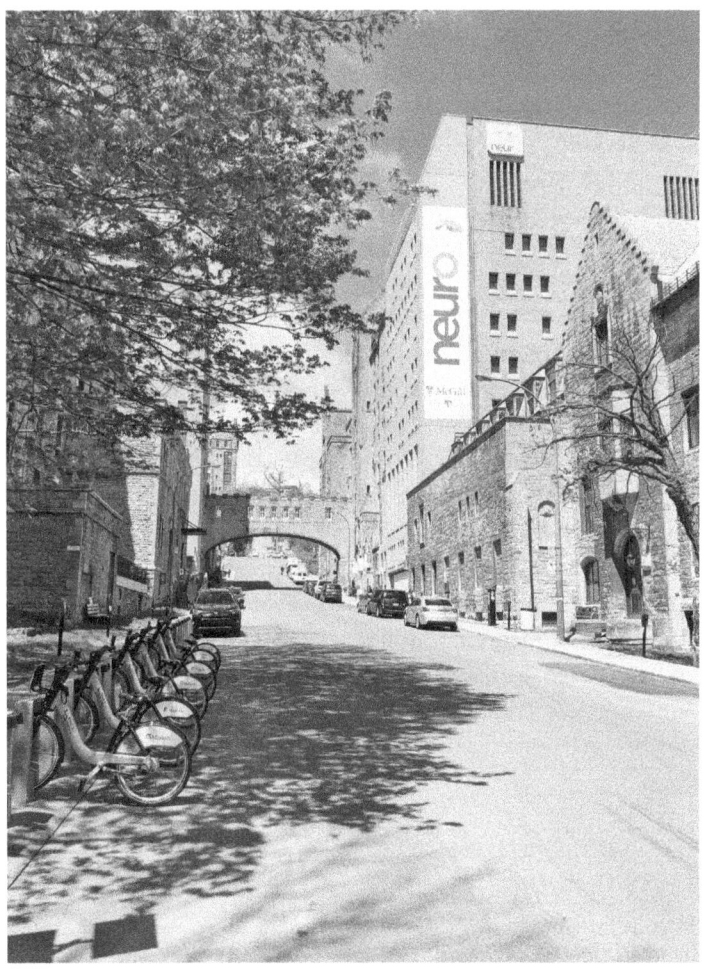

Figure 5.1 The Montreal Neurological Institute (the Neuro).
Source: Courtesy of Richard Leblanc, MD. All rights reserved.

system. In 1928, the Neurological Institute of New York at Columbia–Presbyterian Medical Center opened. Its creation was led by Dr. Charles Elsberg, a neurosurgeon like Penfield. Elsberg's major interest and publications concerned diseases of the spinal cord. The only predecessor to these two institutions was in London. In 1859, the National Hospital for Diseases of the Nervous System including Paralysis and Epilepsy was opened. The name was changed to the National Hospital for Nervous Diseases and more recently to the National Hospital for Neurology and Neurosurgery. This institute is often referred to as "Queen Square" after its location in the center of London. One of the early leaders at Queen Square was Sir Victor Horsley, a neurosurgeon. Drs. Colin Russel and Penfield both spent time at Queen Square before settling in Montreal.

By the end of the first third of the 20th century, Montreal had become a leader in the blossoming fields of neurology and neurosurgery. MNI was a leader in the treatment of epilepsy and brain tumors. MGH had an active neurology program. Dr. David Shirras was the first Professor of Neurology, and he served from 1904 to 1920 at McGill and MGH. At that time, neurology was considered an important component of internal medicine. Dr. Fred McKay became the second Neurology Professor, and Dr. Colin Russel became a well-known neurology consultant. Russel, McKay, Arthur Young, and Norman Peterson established a strong center for neurology at McGill and at MGH and the Royal Vic during the years preceding and after World War I. These physicians and neurologists became strong clinical mentors for Fisher during his time in Montreal.

During the first three-fourths of the 20th century, neurosurgeons were the leaders in caring for patients with nervous system diseases. The predominant conditions treated were brain tumors, spinal cord compression and trauma, and epilepsy. Neurology was predominantly a subdivision of medicine, and strokes, multiple sclerosis, and other nonsurgical conditions were cared for on medical wards mostly by internists. Very few stroke patients were seen in consultation by neurologists. No effective treatment for strokes was recognized or approved. There were few neurologists. Neurologists often practiced what today is called psychiatry, in addition to neurology.

MONTREAL TRAINING, 1945–1947

In July 1945, Fisher returned to the Royal Victoria Hospital to try to resume medical training where he had left off 5 years previously. Initially, he spent time on the metabolic service. He had planned to specialize in diabetes and other metabolic conditions because he had spent time on the diabetic service during his pre-war training. He had been heavily influenced by Dr. Kenneth Evelyn, an expert in biophysics and biochemistry. Evelyn had discovered a way to measure the concentration of various substances in body fluids.

Fisher also spent time on the general medical wards. There, he showed an inkling of his later penchant for thoroughly reviewing the literature, careful thought, and innovation. He was influenced by a published hypothesis that a low-sodium diet could potentially benefit patients with congestive heart failure. The rationale was that the problem was not too much water intake (the explanation at that time) but, rather, retention of electrolyte solutions that carried fluid irreversibly into the extracellular spaces, causing edema, ascites, and pleural effusions. He consulted with his mentor, Evelyn, who agreed with the general principle. They decided to test the hypothesis on a young man who was dying from congestive heart failure due to rheumatic heart disease. Low-sodium diets were not a part of the dietician's library, so Fisher devised one using various food tables. The patient improved on the concocted low-sodium diet, but the attending physician "exploded in wrath at the perpetration of such nonsense and forbade a future trial."[7]

Fisher's perusal of the literature impressed him that patients with rheumatoid arthritis often went into remission when they became jaundiced. He had had the experience in the Royal Canadian Navy that so-called "catarrhal jaundice" (the term then used for infectious hepatitis) was quite benign. He toyed with the idea of giving a patient with rheumatoid arthritis a serum injection of hepatitis. Others were impressed with the dangers of infectious hepatitis, and permission for a single trial was not granted even though the patient was willing.

The 6-month refresher course at the Royal Victoria Hospital included a 6-week rotation on the neurology service at MNI. Fisher commented in his memoirs,

> Although the Montreal Neurological Institute was only about 10 years old, its reputation was worldwide and after World War II young scholars came from all parts of the globe to study and become neurosurgeons, all owing to Dr. Penfield.[8]

A single patient provided a turning point in Fisher's medical career. Fisher examined a high-ranking US Army officer who was admitted to MNI to treat focal epileptic seizures. The seizures began by the patient hearing the beating of tom-tom drums. That night, Fisher sleuthed in the medical library and reviewed the brain anatomy related to hearing. The next day on rounds, Fisher presented the case to Penfield. After the presentation,

Penfield asked Fisher what he thought was going on. Fisher replied that the patient most likely had a tumor that involved the auditory cerebral cortex near Heschl's gyrus in the temporal lobe. Surgical exploration confirmed Fisher's guess. In those days, the only available investigation that was widely used was a skull X-ray. Dr. Walter Dandy (a former trainee of Harvey Cushing) had written about introducing air into the head through a catheter introduced through a burr hole in the skull or through injection into the spinal canal, but this technique was not widely used at that time.[9] Surgical exploration was mainly on the basis of clinical localization from the patient's history and neurological examination. This patient experience and perhaps others impressed Penfield with Fisher's thoroughness, willingness to explore the literature, and willingness to think about his patients. All accounts emphasize the impressiveness and charisma of the persona of Penfield. A young fledgling such as Fisher could not help but be awed by his presence and his domination of the institute. Penfield asked Fisher if he had ever considered a career in neurology, to which Fisher replied he had not. Later during the rotation, Penfield invited Fisher into his office for an interview. One of the questions posed was, "Miller, have you ever done anything really exciting?"[10] Penfield offered Fisher the post of acting

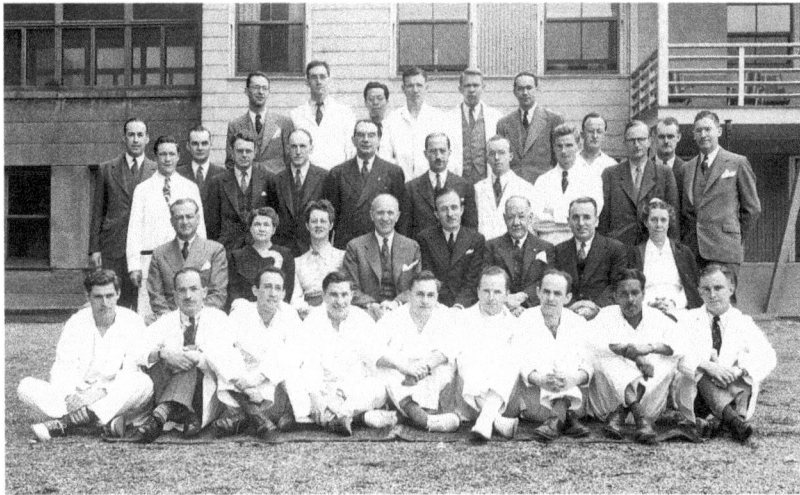

Figure 5.2 The professional staff at the Montreal Neurological Institute, 1945–1946. Fisher is on the far left in the third row. Wilder Penfield is fourth from the left in the second row. Theodore Rasmusen, the second director of the institute, is on the far right in the top row. William Feindel, the third director of the institute, is on the far left in the top row.
Source: Reproduced with permission from W. Feindel and R. Leblanc. *The Wounded Brain Healed—The Golden Age of the Montreal Neurological Institute, 1934–1984*. Montreal, Quebec, Canada: McGill–Queen's University Press, 2016. © Montreal Neurological Institute Archives.

Neurology Registrar while Dr. Preston Robb was away on sabbatical leave. This gave Fisher an opportunity to continue to participate in the neurology ward and clinical services at MNI and Royal Victoria Hospital. One of his responsibilities was to assist Dr. Alan Bailey on the neurology service of the Queen Mary Veterans' Hospital. And, as they say, the rest is history. Fisher never wavered from his dogged enthusiasm and reverence for neurology and neurological diseases. Figure 5.2 shows the professional staff of MNI in 1945–1946, including Penfield and Fisher.

FISHER AT THE MONTREAL NEUROLOGICAL INSTITUTE, 1945–1948

Fisher commented on the circumstances that led him to embrace neurology and to later make contributions to knowledge:

> Entrance into my "chosen field" was largely a matter of chance. This is not an unusual experience judging from the reports of others. What we do within a field, however, is not a matter of chance. I think we are selected to do what we can do rather than selecting to do what we'd like to do. The nervous system loves to do what it can do and is intolerant of what it can't do.[11]

Soon after he began working at the Neuro, Fisher became reacquainted with Dr. Reuben Rabinovitch, also known as gunner Sargent Vosic in the POW camp (see Chapter 4), where Fisher spent most of the war. Fisher commented,

> On occasion I ate at the same table as Dr. Reuben Rabinovitch, a young neurosurgeon in training. He eventually gave up the profession for neurology. Regularly he would say in his gravelly voice. "I know you, we have met before." I was embarrassed not to be able to recall the occasion, although his voice sounded familiar.[12]

One day, Rabinovitch told Fisher the full story, including how he had duped Fisher into believing that he was paraplegic.

During the next few years, Fisher showed proclivities that were to characterize his modus operandi later. He was dedicated to learning by extracting the maximum from each patient encounter. He also liberally used the library facilities to seek and review past reports. He often took nighttime and weekend duty in the emergency department of MNI to be able to examine and follow his patients. He soon recognized that he was not the first person to interview and examine patients who came to the department. One of the full-time MNI personnel often saw patients first and pruned off the "interesting cases," leaving Fisher those thought to be less useful for learning. Fisher later commented, "Several uninteresting cases proved to be important and unique in neurological localization and found their way into the literature. 'Interesting' is in the eye of the beholder."[13] Examples that Fisher gave of such interesting patients were three who presented to the emergency room at MNI with very severe headaches that recurred several times during each 24-hour period, especially during the night but also during the day. The patient, usually a middle-aged man, would arise from bed soon after retiring for the night with a very severe but short-lasting pain on one side of his head and face. The pain would make the sufferer want to go outside or pace. The pain might recur several times each day and night usually during a period of 4–8 weeks. The headache could be precipitated by alcohol intake. Often, there would be redness and tearing of the eye and drooping of the eyelid. Fisher found from his literature search that such patients had previously been described by Wilfred Harris as having "migrainous neuralgia" and by Horton as having histamine-sensitive headache.[14] Later, this headache syndrome was fully characterized by Sir Charles Symonds as a "peculiar type of headache" and referred to as "cluster headache."[15] The same type of clustering of the headaches could recur years later, often during the same season.

Fisher spent much of his time in outpatient clinics. He apparently tried to maximize learning from each patient. Senior attending physicians often became impatient with him and told him not to "dawdle." Fisher commented that "collecting data must be distinguished from dawdling."[16]

Fisher's family was growing during these early years in Montreal (1945–1947). Elizabeth was born in 1941 while Fisher was in the Navy. Peter was born in 1945, and Hugh was born in 1947. Doris and the children joined Fisher as soon as suitable living quarters became available. The family was able to occupy housing in Benny Farms, a residential development in the Notre-Dame-de-Grâce district of Montreal, originally developed in the late 1940s by the government of Canada for returning veterans of World War II and their families. According to all accounts and later observations, Fisher spent virtually all of his time on his medical activities. Doris was the captain of the household and catered to Fisher unselfishly. She assumed the great majority of the child care responsibilities, freeing Fisher to concentrate fully on his medical education and his career.

Fisher became involved in several medical projects. These were forerunners of his later participation in therapeutic trials. One study analyzed the results of sympathectomy to treat severe hypertension. Surgeons posited that interruption of sympathetic nervous system activity might be an effective means of controlling high blood pressure. At that time, there were no effective antihypertensive medications. Hypertension, uncontrolled, was the major risk factor for stroke. The surgery was pioneered by Smithwick in Boston.[17] Surgeons would expose the structures that lay just outside the spinal cord and remove the chain of sympathetic ganglia from the eighth thoracic segment to the second lumbar segment in the mid to low back. Fisher was able to "track down" all 108 consecutive patients who had the surgery. He found that approximately 1 in 5 had some beneficial effect. He presented the information in a talk and penned a 27-page report titled "The Results of Sympathectomy in the Treatment of Hypertension, C. M. Fisher MD and Wilder Penfield MD." This long and very detailed report was never submitted for publication but is included in the third volume of his memoirs.[18]

Fisher also presented thorough discussions on postural hypotension (decrease in blood pressure while standing), hypertensive encephalopathy (findings in the brain in patients with severe uncontrolled hypertension), and syringomyelia (a classic neurological condition in which cysts form in the upper spinal cord and brainstem) to the staff at MNI. Even early in his medical career, Fisher had become accustomed to putting his thoughts and his observations into writing. He was always quite meticulous about his choice of words and his grammatical constructs.

NOTES

1. Fisher CM. *Memoirs of a Neurologist*. Rutland, VT: Academy Books, 1992, Vol. 1, p. 41.
2. Osler's career was described in note 6 in Chapter 2. Two biographies provide extensive details of Osler and his life, career, and accomplishments: Cushing H. *The Life of Sir William Osler*. Oxford, UK: Oxford University Press, 1925; and Bliss M. *William Osler: A Life in Medicine*. New York: Oxford University Press, 1999.
3. Accounts of the history of the Montreal General Hospital and McGill University are found in Gurd FN. *The Montreal General and McGill, a Family Saga*. Edited by D Waugh. Burnstown, Ontario, Canada: General Store Publishing, 1996; Hanaway J, Burgess JH. *A History of the Montreal General Hospital*. Montreal, Quebec, Canada: Montreal General Hospital, 1950; Hanaway J, Cruess R. *McGill Medicine, Volume 1: The First Half Century, 1892–1885*. Montreal, Quebec, Canada: McGill–Queen's University Press, 1996; and Hanaway J, Cruess R, Darragh J. *McGill Medicine, Volume 2: 1885–1936*. Montreal, Quebec, Canada: McGill–Queen's University Press, 2006.
4. Neville T. *The Royal Vic: The Story of Montreal's Royal Victoria Hospital*. Montreal, Quebec, Canada: McGill–Queen's University Press, 1994.
5. Prominent pioneers in the field of nervous system diseases include Kinnier Wilson, Hughlings Jackson, William Gowers, and Gordon Holmes at the National Hospital for Diseases of the Nervous System including Paralysis

and Epilepsy in Queen Square in London; Jean Martin Charcot, Pierre Marie, and Joseph Babinski at the Salpetriere Hospital in Paris; Santiago Ramon y Cajal in Madrid and Barcelona, Spain; and Carl Wernicke, Sigmond Freud, and Moritz Romberg in Germany and Austria. See Garrison FH. *An Introduction to the History of Medicine*, 4th ed. Philadelphia: Saunders, 1929; and McHenry L. *Garrison's History of Neurology*. Springfield, IL: Charles C Thomas, 1969.

6. Penfield's life, career, and accomplishments are described in Eccles J, Feindel W. Wilder Graves Penfield, 1891–1976. *Biological Memoirs of Fellows of the Royal Society* November 1978;24; Penfield W. *No Man Alone: A Surgeon's Life*. Boston: Little, Brown, 1977; and Lewis J. *Something Hidden: A Biography of Wilder Penfield*. Toronto, Ontario, Canada: Doubleday Canada, 1983.

   After matriculating at Princeton University, Penfield won a Rhodes Scholarship to study at Oxford in 1914. Due to the war, he delayed his term at Oxford and began medical studies at the College of Physicians and Surgeons at Columbia University in New York. He began his Rhodes Scholarship by enrolling in the School of Physiology at Oxford in 1915. There, he came under the strong tutelage of Sir Charles Sherrington. Penfield later wrote, "I looked through his [Sherrington's] eyes and came to realize that here in the nervous system was a great unexplored field—the undiscovered country in which the mystery of the mind of man might one day be explored." While at Oxford, Penfield was also greatly influenced by Sir William Osler, then Regius Professor of Medicine at Oxford and a former pathologist and clinician at MGH. Penfield injured his knee when a ship on which he was traveling was torpedoed in the spring of 1916; he stayed at the Osler home while being rehabilitated.

   After obtaining his degree in physiology at Oxford, Penfield returned to the United States and finished his medical school courses at Johns Hopkins University in 1918. During 1918–1919, Penfield served as a surgical intern at the Peter Bent Brigham Hospital in Boston, where he came under the tutelage of Harvey Cushing, a neurosurgical pioneer and then Professor of Surgery. He obtained a fellowship and returned to the United Kingdom at the National Hospital for Neurological Diseases at Queen Square. There, he came under the tutelage of Sir Gordon Holmes in Neurology and Godwin Greenfield in Neuropathology.

7. Fisher CM. *Memoirs of a Neurologist*. Rutland, VT: Academy Books, 1992, Vol. 1, p. 42.
8. Fisher CM. *Memoirs of a Neurologist*. Rutland, VT: Academy Books, 1992, Vol. 1, p. 43.
9. Dandy W. Roentgenography of the brain after the injection of air into the spinal canal. *Annals of Surgery* 1919;70:397–403; Dandy W. Ventriculography following the injection of air into the cerebral ventricles. *Annals of Surgery* 1918;68:5–11.
10. Fisher CM. *Memoirs of a Neurologist*. Rutland, VT: Academy Books, 1992, Vol. 1, p. 44.
11. Fisher CM. *Memoirs of a Neurologist*. Rutland, VT: Academy Books, 1992, Vol. 1, p. 44.
12. The story of Rabinovitch (also known as Vosic) is contained in Feindel W, Leblanc R. *The Wounded Brain Healed: The Golden Age of the Montreal Neurological Institute, 1934–1984*. Montreal, Quebec, Canada: McGill–Queen's University Press, 2016.
13. Fisher CM. *Memoirs of a Neurologist*. Rutland, VT: Academy Books, 1992, Vol. 1, p. 44.

14. Harris W. *Neuritis and Neuralgia*. London: Oxford Publications, 1926; Horton BT. A new syndrome of vascular headache: Report of treatment with histamine: Preliminary report. *Proceedings of the Staff Meetings of the Mayo Clinic, Rochester, MN* 1939;14:257–260; Horton BT. The use of histamine in the treatment of specific types of headache. *Journal of the American Medical Association* 1941;116(5):377–383.
15. Symonds C. A particular variety of headache. *Brain* 1956;79:217–232.
16. Fisher CM. *Memoirs of a Neurologist*. Rutland, VT: Academy Books, 1992, Vol. 1, p. 45.
17. Allen EV. Sympathectomy for essential hypertension. *Circulation* 1952;6:131–140; Smithwick RH, Thompson JE. Splanchnicectomy for essential hypertension: Results in 1,266 cases. *Journal of the American Medical Association* 1953 August 15;152(16):1501–1504.
18. Fisher CM. *Memoirs of a Neurologist*. Rutland, VT: Academy Books, 1992, Vol. 3, pp. 370–397.

PART IV
Neuropathology Fellowship and Experience as a Neurologist Specializing in Stroke

Fisher's experience with neuropathology during a fellowship in Boston in 1949 was instrumental in his lifetime dedication to neuropathology, stroke research, and the care of stroke patients. After his fellowship, he returned to Montreal and avidly began his stroke career.

In 1950, when Fisher returned to Montreal, there was little clinical knowledge or interest in stroke. During the late 19th century and the first quarter of the 20th century, the anatomy of the arteries that supply the brain was studied thoroughly and described in London and Paris.[1] During the 1920s, French physicians analyzed the distribution of brain infarcts in various arterial territories and correlated the anatomy with abnormalities of function found during life.[2] Twentieth-century physicians were taught how to recognize stroke clinically by taking a history and examining patients. However, there was no way during life to visualize either the brain damage or the disease in the heart or blood vessels that supplied the brain that caused the damage. Strokes, like pneumonia, were thought to be the last pathway toward death. No treatments were known or approved. Therapeutic nihilism about caring for stroke patients was rampant. Stroke patients were often relegated to the back wards of hospitals. Few physicians were interested in caring for those who had what was considered a hopeless condition.

When Fisher began his stroke-oriented career, queries abounded in his mind: What was the distribution of atherosclerotic disease among the arteries that supplied the brain? Were there other conditions that affected those blood vessels, and what were their usual locations? When blood vessels became occluded, what was the usual distribution of brain infarction? How did the brain and its supplying blood vessels respond to the occlusions? Was brain embolism a common cause of stroke? What were the sources of emboli to the brain, and where were the usual recipient sites of the emboli? What were the causes and outcomes of patients who had hemorrhages within and around the brain? What were the clinical symptoms and signs in individuals with various cerebrovascular conditions? What were the cerebrovascular conditions that caused reduced consciousness and coma, and how could they be diagnosed clinically? Were there ways to study and image the brain, heart, and blood vessels before death in order to accurately diagnose their conditions? Could doctors recognize conditions that threatened to cause stroke and so provide treatment to prevent a stroke from happening? Was there effective treatment for patients with stroke? He was determined to pursue answers in a neuropathology laboratory and clinically.

After returning to Montreal, during the years 1950–1954, he made sentinel observation about carotid artery disease, transient visual symptoms, the distribution of atherosclerosis in the neck and head, and brain embolism. He began to develop an international academic reputation as a clinician and researcher.

NOTES

1. Vascular anatomy was clarified mostly by Duret in Paris and Stopford in England: Duret H. Sur la distribution des arteres nouricieres du bulbe rachidien. *Archives Physiologie Normale et Pathologique* 1873;2:97–113; Duret H. Recherches anatomiques sur la circulation de l'encephale. *Archives Physiologie Normale et Pathologique* 1874;3:60–91, 316–353; Stopford JS. The anatomy of the pons and medulla oblongata. *Journal of Anatomy and Physiology* 1928;50:225–280.
2. Charles Foix (1882–1927) could well be considered the first stroke neurologist. He died prematurely of pneumonia at age 45 years: Caplan LR. Charles Foix, the first modern stroke neurologist. *Stroke* 1990;21:348–356; Foix C, Hillemand P. Irrigation de la protuberance. *Comptes Rendus des Seances de la Societe de Biologie (Paris)* 1925;92:35–36; Foix C, Hillemand P. Les arteres de l'axe encephalique jusqu'au diencephale inclusivement. *Revue Neurologique (Paris)* 1925;41:705–739; Foix C, Masson A. Le syndrome de l'artere cerebrale posterieure. Presse *Medicale* 1923;31:361–365; Foix C. Hillemand P. Les syndromes de l'artere cerebrale anterieure. *Encephale* 1925;20:209–232;Foix C, Levy M. Les Ramollissements Sylviens. *Revue Neurologique (Paris)* 1927;43:1–51.

CHAPTER 6

Pathology at Boston City Hospital

In 1948, Dr. Wilder Penfield met with Fisher and suggested that Fisher go elsewhere to get post-graduate training in the United Kingdom or the United States. Penfield himself had been widely traveled and educated before settling into a staff position, and he was a great believer in extensive training. One stated goal of the recommended training was to further study the effects of hypertension on the brain, a topic in which Fisher had shown interest and had studied.

Dr. Roy Swank, who had recently been recruited to the Montreal Neurological Institute to head the Multiple Sclerosis Research Unit, convinced Fisher that the best place to obtain further training was the Boston City Hospital (BCH) Harvard Neurological Unit. Swank had spent time at BCH as well as the Peter Bent Brigham Hospital in Boston, which then was affiliated with the Neurological Unit at BCH.[1] Arrangements were made to begin a fellowship in neuropathology at BCH that would include training in pathology at the Mallory Building, a pathology unit that was a part of BCH. Fisher initially was not to receive any stipend or other financial support, but Dr. Francis McNaughton, a neurologist at the Montreal Neurological Institute, intervened and obtained a Multiple Sclerosis Fund fellowship for Fisher that would enable him to go to Boston without causing economic hardship for the family.

Fisher told me that the major reason at the time to go to Boston rather than other sites was the presence of Drs. Derek Denny-Brown and Raymond Adams. He was convinced that these two were among the very few neurologists who "knew everything."[2] Fisher started his neuropathology fellowship at BCH on January 2, 1949.

The experience at BCH proved to be life changing for Fisher. The vigorous academic milieu implemented by the director, Denny-Brown, and the work ethic on the Neurological Unit were new experiences for him. There, he contacted individuals who would prove to be role models, mentors, and colleagues during much of his later career. The Unit at BCH played a major role in neurological research and training during the mid-20th century.[3] Herein, I attempt to convey the working and academic learning environment on the Harvard Neurological Unit during the time that Fisher served his neuropathology fellowship. I also introduce the two key figures in that environment, Drs. Denny-Brown and Adams, each of whom played a key role in Fisher's later career.

BOSTON CITY HOSPITAL AND ITS PLACE IN AMERICAN MEDICINE AND NEUROLOGY DURING THE MID-20TH CENTURY

A cholera epidemic in Boston in 1848 prompted consideration of constructing a hospital for the working poor citizens of the city. At that time, the only large hospital in the city, the Massachusetts General Hospital (MGH), would not accept individuals with tuberculosis, chronic diseases, or postpartum illness. The newly planned hospital was intended "for persons of temperate and industrious habit who by sickness or accident require that attention for which they are unable to pay."[4] Funds were gathered, plans were made, and the first patient was admitted to BCH on June 1, 1864. The construction was based on similar public hospitals in Europe. The area consisted of a central building and separate pavilions spaced over a large enclosed area in downtown Boston. Figure 6.1 shows the hospital complex as it appeared in 1960, a decade after Fisher arrived.

Nervous system disease (now classed as neurological and psychiatric) was a component of care even during the early years of BCH. Following publications of clinical research in Paris, electric currents were used to treat patients with neuromuscular conditions. During the last quarter of the 19th century, a "nerve service" at the hospital was created. The hospital administration appointed Dr. Samuel Gilbert Webber, who was adept at electrical treatments, to a position titled Electrician and another individual, Dr. Morton Prince, as Physician for Nervous Disease. Prince was to lead the new service.[5]

During the 1920s, the Rockefeller Foundation became committed to developing institutions in major cities that were dedicated to research on the brain and nervous system and to the care of patients with nervous system diseases. Chapter 5 presented the story of the role that the foundation

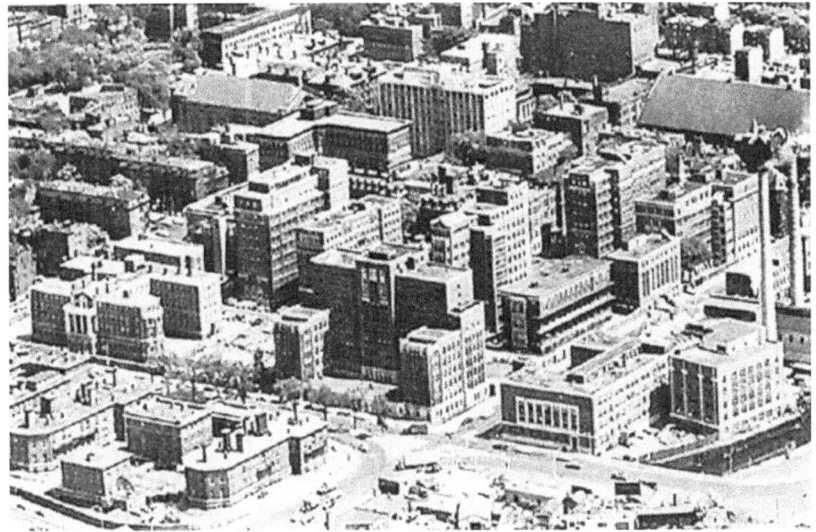

Figure 6.1 Boston City Hospital complex in 1963.
Source: Photograph by Dr. Thomas Sabin.

played in the funding of the Montreal Neurological Institute. The same strategies were applied in Boston. In the late 1920s, the Rockefeller Foundation decided to build an institute for neurological diseases in Boston or Philadelphia. Before making a decision regarding the location, Dr. Allan Gregg was invited to Montreal to hear a proposal put forward by Penfield. Convinced that Penfield had a germinal idea for a clinical and research center, the foundation funded Penfield's further education abroad and then was instrumental in his appointment as director of the Montreal Neurological Institute. The foundation gave McGill University funds to defray building costs and an endowment years later.

In Boston, the designated individual to lead the neurological center was Dr. Stanley Cobb. Cobb was born in Brookline, Massachusetts, in 1887. Early in life, he became interested in natural history and the nervous system.[6] He had a lifelong stammer that might have stimulated his interest in the brain. He studied biology at Harvard College and medicine at Harvard Medical School. After serving in the army, he completed a residency at Johns Hopkins University. In 1919, he accepted a position at Harvard Medical School, where he was expected to teach neurology. His initial interest was to study epileptic patients (as had been the case with Penfield in Montreal). The Rockefeller Foundation supported Cobb for 2 years of study in Europe to heighten his background in neurology. In 1925, when he returned from Europe, he was appointed the Bullard Professor of Neuropathology at

Harvard Medical School, and he was asked to develop a neurological unit at BCH. The Rockefeller Foundation offered Harvard University a substantial gift to "establish an academic department of Neurology" if the university would add a moderate amount to what it was already spending annually for neurology to equal the amount of the foundation's gift.[6] A neurological unit was to be built at BCH along with the construction of new medical wards. Cobb and Dr. Abraham Myerson (then Professor of Neurology at Tufts Medical School) were appointed as visiting physicians to the 40-bed neurological ward. The grant from the foundation also stipulated that there would be laboratories for animal experimentation and office space for the full-time staff of the Neurological Unit. BCH agreed to supply the buildings and the upkeep and expense for care of the patients, and Harvard Medical School agreed to supply the salaries for the personnel and the cost of research and teaching at the Neurological Unit. Dr. Donald Munro was appointed head of neurosurgical services, and Dr. Tracy Putnam was appointed to direct neurosurgical and neurological research.[7]

Under Cobb's direction, the Harvard Neurological Unit at BCH became the pre-eminent center for neurological research in the United States during the 1930s and 1940s.[3] Active research on the spinal fluid that surrounds the nervous system was led by Dr. Freemont-Smith. Drs. William Lennox and Frederick and Erna Gibbs were pioneers in the use of electroencephalography and in the diagnosis and treatment of epilepsy. Drs. Tracy Putnam and Houston Merritt developed the first anti-epileptic drug Dilantin. Merritt later moved to New York City, where he chaired the Neurology Department at Columbia University from 1948 through 1967.[7]

Beginning in 1939, the dean and leaders at Harvard Medical School began to explore with Gregg of the Rockefeller Foundation the appointment of a world leader to head the Neurological Unit. Putnam had expressed his desire to move to New York City, and the position of director of the unit would soon be open. Gregg opined that neurology was much stronger scientifically in England and Europe than in the United States. He suggested appointing a leader from abroad and recommended several outstanding individuals, some of whom had been funded by the Rockefeller Foundation. After much discussion about potential internal and external candidates, the dean and committee of professors decided to offer the position to Denny-Brown. They asked him to visit the hospital and medical school and to seriously consider the offer.[8]

Denny-Brown was one of the two most prominent candidates suggested by Gregg of the Rockefeller Foundation. Originally from New Zealand, Denny-Brown had spent several years learning physiology under the tutelage of Sir Charles Sherrington, a Nobel Laureate in Medicine and

Physiology in 1929. After receiving his DPhil in neurophysiology, he received a Rockefeller Foundation fellowship for further training in neurophysiology at Yale University with Dr. John Fulton. His clinical position was as a consultant to St. Bartholomew's Hospital and to the National Hospital for Neurological Diseases at Queen Square in London. When approached about the Harvard position, he appeared enthusiastic and agreed to visit Boston.[8]

Then the war happened. Germany had invaded Poland, and Great Britain had declared war. Denny-Brown wrote of a "very unpleasant" trip home from Boston after visiting BCH in 1939, navigating through waters under constant threat of a German U-boat submarine attack. He accepted the Harvard offer but emphasized that he could not come to Boston until the war situation was clarified. He was at that time commissioned as an officer assigned to Oxford, UK, and was given the rank of a Brigadier General. Denny-Brown wrote, "It is difficult to resign a commission without the opprobrium of shirking one's responsibilities."[8] He recognized that Harvard would not wait indefinitely for him to assume the position in Boston.

In June 1940, President Franklin Roosevelt appointed James Conant, President of Harvard University, as the wartime head of the Office of Scientific Research and Development. Conant was a chemist and scientist by training. He had been heavily involved in the proposed appointment of Denny-Brown. Conant and his committee met with Winston Churchill several times, delivering salutary news about US support of the war effort. After one meeting, Churchill was reported to have turned to Conant and say, "Mr. Conant you have been very good to us. Is there anything I can do for you."[8] The reply was to request that General Denny-Brown be released from his war duties and be allowed to move to Boston to take up the Harvard position. Churchill then turned to the appropriate British Cabinet secretary and said, "Hankey, see to it."[8] Lord Hankey sent an official letter informing Denny-Brown that he would not have to give up his commission and noted that "I can assure you that you would be rendering a very valuable service by accepting Dr. Conant's invitation." Denny-Brown responded,

> In view of your assurance that I would not be required to resign my commission . . . and that my service in Boston would outweigh my usefulness here, I have no longer any objection to proceeding to Harvard. . . . I presume the war office will instruct me.[8]

Denny-Brown came to Boston in 1941 to assume leadership of the Harvard Neurological Unit, but he was recalled to active military duty in 1944 and was stationed in India and the Far East. He did not return to Boston until the end of the war in 1945.

Denny-Brown and Adams were central figures in the career of Fisher, and these authoritative figures were also major leaders in 20th-century neurology and stroke.

DEREK DENNY-BROWN AND THE NEUROLOGICAL UNIT

Denny-Brown, also known as Denny, was an imposing figure (Figure 6.2). Tall and well groomed, he had a carefully trimmed mustache, his countenance was characteristically stern and serious, and he spoke authoritatively but often mumbled. His thick New Zealand accent and frequent mumbling often made his discussions difficult to follow unless one was close by and listened intently. He has been described as the "quintessential man of science whose great interest in both Neurology and Medicine led him into Neurology. He was constantly curious about all aspects of Neurology and tackled virtually all of them in his clinical observations and basic research."[8]

Denny-Brown ran the Neurological Unit with an iron hand. He was well known for dedication to his work and for his intellect. He had been trained by pioneers in physiology and neurology and was well versed in the history and evolution of ideas in all of the various branches of neurology—muscle disease, peripheral nerve disease, spinal cord abnormalities, cognitive and

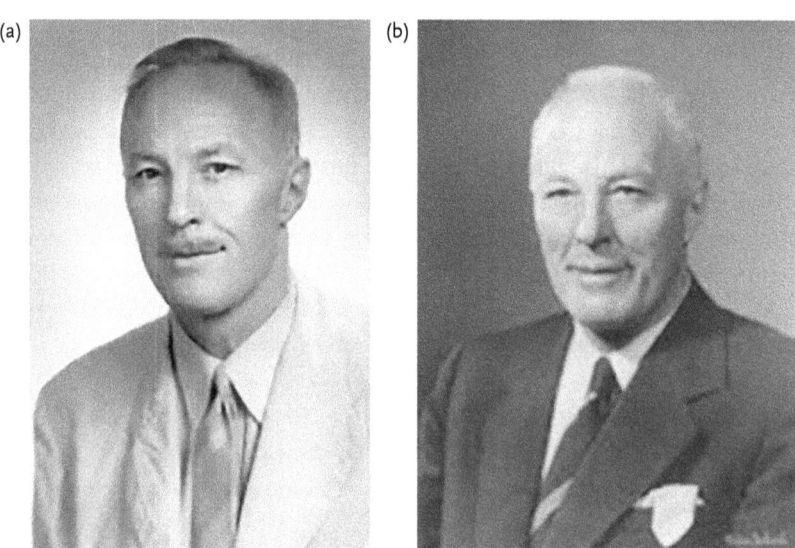

Figure 6.2 (A) Derek Denny-Brown soon after arriving at Boston City Hospital. (B) Later portrait of Denny-Brown.
Sources: A, photograph at Boston City Hospital kindly provided by Dr. Thomas Sabin; B, provided and signed by Dr. Denny-Brown.

behavioral disorders, cerebrovascular disease, epilepsy, etc. His special interest was in the physiology of movement disorders and diseases of the extrapyramidal system (the so-called basal ganglia—the caudate nucleus, putamen, and globus pallidus within the deeper regions of the cerebral hemispheres). He was also known for his irascibility, rigidity, and temper.

Because the Neurological Unit at BCH and Harvard was one of the foremost training grounds for young neurologists, the program attracted students, residents, and fellows from throughout the world but especially from Canada and the United Kingdom. The Neurological Unit contained 15 neurology residents, 5 in each of the 3 years of the neurology residency training program. One resident from each of the three Boston Medical School medical services (Harvard, Tufts, and Boston University) rotated for 4–6 weeks on the Neurological Unit. Fellows who had completed their neurology residency training and were interested in further concentrating on various selected aspects of neurology and neuropathology were also attached to the unit. Fisher was one of the fellows in neuropathology. He and the other fellows also attended many of the teaching rounds of the unit. Trainees and even junior staff were fearful of Denny-Brown's discipline and temper, and they became quite anxious when presenting cases to him.

All the trainees had great respect for Denny-Brown's knowledge and experience. He was a perfectionist who expected and demanded the highest level of care for patients on the unit. He also believed it was important to learn from patients how their symptoms and findings on neurological examination helped increase the understanding of the human nervous system and also the condition and diseases of the patients. The patient was the laboratory. He had high expectations for his residents.[9] When his residents had completed the training program, he expected that they would be able to spontaneously discuss any neurological problem in depth, including the history of that condition, its manifestations, and its management. His way of training residents was based on his experience with Sherrington. During the first year of training, he would rarely acknowledge the presence of the resident except to render criticism. During the second year, he was more circumspect and would call the resident aside or criticize only privately. By the third year, he would speak more familiarly with the resident, and after training, the former resident became a trusted colleague whom Denny-Brown would promote and loyally defend. Full knowledge of the medical and neurological literature was emphasized. Residents and fellows were expected to have read prior reports and reviews of neurological conditions that were published in medical journals and books.[10]

During his neuropathology experience at BCH, Fisher spent considerable time on the clinical units, attending rounds and observing research and patient care. The Neurological Unit was located on the top floors of the medical building. Floor 7 was a ward for men, and floor 8 housed women patients. The head nurses (Grace McKay and Norma Richards) were instrumental in maintaining a standard and a discipline that ensured good nursing care, much like the tradition of nursing sisters in the United Kingdom who were very much in charge of their wards. Floor 9 contained the neurological library, meeting rooms, administrative offices, and clinical laboratories (electroencephalography, electromyography, and spinal fluid). Basic research and animal study laboratories were located on the 10th floor.

The task of the neurology resident on the consultation service was to choose one patient each day from the emergency room or the medical and surgical wards to be transferred to the Neurological Unit for further study and treatment. That patient would be assigned for thorough evaluation to one of the neurology junior residents who were assigned to the ward service or one of the three rotating residents. Six new patients were admitted to the Neurological Unit each week. At that time, there was no push from authorities to move patients out quickly. Many patients stayed for weeks or months and some even for years. Denny-Brown only allowed his neurology residents to care for his own occasional private patient. The junior residents and rotators had only one new patient to study during the week, in addition to continuing to care for their other patients who were still on the neurology ward. A second-year senior neurology resident also examined each patient and mentored the junior trainees. Each patient's history, general examination, neurological examination, and investigations were extensively documented in the hospital record. The reporting rigidly followed directions in a handbook written by Denny-Brown.[11]

Every month, an experienced staff neurologist was assigned to be the responsible attending physician and to give teaching rounds for the entire month. These rounds occurred on each weekday morning. Denny-Brown was the attending physician during 2 months of the year. During Fisher's time at BCH, Adams would be the attending physician for 2 months, and during those months Fisher would often attend Adams' daily ward rounds. Grand rounds were held each Tuesday morning. During the grand rounds, three or four of the new patients admitted the previous week were presented to Denny-Brown at the patients' bedside. He also rounded on all of the patients who had been previously presented who were still on the ward. The neuropathology staff and fellows always attended grand rounds. During the month that he was the attending physician, one of the more senior attending physicians (e.g., Drs. Joseph Foley, Raymond Adams, or Flaviau Romanul) would hold the grand rounds and Denny-Brown would also be present and would make comments.

On the Tuesday mornings of the grand rounds, all of the residents and students, as well as the junior and senior neurology attending physicians and any visitors, would congregate in the Neurological Library and wait for Denny-Brown. When he appeared, often quite a bit after the usual starting time, all present would stand. The group would proceed to the bedside of the first patient to be presented housed on Medical 7 or 8. The march was very hierarchical, with Denny-Brown in the lead, followed by the senior attendings, junior attendings, visiting senior physicians, senior residents and fellows, and junior residents. Students would bring up the rear. The group would wind up in a large circle around the patient to be presented. The senior resident and attending physician for the month would usually have chosen the most interesting or challenging patient for the first case. The resident who was assigned to the patient would present the history and findings to the senior physician holding the round (most often Denny-Brown). Before presenting the case, almost always that resident would have practiced the presentation under the aegis of the senior resident. The neurological findings had to be told in a precise order. The cognitive and behavioral testing came first, followed by examination of the structures innervated by the nerves that supplied the structures within the head (the cranial nerves), then movement, strength, and coordination of the arms and legs, then deep tendon and superficial reflexes, and finally sensation. The reflexes were quantified and displayed on a chart. Sensation was also shown on a chart, meticulously filled in by the resident. The responses to various sensory stimuli on the limbs and the torso (cotton touch, pin, temperature, vibration, and position sense) were quantified according to the patient's responses. Figure 6.3 is an example of a sensory chart created after examining one patient.[11] The senior resident would stand near Denny-Brown, holding a box that contained various equipment used in the examination—cotton wool, test tubes with graded temperatures of water, a reflex hammer, vibration fork, etc. These would be handed to the examiner on request.

The attending physician holding grand rounds (Denny-Brown for 10 months of the year) would go over key points in the history with the patient, examine him or her, and then deliver a detailed erudite analysis emphasizing what could be learned from some features or aspects of that patient's condition. Further investigations and management would also be discussed. Other senior physicians attending the round would be asked for their opinion. The new patients would be seen in turn, followed by those patients who had been previously presented and discussed and were still available on the ward. These latter patients would be seen cursorily by Denny-Brown after interim progress had been reported on their case.

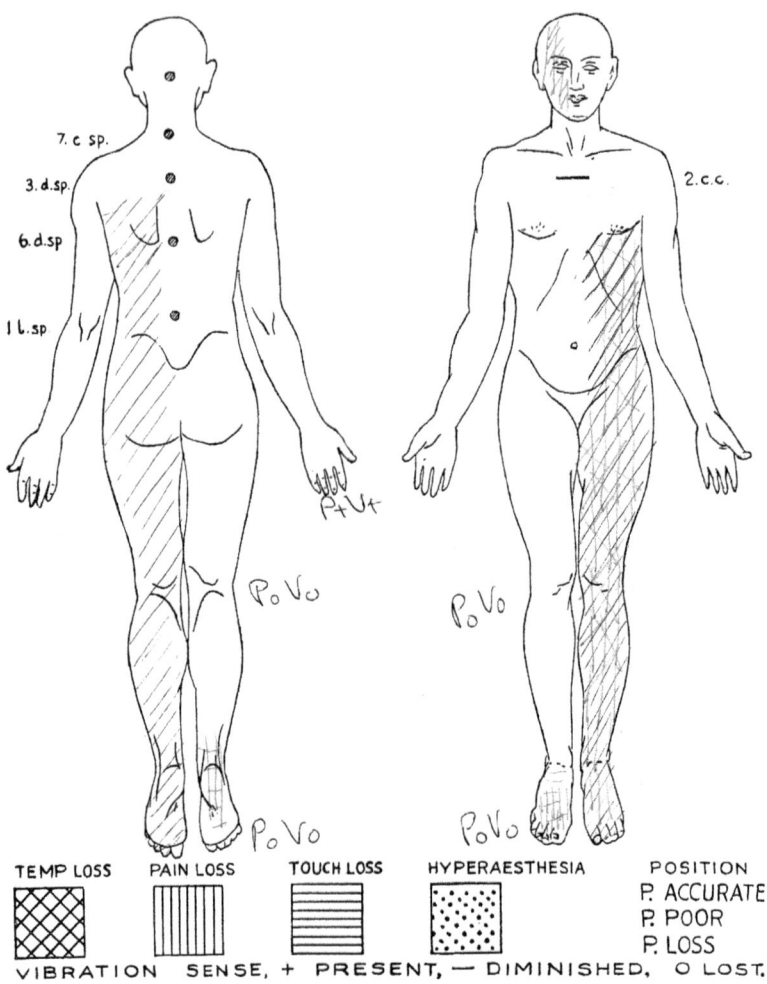

Figure 6.3 A sensory chart of a patient with a brainstem stroke who also had a peripheral neuropathy. The chart shows a loss of pain and temperature sensation on the right face and left body sparing the arm and a loss of touch, pain, position, and vibration sense on the feet. This chart is available in the neurological library at BCH.

A conference was held each Saturday morning during which the other two new patients who had not been presented at Tuesday's grand rounds were presented to Denny-Brown in a conference room on Medical 9. The walls of the room were covered with anatomical drawings of the brain and other parts of the nervous system. The room was imposing for trainees. The patients would be brought to the conference room, and the presentations, examinations, and discussions would proceed in a pattern similar to that followed during grand rounds. Denny-Brown would hear the history and then examine the patient. Figure 6.4 is a photograph of Denny-Brown examining an infant during a Saturday morning conference. Neurologists from throughout Boston often attended these meetings. Denny-Brown would invite comments and discussion from attendees after he had finished his analysis of the case and its main teaching points.

Denny-Brown would criticize, castigate, or berate a resident whom he thought had missed an important sign or had not recorded the findings accurately. He was known to tear up sensory charts that he found inaccurate. For that reason, residents were accustomed to making carbon copies of all of their charts in case they had to redo any of them. Residents and all members of the Neurological Unit recognized that each patient had to be thoroughly and completely studied, and the findings had to be accurately recorded and correctly interpreted.

A neuropathology conference was held on each Thursday afternoon. This teaching session was usually the highlight of the week's academic schedule for the attendees. During the last year of the 3-year neurology training program, most senior residents were trained in neuropathology. Fellows such as Fisher were also trained and would occasionally be called on to enter the discussion of

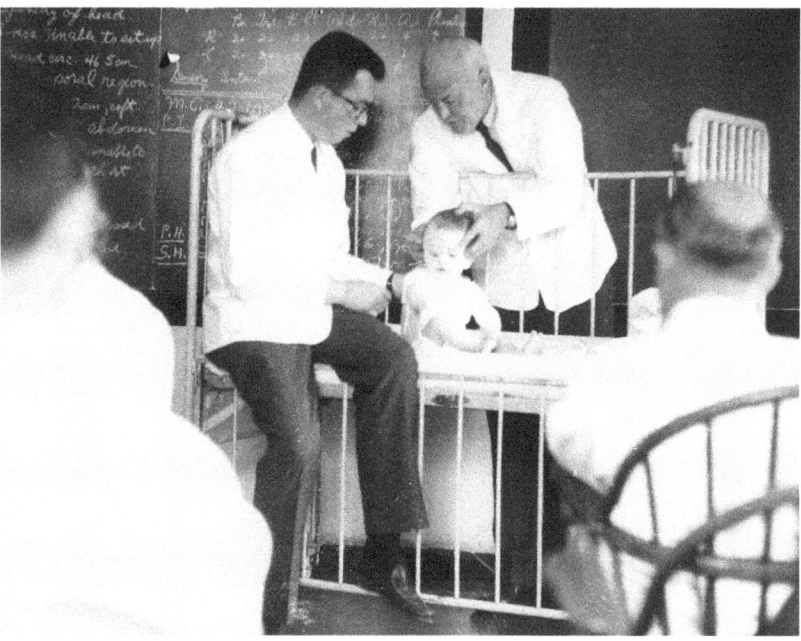

Figure 6.4 Denny-Brown examining an infant during a Saturday morning conference.
Source: Photograph provided by Dr. Thomas Sabin.

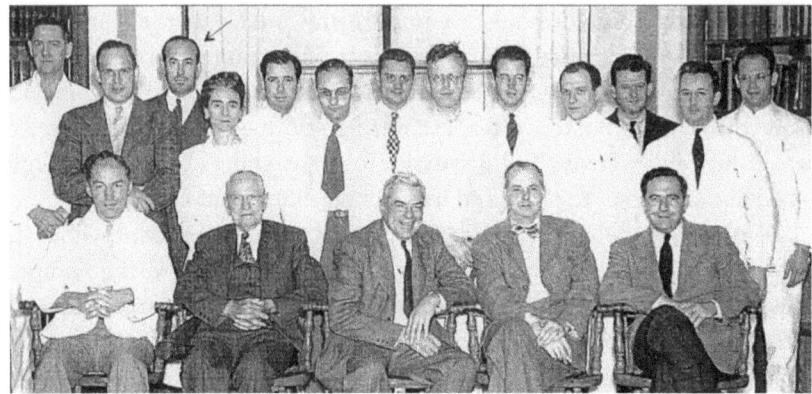

Figure 6.5 Photograph of the staff of the Mallory Pathology Department in 1949. Raymond Adams is seated in the first row at the far left. Fisher is standing in the rear (arrow).
Source: Mallory Institute of Pathology at BCH.

the neuropathology at these weekly conferences. The pathology laboratories and conference rooms were located in the Mallory Building within the campus of BCH. Neuropathology was under the direction of Raymond Adams. Fisher was a visiting fellow in neuropathology during 1949–1950 (Figures 6.5 and 6.6). Formal printed protocols describing the clinical information concerning

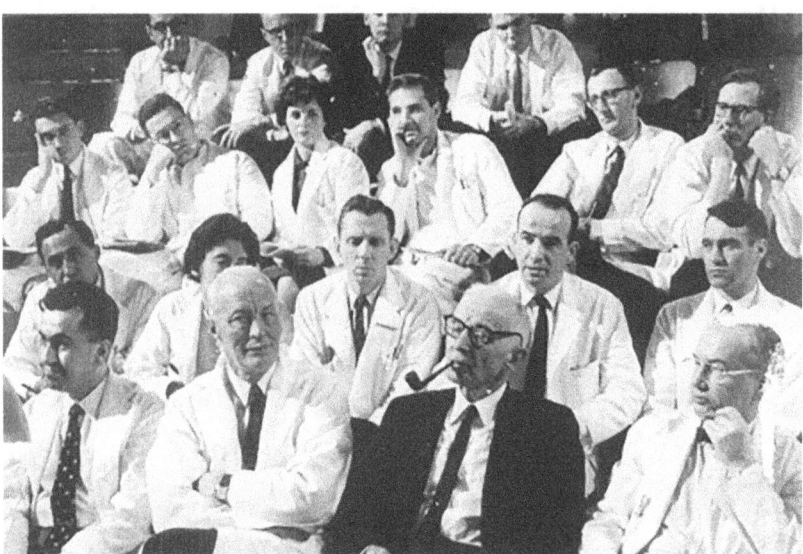

Figure 6.6 Photograph taken at a brain cutting session. Denny-Brown is seated in a white coat second from the left in the front row. Paul Yakovlev is the gentleman with a pipe seated to the right of Denny-Brown.
Source: Photograph provided by Dr. Thomas Sabin.

[94]   *Fellowship and Experience as a Neurologist*

two patients were handed out in the conference room at 4 p.m. sharp. At approximately 4:20 p.m., the session began. Denny-Brown would call on one of his junior Harvard neurology residents to briefly discuss case 1 and to render a diagnosis and speculate on what would be found within the brain. This would be followed by Denny-Brown choosing a second junior neurology resident to add to or disagree with the first discussant's diagnosis and speculation. Senior residents and junior attendings would then be asked for their comments. These would be followed by remarks from the neuropathologist, Adams. The neuropathologist had not cut the brain in sections but had viewed the brain from the outside. Figure 6.7 shows Adams about to section the brain at one of these conferences. Finally, Denny-Brown would comment. Adams would then cut the brain in fine sections, and the brain sections could be viewed by all those at the conference. Final remarks that summarized the main teaching points of the case would conclude case 1. Discussion of case 2 would then follow. These clinical–neuropathology conferences provided an opportunity for Fisher and the other neuropathology trainees to fully interact with the clinical staff at BCH.

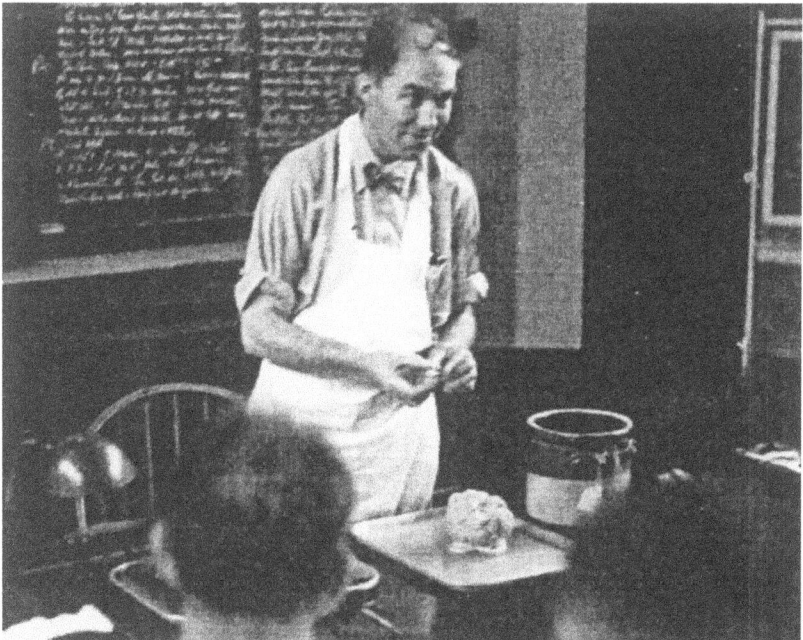

Figure 6.7 Raymond Adams at a brain cutting session early in his career at Boston City Hospital. The brain is in front of him on a pan ready to be cut. The receptacle in which the brain was fixed is on the side of the brain.
Source: From with permission Robert Loreno. *Raymond D. Adams: A Life of Brain and Muscle*. New York: Oxford University Press, 2009.

RAYMOND DELANCEY ADAMS AND NEUROPATHOLOGY AT BOSTON CITY HOSPITAL

One of the main considerations that led Fisher to come to Boston in 1949 was the presence of Dr. Ray Adams. By that time, Adams had attained a strong national and international reputation. The aristocratic demeanor Adams displayed in his later years belied his very humble background. Adams was born February 13, 1911, in Portland, Oregon. His early life was marked by poverty and hardship.[12]

After college, Adams entered a master's degree program in psychology. He became dissatisfied with the way psychology was trending:

> *I saw the weakness of psychology in general and the difficulty in doing experimental work. That influenced my decision to get a sound grounding in nervous system anatomy, physiology, and pharmacology and to get a medical degree rather than a doctorate in psychology.*[13]

His master's thesis was on various tests to detect tremor and ataxia as an aid to selecting factory workers. It was titled "The Importance of Steadiness in Marksmanship and Several Other Practical Skills."

Adams happened on a catalogue that contained an announcement that Duke University was accepting medical school applicants. He sent an application to the dean, Wilburt Davidson, explaining that he "wanted to study medicine to find out more about the nervous system."[6,14] He soon got the response "Come Along." He was the last of 60 students admitted to the third class at Duke Medical School. During medical school, Adams found the 3-month course in neuroanatomy very stimulating and appealing. Also during this time, he spent vacation time at a tuberculosis sanitarium in Winston-Salem, where he received mentoring in identifying abnormalities that he heard while listening to the lungs of patients with a stethoscope and in performing chest fluoroscopy.

By going to summer school, he was able to finish medical school in 3 years, graduating in 1937. After medical school graduation, Adams began a residency in medicine at Duke. He had applied for a neurology residency position at Massachusetts General Hospital (MGH) in Bosotn but had not yet received a reply. At that time, there were few neurology residency positions, and Boston medicine was already receiving acclaim. While a medical service intern, he impressed the chair of medicine, Dr. Hanes, who was able to obtain for Adams a 3-year Rockefeller fellowship in psychiatry. When he heard affirmatively about the neurology residency position at MGH, Hanes released Adams from the medicine training program to accept the neurology training position. Neurology training was planned to occur during the first year, followed by training in psychiatry during the succeeding 2 years. It was understood that Adams would return to Duke as a staff psychiatrist after the fellowship.[15]

The MGH neurology residency program was in its sixth year. Adams was one of two residents. Dr. Ayer, the Chair of Neurology, paid half his salary, and the Rockefeller Foundation paid the other half. During the year, Adams received accolades from Ayer. A group of medical students and trainees asked Ayer if he could arrange for Adams to spend more time with them. Ayer was quoted as saying that this proved Adams' ability as a teacher because it was rare to find someone who could correlate neurology, chemistry, pathology, and anatomy as well as Adams.[16] After the neurology year, Adams stayed at MGH in the psychiatry department under Stanley Cobb but also did neuropathology with Dr. Charles Kubik and attended Dr. Paul Yakovlev's weekly neuroanatomy discussions at the Fernald School. Adams was stimulated by these sessions with Yakovlev, who had originally studied in Russia. One night a week, Yakovlev would put on display whole brains that were cut in serial sections. One week he would describe the thalamus and its connections in great detail, and another week he would highlight a different brain region and its connections. Yakovlev's sessions would begin at 9 p.m., and the discussions and lectures would often continue until 3 or 4 a.m. According to Adams, Yakovlev had much to say about Russian, French, Swiss, and German neuroanatomy. Adams' third and last year of psychiatry fellowship was at Yale University, where he was exposed to John Fulton, the neurophysiologist. Recall that Denny-Brown had also spent time with Fulton, the acknowledged American leader in neurophysiology research at that time.

After his third year as a Rockefeller fellow, Adams was scheduled to join the Psychiatry Department at Duke University. The prospect did not appeal to him because he was by then more attracted to neurology and neuropathology than to psychiatry. In 1941, Adams received an invitation from Houston Merritt to join the Neurological Research Unit at BCH; Adams promptly accepted. BCH had 1,800 patients at that time. Adams began work under the tutelage of Merritt, who was by all accounts a diligent and skilled neurologist and a very active researcher and clinician.[7] There were only two salaries for staff on the Harvard Neurological Unit—one for Merritt and a smaller stipend for Adams. When Denny-Brown arrived to become the head of the unit, of course he was given one of the two available stipends. Merritt retained the other salary. Adams was appointed neuropathologist for the hospital at the Mallory Institute in order to continue to fund his salary. Before that time, Adams had had no formal training in pathology or neuropathology. During the next years, Adams trained in general pathology and neuropathology. He performed general and nervous system autopsies and became the chief neuropathologist of the hospital. He also worked part-time in neurology on the hospital neurology wards and in the clinic.

Adams decided to study all of the brains of patients that were examined at autopsy (800–900 per year) and the clinical notes concerning these patients. He initiated brain cuttings each Tuesday afternoon. Doctors from MGH, Brigham, Beth Israel, and elsewhere would often attend. When Denny-Brown assumed his position, these sessions became even more popular. As his reputation as a neuropathologist grew, formalin-fixed brains (uncut—approximately 100 per year) would be sent to Adams for his opinion. In 1949, Fisher came as a fellow to the Neuropathology Unit at BCH to study under Adams and Denny-Brown.

Fisher described Adams as "calm, indefatigable, knowledgeable beyond human expectations, and completely devoted to teaching and demonstration. His extemporaneous presentations flowed in perfectly arranged sentences, clear, concise, and authoritative, often to the amazement of his audience."[17] Figure 6.8 shows Adams later in his career. The fellowship time

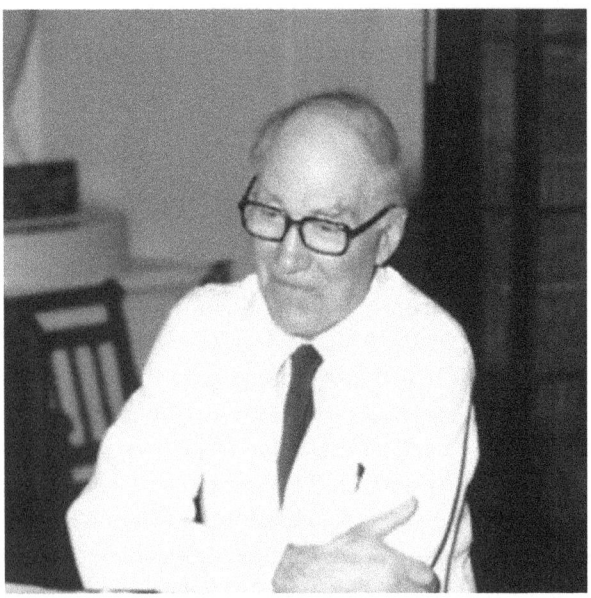

Figure 6.8 Photograph of Adams later in his career.
Source: Provided by Dr. Raymond Adams.

in 1949–1950 was the beginning of a half century of a very close collegial relationship between Fisher and Adams.

FISHER'S YEAR AT BOSTON CITY HOSPITAL AND NEUROPATHOLOGY

Fisher's exposure to the two giants, Denny-Brown and Adams, and to the academic milieu at BCH cemented his determination to be a productive contributor to future knowledge about neurology and about caring for patients with neurological conditions. His discoveries with Adams during this fellowship concerning the abnormalities found in the brains of patients with strokes made it clear that cerebrovascular disease and stroke were to be his life's work.

Fisher was clearly awed by both Denny-Brown and Adams. He wrote,

> *It was a two man show. Dr. Derek Denny-Brown, handsome, dignified, polished, articulate, autocratic, authoritative, betimes choleric. After attending one of his lectures, medical students all aspired to be neurologists. Dr. Adams, equally articulate was a model of tolerance. Dr. Denny-Brown had been a household name in Neurology for many years and was to become even more famous. Dr. Raymond Adams was relatively unknown except in Boston where he already was recognized as the premier clinical neurologist. Still in his 30s, his star was ascending steeply.*[18]

In his memoirs, Fisher first commented on the milieu he found in Boston:[7] "There was an air of hustle and bustle, vigor, enthusiasm, excitement and cockiness. It was medicine in depth, painstaking, penetrating, inquiring, competing."[19]

Fisher noted that many staff members lived in dormitories on the campus. In the spacious dining room, each linen-covered table could seat six to eight individuals; waitresses served the diners. Interns and residents and fellows mingled at meals with junior and senior staff physicians. Fisher commented that during one lunch, he sat at a table with Denny-Brown and a distinguished guest from London, Sir Charles Symonds. Much teaching and discussion permeated the dining room. Staff and trainees from different disciplines—medicine, surgery, obstetrics, and neurology—all mingled and shared ideas, observations, and concerns.

At BCH, Fisher's immersion in pathology and neuropathology cemented a lifelong adoration and dedication to neuropathology. After his training at BCH, he maintained a neuropathology laboratory during his entire career. Later, during his career at MGH, when asked about his profession, he would respond proudly that he was a neuropathologist. Just weeks before his death, during a visit with me, he repeatedly emphasized that "we need more neuropathology." In his memoirs, he commented on the importance of the visual aspect of neuropathology:

> *Ultimately my exposure to the anatomy and neuropathology of neurological disease under Dr. Adams gave me the feeling that prior to that time, I had not really lived, neurologically. Having learned basic neurology without immersion in Neuropathology, I may justifiably claim that achieving a visuospatial basis for thought is not only fundamental, it is the only method.*[20]

During Fisher's time at BCH, necropsy examinations of the body and brain were very prevalent after the death of patients. Investigations during life often did not clarify the nature of a patient's disease, and the autopsy was the major way that physicians could learn of the nature of the condition and the location and extent of involvement. They could correlate the patient's symptoms and findings with the condition. This type of knowledge was indispensable for allowing correct diagnosis and management of future patients with the same condition.

In 1949, the pathology department at BCH performed approximately 1,000 autopsies each year, and in most cases, the brains of these patients were available for study. Approximately 700 brains from these autopsies were examined by the Neuropathology Department each year. In some patients in whom there was evidence that the condition was spinal, the spinal cord and attached nerve roots were also removed from the body. Because of his interest and experience, Adams was also sent approximately 2 brains each week from other hospitals for examination.

Removing the brains from the body, sectioning them, and examining the cut sections under the microscope comprised a full-time job for the two neuropathology fellows, Fisher and David McDougall. McDougal, who was senior to Fisher, had a formalin-related dermatitis, so he did not place brains in formalin or cut the formalin-fixed brains. Fisher sectioned all of the brains, with his senior colleague observing over his shoulder. Ultimately, Adams supervised and signed out each of the neuropathology reports, teaching the fellows as they reviewed the sectioned brains and the subsequent microscopic examinations.

Two brains or brains and spinal cords were not sectioned but, rather, were reserved for the brain-cutting teaching session that occurred each Thursday afternoon. These usually were from patients who were thoroughly studied neurologically during their clinical course and had well-described symptoms and neurological abnormalities.

Fisher commented on what made his sojourn and training at BCH such a fruitful and stimulating experience:

> Every case, every inquiry, was the occasion for a penetrating yet wide-ranging account into every facet of a problem. In some areas Dr. Denny-Brown was superior and in many areas it was Dr. Adams, but together it was a performance that bordered on the amazing, one that left visitors incredulous. Vague muddleheaded pronouncements were not tolerated. There is no substitute for experience and knowledge in depth. Guided by the facts of neuropathology, Dr. Adams methodical measured expositions delivered in beautiful flowing English were models of practical information that had the ring of permanence, even that early. He made it all look easy. . . . Here were two giants whose like I would not meet again. Dr. Penfield I had already met.[21]

While working in the neuropathology and clinical neurology departments at BCH, Fisher was exposed to experimental research and its techniques. Diphtheria was prevalent in Boston at the time, and Fisher, with Adams and their colleagues, had the opportunity to examine the nerve roots and peripheral nerves of 10 patients who died from this disease. Experimental studies on the mechanism of the nerve damage were performed in guinea pigs injected with diphtheria toxin at BCH. Anatomical studies on the brains that were injected with opacifying dyes gave insight into the most vulnerable brain regions that were deprived of blood flow when the blood pressure was low or the heart stopped pumping normally. These were labeled "border-zone regions" of blood supply because they lay between the main flow of the major arteries that supplied the brain.

Fisher was taught various techniques for optimally studying the regions of brain damage due to stroke and visualizing any abnormality within the blood vessels that supplied these zones. Cutting the brain in sections in a plane horizontal to the ground proved superior to using vertical plane sections in viewing the blood vessels.

Louis Pasteur commented that "fortune favored the prepared mind,"[22] and so it was with Fisher. In his memoir, Fisher opined that the discoveries he made on one afternoon determined his entire future career in medicine and neurology.[23] Soon after his arrival in Boston, after cutting brains in section and examining the blood vessels that supplied the areas of damage in these brains, he wrote,

> The first specimen showed a typical large hemorrhagic infarction . . . I carefully examined the cerebral arteries supplying the infarcted region looking for any blockage. None was found. Specimen number two for the day disclosed another large hemorrhagic infarct . . . again there was no arterial obstruction. . . . Later in the afternoon

a third specimen revealed another hemorrhagic infarct again without any sign of occlusion in the artery of supply which itself appeared free of disease. All three of the patients with hemorrhagic infarction had atrial fibrillation and there were infarcts in spleen and kidneys suggesting emboli to those organs. Presumably the cerebral infarcts were also embolic.[24]

Four aspects of these observations were important and represented new information. First, in the medical literature up to that time, it was assumed that most ischemic strokes (i.e., those attributable to loss of blood supply) were caused by degenerative changes within the arteries that supplied the brain. Infarction is the term used to describe brain tissue that has died because of insufficient supply of blood. Embolism (material that arose in one region and traveled to another) was considered a very unusual or rare cause of ischemic strokes. Embolism was known to occur in individuals with heart valves damaged by rheumatic fever and infection (bacterial endocarditis). These known embolic circumstances were estimated to account for only approximately 5% of ischemic strokes. And yet it struck Fisher as important that he had found on three occasions in one day embolism as the cause of brain damage in patients who did not have heart valve disease. Were the prior assumptions about embolism dead wrong? Second, a key feature of the regions of damage was that they contained regions of bleeding. They were so-called hemorrhagic infarctions. Little had been written about hemorrhagic infarcts, so this observation sparked interest in how and why the bleeding developed. Third, all three patients had atrial fibrillation. At that time, atrial fibrillation (erratic contraction of the atrial regions of the heart) was neither a known nor a posited cause of stroke. Fourth, emboli could block an artery long enough to cause infarction and then somehow pass through the system and not be evident at necropsy.

Fisher wrote,

From these observations it was speculated that embolic material must have obstructed the flow of blood causing infarction and then disappeared from the expected site, migrating distally or undergoing lysis. Based on one afternoon's work, the proposition of dissolution of emboli was formulated and the association of cerebral hemorrhagic infarction with embolism was recognized.[25]

When Fisher left Boston after his fellowship to return to Montreal, he was determined to chase further the queries raised by the three patients and to devote his career to research and care of stroke patients. He also realized that thorough review of past knowledge as contained in the medical literature was crucial to making progress. Clinicians and researchers had to be familiar with the past and the present in order to guide progress in the future. What were past assumptions and were they well grounded in evidence? What did physicians practicing at the time do, and was their information that supported the safety and efficacy of the present practices? Fisher, always the serious student, was determined to make progress not only academically but also in helping benefit patients he and others would see.

NOTES

1. Swank later became the first Chairman of Neurology at Oregon University. His major contribution related to dietary treatment of multiple sclerosis. The career of Swank is outlined in Bourdette, D. Roy Laver Swank, MD, PhD (1909–2008): In memoriam. *Neurology* 2009;72:1120.
2. Remarks during an interview of Fisher by me for the American Association of Neurological Surgeons in 1984 (available on YouTube).
3. Dawson DM, Sabin TD (Eds.). *The Cradle of American Neurology: The Harvard Neurological Unit at the Boston City Hospital*. Hollis, NH: Hollis, 2011.
4. Accounts of the early years of Boston City Hospital are found in Dawson D. Boston City Hospital: The first 50 years. In Dawson DM, Sabin TD (Eds.), *The Cradle of American Neurology: The Harvard Neurological Unit at the Boston City Hospital*. Hollis, NH: Hollis, 2011, pp. 1–16; Byrne JJ, et al. *History of the Boston City Hospital, 1905–1964*. London: Sheldon Press, 1965.
5. After training in Europe, Prince, the son of a mayor of Boston, was appointed as Physician for Nervous Disease. He held that position from 1885 until 1913 and remained a consulting physician at the hospital until 1929. His work mostly concerned psychological and psychiatric aspects of illness.
6. Cobb S, Munro D. Neurological unit at the Boston City Hospital, Bulletin of the Harvard Medical School Alumni Association. In Dawson DM, Sabin TD (Eds.), *The Cradle of American Neurology: The Harvard Neurological Unit at the Boston City Hospital*. Hollis, NH: Hollis, 2011, pp. 18–25.
7. The lives and careers of Putnam and Merritt and their activities at Boston City Hospital are described in Rowland L. *The Legacy of Tracy J. Putnam and H. Houston Merritt: Modern Neurology in the United States*. New York: Oxford University Press, 2009.
8. Accounts of the recruitment of Denny-Brown and his activities in the Neurological Unit are found in Tyler KL, Tyler HR. The appointment of Derek Denny-Brown (DDB) as head of the Neurological Unit at the Boston City Hospital and Harvard Medical School. In Dawson DM, Sabin TD (Eds.), *The Cradle of American Neurology: The Harvard Neurological Unit at the Boston City Hospital*. Hollis, NH: Hollis, 2011, pp. 63–81; Gilman S, Vilensky JA. Derek Ernest Denny-Brown (1901–1981): The man and his role in twentieth century neurology. In Dawson DM, Sabin TD (Eds.), *The Cradle of American Neurology: The Harvard Neurological Unit at the Boston City Hospital*. Hollis, NH: Hollis, 2011, pp. 93–104.

9. I was among the last group of residents trained by Denny-Brown.
10. I was able to read in the Neurological Library all the editions of the journal *Brain* from 1900 to 1966 while on call during my 3-year residency training.
11. Denny-Brown D. *Handbook of Neurological Examination and Case Recording*. Cambridge, MA: Harvard University Press, 1942.
12. An account of Adams' early life and career is found in Loreno R. *Raymond Adams: A Life of Brain and Muscle*. New York: Oxford University Press, 2009. His father had built the house in which Adams was born. The home had no gaslight or electricity. It was heated with logs and a furnace, and oil lamps were placed in each room for illumination. Adams' father's family were farmers; none had attended high school. They read little. There were few, if any, books in the home. Adams' father ran a farm and delivered oil for the Standard Oil Company. He used a tank wagon that was pulled by horses to deliver the oil in tanks to gas stations and businesses that used it for heating. Later, he worked for the railroad as a baggage handler. When Adams was young, he had to walk a mile to get to elementary school. During high school, he had many after-school hours jobs to help with family finances. His grades in high school were only average. Adams later commented, "I was a rather mediocre student in high school. I would always pass easily, but I didn't make any great effort. The children that I grew up with disdained scholarship and study."

    After high school and before college, Adams signed on for $30 a month to work on an oil tanker (the *S.S. Moffett*) that sailed from Alaska to San Diego and San Salvador and back. As a seaman he scrubbed decks, took turns at watch, and performed other tasks on board. He said that it was during this time that he was exposed to the "rather seamy side of life." He enrolled at the University of Oregon and became a member of the university's tennis team; he was also very active in other sports. During his early college days, he was not an avid student. He opined years later, in retrospect, that he was slow in finding courses that interested him and had difficulty avoiding distractions that were more interesting than the coursework. He did become very interested and stimulated by courses in physiology and psychology during his last 2 years in college. He supported himself at college by working at a fraternity house and library. His other work involved serving on a construction crew digging ditches and performing hard labor. During his college years, he met and married Margaret Elinor Clark, who was a student at Monmouth Teachers College. He was encouraged by her to pursue more academic inquiry.

    Because he was the son of a baggage handler, Adams was able to travel free by train from Portland to North Carolina to attend Duke University School of Medical. During the entire 3-day train ride, he sat straight up. The last leg of the trip to Durham and Duke University was on a one-car freight train that had a few seats at one end. He only had funds to pay for 1 year of the medical school tuition. He could not afford to room in the dormitory, so he lived in a janitor's closet under the auditorium. The room and $1 a day were his compensation for delivering ice. He had to arrive at the hospital at 6 a.m. to deliver the large cakes of ice. Adams would push the ice wagon to each ward and scoop out ice cakes for the kitchens that distributed food.
13. Loreno R. *Raymond Adams: A Life of Brain and Muscle*. New York: Oxford University Press, 2009, p. 27.
14. Loreno R. *Raymond Adams: A Life of Brain and Muscle*. New York: Oxford University Press, 2009, p 27.

15. Loreno R. *Raymond Adams: A Life of Brain and Muscle.* New York: Oxford University Press, 2009, p. 36.
16. Loreno R. *Raymond Adams: A Life of Brain and Muscle.* New York: Oxford University Press, 2009, p. 39.
17. Fisher CM. *Memoirs of a Neurologist.* Rutland, VT: Sharp, 2006, Vol. 1, p. 165.
18. Fisher CM. *Memoirs of a Neurologist.* Rutland, VT: Sharp, 2006, Vol. 1, p. 47.
19. Fisher CM. *Memoirs of a Neurologist.* Rutland, VT: Sharp, 2006, Vol. 1, p. 47.
20. Fisher CM. *Memoirs of a Neurologist.* Rutland, VT: Sharp, 2006, Vol. 1, p. 47.
21. Fisher CM. *Memoirs of a Neurologist.* Rutland, VT: Sharp, 2006, Vol. 1, pp. 49–50.
22. Pasteur L. Address to the Fraternal Association of Former Students of the École Centrale des Arts et Manufactures, Paris, May 15, 1884.
23. Fisher CM. *Memoirs of a Neurologist.* Rutland, VT: Sharp, 2006, Vol. 1, p. 48.
24. Fisher CM. *Memoirs of a Neurologist.* Rutland, VT: Sharp, 2006, Vol. 1, p. 48.
25. Fisher CM. *Memoirs of a Neurologist.* Rutland, VT: Sharp, 2006, Vol. 1, pp. 48–49.

CHAPTER 7
Montreal, 1950–1954

When the Fishers first returned to Montreal in 1949, they lived in a third-floor apartment in a veterans housing complex. Elizabeth, the oldest of his 3 children, recalls that there were at least 16 young children in the neighborhood. Miller was later able to locate a home for his family in Montreal West at 135 Ballantine Avenue North (Figure 7.1). Montreal West was a small residential district approximately ½ mile wide and almost 1 mile long in which lived mostly English-speaking families. Doris had her hands full managing the house and the children as Elizabeth was 8, Peter was 4, and Hugh was 2 years old. Figure 7.2 shows photographs of family scenes taken during the time the family was in Montreal.

Fisher anticipated that Montreal would be his permanent home. Armed with the knowledge and experience gained from his Boston neuropathology fellowship, he was excited and passionate about getting on with his career. He had chosen cerebrovascular disease and stroke as his life's work. Almost all of his time was spent pursuing his goals and his work; once again, Doris was the captain of the home.

Arrangements were made for Fisher to set up a neuropathology laboratory at the Montreal General Hospital (MGH) that would be dedicated to the study of strokes. Dr. Francis McNaughton, the head of neurology at MGH, and Dr. Harold Elliot, the chief neurosurgeon at the hospital, facilitated the appointment and supported Fisher fully during his time in Montreal. The dean of McGill Medical School, Professor Lyman Duff, supported Fisher's scholarly activities and functions at the medical school. Dr. Bea Johnston, the superintendent at MGH, helped arrange funding and support of the neuropathology laboratory. Fisher was appointed Clinical Assistant

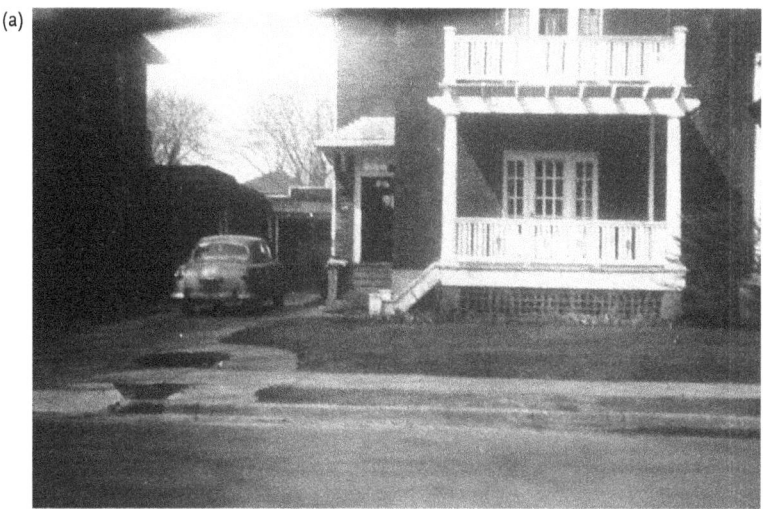

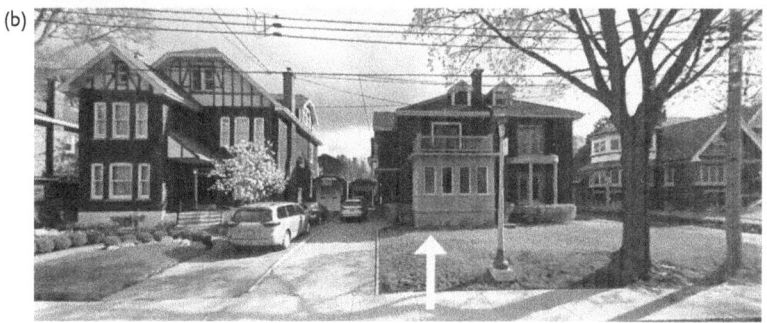

Figure 7.1 Fisher's home in Montreal. (A) Photograph taken at the time of residence. (B) Photograph of the area in 2018. The arrow points to the home.

Neurologist to MGH in 1950. He was promoted to Assistant Neurologist in 1951 and to Associate Neurologist in 1953. He attended conferences at the hospital but was not active in the outpatient clinics or wards. He also served as a consultant to Dr. Kenneth Evelyn's hypertension clinic held at the Royal Victoria Hospital.

Fisher also received an appointment at the Queen Mary Veterans' Hospital, where he agreed to attend 2 half days in the neurology outpatient clinic and 2 half days each week as a neurological consultant for inpatients. Soon after beginning his clinical work at Queen Mary, he requested and was granted permission to fulfill the 4 half-days requirement for work at the hospital contained in his original contract by working 1 day a week from 8 a.m. until midnight or later. He also saw patients at St. Anne's Hospital in Sainte-Anne-de-Bellevue near Montreal, approximately 25–30 miles away

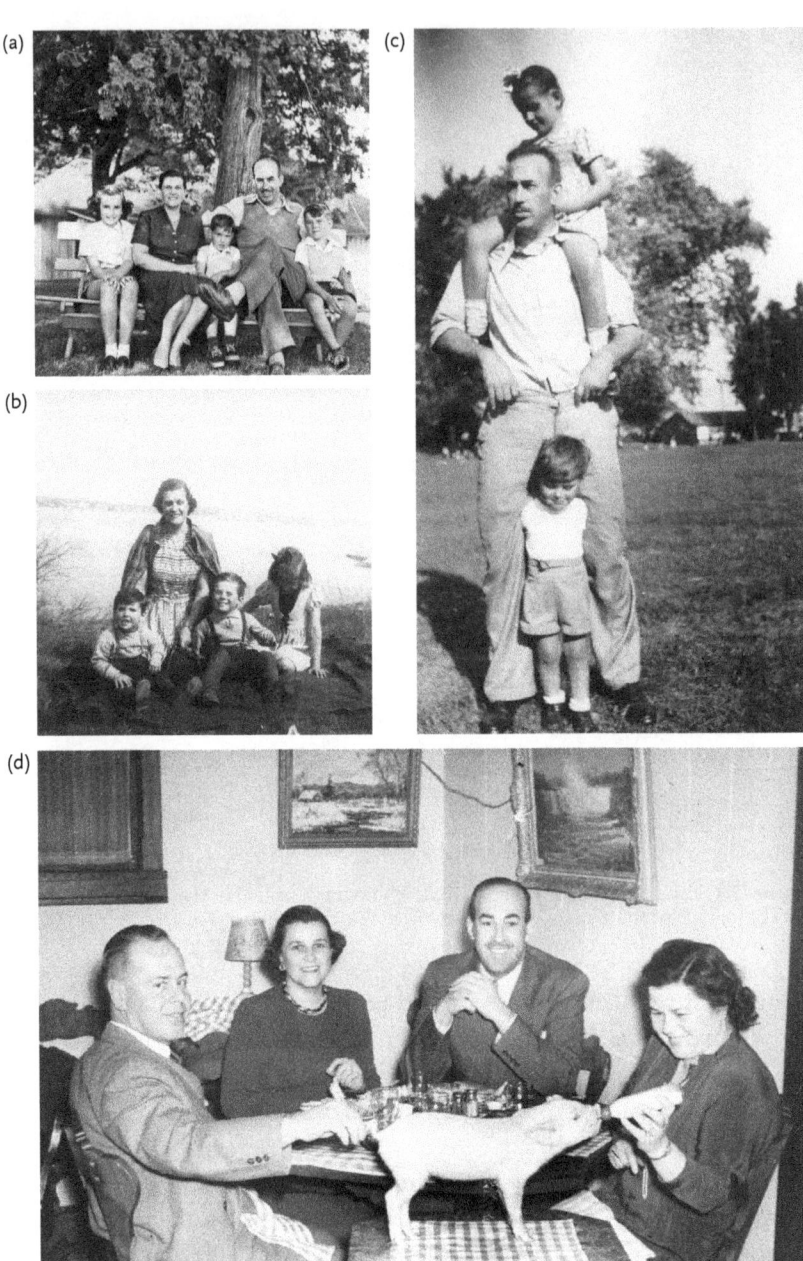

Figure 7.2 Family scenes in Montreal. (A) Fisher and Doris with Elizabeth, Peter, and Hugh. (B) Doris and the children at the seaside. (C) Fisher with Elizabeth and Hugh. (D) A dinner with friends.

from his home. This hospital primarily served veterans of the Canadian Armed Forces and specialized in long-term and geriatric care. Fisher shared responsibility for covering the consults at St. Anne's Hospital with Dr. Norman Peterson. He would visit St. Anne's several times a month. His income was mostly based on a salary from Queen Mary Veteran's Hospital and a stipend for performing pathology at MGH. He could also collect fees by billing consults at private hospitals in Montreal. His home in Montreal West was quite far from MGH, which was located in downtown Montreal. He had to either take a train to Windsor Station and then a bus to the hospital or drive the family car directly to and from the hospital or to Queen Mary Hospital.

During most weeks, Fisher spent 6 days and many nights a week at work in the neuropathology laboratory at MGH. He was effusive in his praise for MGH, especially the pathology and neuropathology labs and their personnel. Dr. William Osler, a Canadian like Fisher, had created the pathology department at MGH (1876–1884) and performed more than 800 autopsies while in Montreal. Dr. Joseph Pritchard was Chief of Pathology at MGH when Fisher worked there. Fisher commented that Pritchard "was most kind to me and provided every facility asked for."[1]

FISHER'S FIRST MAJOR CONTRIBUTIONS: CAROTID ARTERY DISEASE AND TRANSIENT ISCHEMIC ATTACKS

Serendipity and luck play a role in many, if not most, discoveries. So it was with Fisher. He was eager to get on with his work on stroke. He wrote in his memoirs, "Hardly had my family and I settled back in Montreal when in the clinic at Queen Mary Veterans' Hospital I examined an unfortunate veteran who had suffered a rather severe left hemiplegia two-and-a-half years before."[2] This disabled man who had preserved intellect but severe paralysis of his left limbs related a story to Fisher that would have a profound influence on his career and for the diagnosis and treatment of patients with stroke. As Pasteur had written, "Dans les champs de l'observation le hasard ne favorise que les esprits préparés," which translates to "In the fields of observation, chance favors only the prepared mind."[3]

The veteran told Fisher that during the weeks before the stroke, he had had several attacks of temporary blindness in one eye. While Fisher was writing his consultation note, the veteran remarked, "Isn't it funny, I went blind in the wrong eye. I am paralyzed on the left side and I went blind in the right eye."[4] One week later, another veteran told Fisher a similar story. He said that before he had his stroke, he was in his favorite tavern when he went blind in one eye. His friends who were with him reassured him that it would go away in a minute and that everybody had those things. They told him that he may be drinking the wrong booze. The eye symptoms recurred several times before the stroke. Again, the blindness was on the wrong side. The temporary blindness involved the eye on one side and the paralysis affected the limbs on the other side of the body.

These two patients' histories stimulated Fisher to review the anatomy of the blood vessels that supply the brain. The transient blindness could best be explained by a lack of blood flow to the eye because the eye is supplied by blood through the ophthalmic artery, a branch of the internal carotid artery. The ophthalmic artery is most often the very first branch of the artery originating just after the internal carotid artery enters the cranium. Figure 7.3 shows diagrams of the anatomy of the carotid artery. The internal carotid artery then gives off branches that supply the cerebral hemispheres on the same side. There are two cerebral hemispheres. Each contains nerve cells that control movement and feeling in the face and limbs on the opposite side of the body. So, in the first veteran described, the most likely explanation for his symptoms was an obstruction of blood flow in the right internal carotid artery. This could lead to a lack of blood flow to the right eye and ischemic damage to the right side of the brain causing paralysis of the left limbs. The blockage in the carotid artery was most likely a clot that could break off and land in its branches (the anterior and middle cerebral arteries) in the head. The presence and location of a carotid artery lesion as the cause of the strokes in the two patients were speculative and unproven. It was a hypothesis that floated in Fisher's mind and thoughts.

The stories told by the two veterans also raised the question in Fisher's mind of how often stroke patients have temporary minor episodes that precede the stroke and provide a warning that a stroke might develop. He began to assiduously question stroke patients as to whether they too had had any temporary neurological dysfunctions before their strokes occurred. He wrote,

Patients at the Queen Mary Veterans Hospital and St. Anne's Hospital who had had strokes were then asked about the occurrence of premonitory symptoms. Saturday and Sunday afternoons were good times to inquire as families were visiting the patients. It was amazing how often transient prodromal symptoms were reported.[5]

Fisher recognized that stroke patients often did not report all their symptoms accurately. Some forgot them; others, especially those with strokes that affected the language regions of the left side of the brain, had impaired cognitive and communication abilities so that they could not

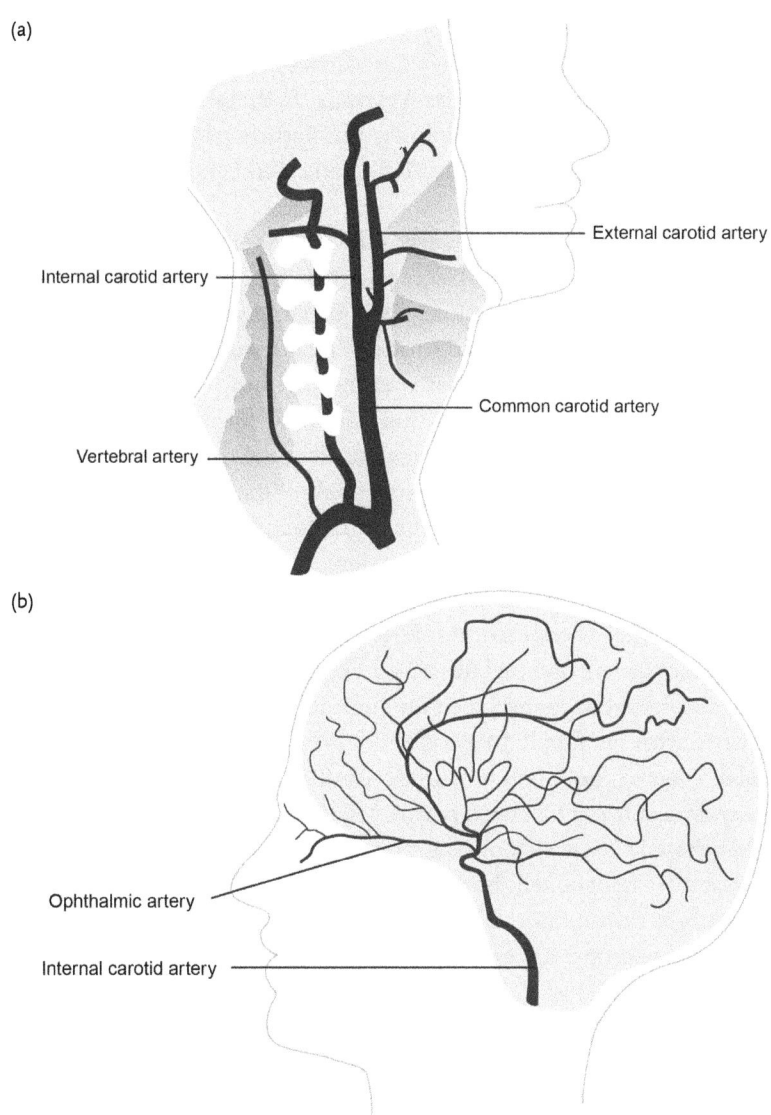

Figure 7.3 The anatomy of the carotid artery: (A) portion within the neck; (B) portion within the cranium.
Source: Modified with permission from Caplan LR. *Caplan's Stroke* (5th ed.). Cambridge, UK: Cambridge University Press, 2016.

relate symptoms accurately. Family members, on the other hand, often reported incidents that had not been described by the patients. His 1-day per week arrangement with St. Mary Veterans' Hospital quickly turned into 1 day plus considerable weekend time. This pattern of visiting the hospital on weekends and evenings to question family members was to continue for the remainder of his career.

During the next weeks after seeing the two veterans, Fisher exacted detailed histories from stroke patients and their spouses and visitors. Always a stickler for details, the questions abounded in his mind.

For patients who had warning attacks, Fisher would inquire: How often did warning attacks occur? What was their nature? How long before the stroke? How many attacks? How long did each warning attack last? and Were the symptoms the same in each attack or did they vary? For patients with blindness or visual loss, he would ask, What was the nature of the change in vision? He also read the medical literature to determine if others had observed and written about transient attacks that preceded strokes. In addition, he was curious about disease of the carotid artery. Were there previous writings about carotid artery disease?

The first patient who had described his transient visual loss and stroke developed colon cancer and died on June 16, 1950. Fisher was away from Montreal with his family that weekend. When he returned to the city on Sunday evening, he found a message notifying him that the patient had died and no autopsy had been performed. He later learned that the family had requested a postmortem examination but had been told that it was not necessary. He telephoned the widow, and she readily gave permission for a postmortem examination. He called the funeral director, who told Fisher that he was welcome to perform the examination. At 11 p.m. that Sunday night, after visiting hours, the funeral director and Fisher performed a limited autopsy that included examination of the right carotid artery in the neck. At that time, postmortem removal of the carotid arteries in the neck was usually forbidden by undertakers, who depended on these vessels for embalming the head. Despite this custom and dictum, this particular funeral director was fully cooperative and went out of his way to help Fisher obtain the information Fisher needed. Fisher told me that when he cut down on the artery and found that it was totally occluded, he felt a wave of emotion. The hypothesis of a young, inexperienced, clinically naive individual that the responsible lesion must be in that carotid artery in the neck had proven to be correct.

He then focused intently during his clinical encounters at the veterans hospitals, and in medical libraries, on transient loss of vision in one eye, on warnings before strokes, and on carotid artery disease. He collected clinical information from patients and pathological data from his autopsies performed at MGH. As would be true throughout his later career, once he had convinced himself that he had accumulated enough information to share his observations with others, he reported his findings at medical meetings and authored reports. In 1951, he presented a report titled "Transient Monocular Blindness Associated with Hemiplegia" at a meeting of the American Neurological Association in Atlantic City, New Jersey. Many senior neurologists and neurosurgeons who practiced in the United States and Canada were present at this meeting. Fisher's report was subsequently printed in the transactions of the meeting.[6] In the presentation, he described seven patients in whom paralysis on one side of the body was preceded by attacks of temporary loss of vision involving the opposite eye. In only one of these patients had Fisher confirmed by postmortem that the carotid artery on the side of the affected eye was occluded. In another patient, the carotid artery occlusion was visualized during angiography, and in the others the diagnosis of carotid artery disease in the neck was supported by Fisher being unable to feel a pulse in the carotid artery in the neck.

Fisher wrote a more detailed report that was published later in 1951 in the *American Medical Association Archives of Neurology and Psychiatry* titled "Occlusion of the Internal Carotid Artery."[7] This 31-page paper described eight patients in detail. One patient had been added since the original report. In four patients, the occlusion of the carotid artery was confirmed at autopsy, in two patients it was confirmed by angiography, and in the two other patients the diagnosis was based on the clinical findings only. In this report, Fisher included photographs and diagrams of the findings in the brain and the arteries, including a diagram that showed the location of a long blood clot that began at the origin of the right internal carotid artery and extended into the portion of the carotid artery within the cranium.

Fisher's postmortem studies of the carotid arteries caused some initial problems for him.[8] His technique of removing the common carotid artery bifurcation in the neck at autopsy made it impossible for morticians to perfuse the face through the external carotid artery, precluding an open casket for the families. Complaints from undertakers eventually reached the dean of McGill Medical School. A solution had to be found if Fisher was to continue his pathology studies on the carotid artery. With the resourcefulness of an ex prisoner-of-war camp survivor, he inserted one end of a red rubber catheter in the stump of the common carotid artery and another catheter into the external carotid artery. This allowed the undertaker to use the external carotid artery to perfuse the face with fixative even when the carotid bifurcation was removed.[8]

At the time when Fisher was investigating carotid artery disease in Montreal, angiography had only recently been introduced into patient care. During the 1940s and 1950s, angiography was considered a rather dangerous surgical procedure and was seldom performed in the United States. Dr. Egaz Moniz, a neurologist who later received the Nobel Prize in Medicine for his work on frontal lobotomies, published his angiography results during the 1930s.[9] He was the first person to successfully visualize the brain using radiopaque substances. The procedure was performed at that time by a surgeon making an incision in the neck and inserting a catheter into the common carotid artery and injecting dye. Some of the first dye substances used proved very harmful to the brain. During the following years, Moniz and co-workers pursued their investigations in Lisbon, and a growing number of examinations were performed. They had not expected that many of the patients injected would later die of radiation poisoning.

The aim of angiography was to identify intracranial tumors by interpreting the distortions of the normal images of the brain's blood vessels. Moniz and co-workers soon learned not only that cerebral angiography was a way to identify space-occupying lesions but also that the vessels deserved attention because findings such as aneurysms and vascular malformations were discovered.

Other previously unknown conditions, such as internal carotid artery occlusions, were also found. Remarkably, those conditions had not been described in the past, despite the long history of anatomical dissections. Moniz's first case of internal carotid artery occlusion was identified in October 1931.[10] A 52-year-old man had had headaches, seizures, speech disturbances, and a few transient episodes of right arm and leg weakness leading to hemiplegia (paralysis of the limbs on one side of the body) for a few days. A brain tumor was suspected, and angiography was performed. During the procedure, Moniz was surprised that only branches of the left external carotid artery were identified and no left internal carotid artery was shown. He also noted that when the right carotid artery was injected, the contrast material crossed to the left hemisphere through the anterior communicating artery, indicting a low-flow state in the left cerebral hemisphere.

It was not until September 1934 that Moniz's angiography showed a second instance of carotid artery occlusion. A 46-year-old man who had known syphilis had a history of sudden loss of vision in his right eye followed, a few months later, by episodes of left side arm and leg weakness. The angiography showed a right internal carotid artery occlusion. Moniz was the first to describe and report carotid artery occlusion during life, but he considered the condition very rare.[11]

In the second paragraph of his 1951 report on occlusion of the internal carotid artery,[7] Fisher commented on the accepted dictum at that time that most brain infarcts were caused by disease of the arteries within the head, especially the middle cerebral artery. He noted that in his prior experience in Boston working with Raymond Adams, among 200 autopsies performed in patients with cerebrovascular disease, not a single instance of disease of the middle cerebral artery was found. The common clinical impression in these patients before death was occlusion of the middle cerebral artery. He then reviewed the past literature concerning carotid artery disease, emphasizing that this diagnosis had seldom been considered or confirmed in the past and likely accounted for many cases of stroke that had been attributed to disease of the middle cerebral artery, the main branch of the internal carotid artery in the head. During autopsies, the arteries in the neck had been rarely examined in detail. He cited 16 reports mostly published in the 1940s that included 69 patients who had carotid artery disease. Of these reports, 6 were in German and 2 were in French. He had learned German during his prisoner-of-war experience.[12]

During his exhaustive search of the literature, Fisher uncovered an original report by Dr. Hans Chiari, a physician born in Vienna, Austria, who was Professor of Pathology at the German University in Prague at the time of his publication on carotid artery disease in 1905.[13] Chiari's attention to the carotid artery was stimulated by one case. In this patient, Chiari found at postmortem a brain infarct, and he searched for a cause in the usual places—the heart and aorta—but found nothing wrong in those organs. He then examined the neck arteries and was surprised to find severe arteriosclerosis of the carotid artery on the side of the brain infarct. A long thrombus that blocked the common carotid artery that extended into the internal carotid artery was found. A piece of that clot had broken off and went into the middle cerebral artery, causing the brain infarct. Chiari commented that he had dissected in great detail the aortic system in approximately 400 subjects with special regard to the carotid arteries and their branches. He found only seven examples of severe partial or complete occlusion of the carotid arteries in the neck, sometimes on both sides. The aim of his report was to call attention to examination of the arteries in the neck at postmortem. He opined that atherosclerotic disease of the internal carotid artery at its origin from the common carotid artery was common and only surpassed by atherosclerosis of the thoracic and abdominal aorta. Fisher also cited one other report, again in German and published in 1942, of an example of an occluded internal carotid artery in the neck giving rise to an embolus that caused a stroke.[14] Prior to Fisher's detailed report, the literature describing carotid artery pathology was very scanty; the great majority of reported cases were recognized by angiography or only suspected clinically.

In his detailed 1951 report, as would be his practice throughout his career, Fisher described the history and findings in simple English and often quoted the words used by the patients or others.[7] A typical example was in the description of a 68-year-old man who, during the 2 months before a stroke, had had five or six episodes of transient blindness in the right eye, each lasting approximately 3 minutes: "It was if a blind had been pulled down." During the same time period, the patient often remarked to his wife, "I don't seem to have much feeling in my left hand." Another patient who had had many attacks of numbness and weakness of the right hand remarked to his wife, "I just had a scare—I couldn't talk." One attack of inability to speak occurred while he was with visitors. He excused himself with a gesture and went to tend the furnaces. When he returned from that task, he could speak normally.[7]

Fisher focused his initial report about carotid artery disease on the typical clinical findings. He hoped to attract interest among pathologists and clinicians in recognizing disease of the carotid artery in the neck. He emphasized the key diagnostic findings that pointed to carotid artery occlusion: temporary episodes of loss of vision in one eye; headaches unusual for the patient and often localized above the symptomatic eye; brief, often multiple, varied attacks of loss of brain function involving the limbs on the side of the body opposite the eye with the visual loss and sometimes affecting cognitive functions such as speech that are localized to the cerebral hemisphere on the same side as the visual loss; and culminating in the development of paralysis of the limbs on the side of the body opposite to the visual loss. The transient episodes preceded the paralysis and usually ceased once the paralysis occurred.

At the time of Fisher's report, there had been very few brief comments in the literature about transient attacks that occurred before strokes. Sir Thomas Willis, a physician practicing in Elizabethan England, is often given credit for calling attention to warning spells, but his 1679 description is anything but precise: "The irradiation of the spirits is wont to be interrupted with little clouds, as it were, scattered here and there but in the former, the same is forthwith wholly darkened and undergoes total eclipse."[15] Sir William Gowers wrote in his widely read textbook of neurology published in 1888, "The symptoms produced by the occlusion of an artery . . . being of two classes, one transient, the result of the sudden interruption with the functions of the brain, the other more or less permanent."[16] Sir William Osler, a fellow Canadian whose pathology laboratory at MGH Fisher now occupied, in his classic medical text first published in 1892 included one sentence under the heading arterio-sclerosis": "Transient hemiplegia, monoplegia, or aphasia may occur in advanced Arterio-sclerosis."[17] In an article in 1911, Osler called attention to attacks of weakness, loss of speech, and sensory disturbances that improve or completely abate in patients with high blood pressure and arteriosclerosis.[18] Osler speculated on the cause—perhaps a vascular spasm—and did not note any relation to further strokes or to any specific arterial lesions. Fisher, in his 1951 paper on internal carotid artery disease, was the first to emphasize the importance of these warning attacks: "Prodromal fleeting attacks of paralysis, numbness, tingling, speechlessness, unilateral blindness, or dizziness" often preceded and warned of impending strokes in patients with carotid artery disease.[7] Transient ischemic attack was not adopted as the term for these attacks until 1965, 14 years after Fisher's classic report.[19]

Before Fisher finished his report, he had lunch with a Montreal colleague, Dr. R. R. Fitzgerald, who had just returned from a national surgical meeting in New Orleans. Fisher was told about the remarkable surgical procedures that were being performed on arteries. Fitzgerald and Fisher posited that "the carotid plaque because of its strictly focal extent should be amenable to a surgical bypass procedure."[20] Fisher concluded his 1951 report with comments on treatment. He noted, "On that subject there is little definitive to state," but he speculated, "It is even conceivable that some day vascular surgery will find a way to bypass the occluded portion of the artery during the period of ominous fleeting symptoms."[7] He also noted that "prolonged use of anticoagulants (heparin and dicoumarol) is at present being tried when the patient is seen at the stage of intermittent symptoms."[7] Even when presenting very detailed analyses on pathology and mechanism, he always kept his mind on treating the individual patient, hoping that the information in his reports would lead to therapeutic advances.

In 1952, Fisher presented his research on carotid artery disease at a meeting of physicians and surgeons in his native Canada.[21] This communication was awarded the 1952 prize in Medicine of the Royal College of Physicians and Surgeons in Canada. During the same year, he published a 36-page report in the *Archives of Ophthalmology*.[22] His intent was to make eye doctors aware of the significance of transient loss of vision in one eye. This communication began with a short rationale for the report:

> *I have encountered several cases of transient monocular blindness associated with contralateral hemiplegia, the attacks of blindness usually preceding the stroke as a sort of warning that disaster threatened. A prominent finding on examination has been occlusion of the internal carotid artery on the side of the affected eye. Attention has not previously been drawn to this clinical syndrome.*[22]

He then described the 150 prior literature reports of transient visual symptoms localizable to one eye; many of these reports were written in French and German. Fishers review consumed a full 18 pages of text. In this report, he included more detail about the visual loss:

> *The blindness most commonly comes on as though a blind were being lowered or raised and vision returns from the opposite direction. In one case the blindness was described as a "fog rolling in."* . . . *The attacks last from a minute or so up to seven minutes or more. They may occur with almost any frequency from once a month to once or twice a day. The onset as well as the recovery may be sudden or gradual. Usually blindness is total at the height of the attack.*[22]

In the remainder of the report, Fisher speculated about the mechanism of the visual loss. During the next 2 years, he continued to work exhaustively on the pathology and clinical findings in patients with carotid artery disease, and in 1954 he published another report titled "Occlusion of the Carotid Arteries: Further Experiences."[23]

By the time of the second report, Fisher had performed 432 autopsies in which he had examined the brains and the arteries within the neck and head. He discovered among these cases that 28 patients had complete occlusion of one or both internal carotid arteries, and another 13 had very severe narrowing of these arteries. Many other patients had plaques within the carotid arteries in the neck that did not lead to severe narrowing. This second long report focused on the pathology that he found in the arteries.

The pathology began with plaque formations that consisted of atherosclerotic deposits within the arterial wall at the origin of the internal carotid artery from the common carotid artery. The plaques could enlarge until they virtually occluded the artery or a thrombus might be deposited upon the plaque and result in occlusion of the artery. Sometimes hemorrhages developed within the plaques, causing swelling of the vessel wall and further narrowing of the artery. Plaques tended to ulcerate and form a superimposed thrombus attached to the region of ulceration. A clot could extend toward the brain. The blood clot often became organized and changed into a solid yellow cord. Fisher often found thrombi beyond the occluded artery within the neck and also within the branches of the artery within the head. The internal carotid artery within the pharynx before entering the skull almost never showed atherosclerosis. In four patients, the disease began in the carotid artery within the head. When the intracranial artery became blocked, there was no blood flow beyond the block so that thrombus developed in the blood that stagnated within the artery in the neck. The clot often extended downward to near the internal carotid origin.

Fisher emphasized that many of the patients who had severe carotid artery disease did not show the typical clinical symptoms and findings that he had described in his earlier report on carotid artery disease. Seven patients whose carotid artery was occluded on one side had no symptoms. Some with unilateral and bilateral carotid artery occlusions had dementia. Fisher wrote,

> *The clinical picture in the present series of cases differs from that described in the literature. . . . The present group of patients was much older, the cases being scattered evenly between 60 to 85; the onset in most cases took place during a relatively short period (a day or so), and prodromal warnings in the form of transient attacks were few.*[23]

One-fourth of the patients died during the acute phase of a stroke. Fisher concluded his report by commenting on treatment:

> *From a therapeutic point of view no concrete suggestions can be made at this time but it is anticipated that knowledge of the pathological basis and delineation of the clinical picture, which must always precede logical and orderly advance in therapy will lead to helpful measures in these cases.*[23]

Several months after Fisher's 1951 report on carotid artery disease was published, he visited the National Neurological Hospital located in Queen Square in London. During clinical rounds, Sir Charles Symonds, a well-known senior neurologist, asked Fisher, "Are you the one that wrote the paper on blocked carotid artery and transient blindness?"[24] This conversation astounded Fisher. He had no idea that scientific publications had such widespread audiences and quickly affected clinical practice. Soon after the carotid artery report was published, a neurologist in Mendoza, Argentina, was consulted about a patient who became blind in the left eye and had right limb paralysis. He referred the patient to Dr. Raul Carrea, a neurosurgeon who had been in New York and had read Fisher's report on carotid artery disease. Carrea, with Dr. Mahels Molins, performed the first known surgery on the carotid artery in 1951.[25] The surgeons first made a cut approximately 5 mm beyond the diseased portion of the internal carotid artery. They then made a cut in the external carotid artery, which was located near the side of the internal carotid artery at approximately the same level and attached the cut end of the external carotid artery to the internal carotid artery above the region of blockage. The surgery created a bypass that Fisher had mentioned in his report. Blood flowed from the common carotid artery through the external carotid artery into the internal carotid artery above the diseased segment—a detour. The patient was followed for

27 years. He remained blind in the left eye, but his strength improved on the right side. Carrea and colleagues published the report of this case in 1955.[26]

Soon after Fisher's 1954 report, Dr. George White Pickering, a professor of medicine at St. Mary's Hospital in London, examined a 66-year-old woman who had intermittent attacks of right limb paralysis and visual loss in the left eye. He referred the patient to Dr. Charles Robb, the chief of surgery at the hospital. Dr. Felix Eastcott, the assistant director in the surgery department, under Robb's supervision then performed a surgical procedure—a bypass similar to that performed by Carrea in Argentina. Robb was from Montreal and clearly knew of Fisher's reports. Eastman, Pickering, and Robb reported their surgery in a widely read British journal, *Lancet*, in 1954.[27]

Vascular surgeons soon began to perform a different surgical procedure, endarterectomy, on large blood vessels. This involved operating directly on the diseased portion of the artery—clearing away the region of blockage and by doing so restoring good blood flow. This was direct surgery on severely narrowed arteries rather than a bypass as had been performed by Carrea and by Eastcott and Robb.[28]

OTHER PROJECTS
Lacunes

While performing autopsies on elderly patients in Montreal, Fisher became struck by differences in the brains of demented individuals compared to those of nondemented patients of roughly the same age. The brains of many of the individuals who had been hypertensive in life harbored small cavities that had been called lacunes in the French literature. As was his custom, Fisher spent much time exploring this topic in the libraries at McGill and the various hospitals in Montreal and reviewed the French reports.

Durand-Fardel first introduced the term *lacunes* in 1843 to describe small holes, usually found in the deep gray matter within the cerebral hemispheres, which contain a fine meshwork of tissues and vessels.[29] The clinical findings in patients with these lacunes were first described by Dr. Ferrand, working in Paris in the laboratory of Dr. Pierre Marie, Professor of Neurology, and by Marie himself. These French authors noted the usual locations of these lacunes within the cerebral hemispheres and the brainstem. Paralysis of the limbs on one side of the body, hemiplegia, was the major finding in patients who had developed recent lacunes. The clinical condition of multiple lacunes was termed "état lacunaire" (*lacunar state*) by Marie, and it was characterized by slurred speech, difficulty swallowing, and an abnormal small-stepped gait.[30]

The French authors recognized that these lacunar cavities were infarctions caused by insufficient supply of blood, but they had not characterized the cause within the blood vessels that supplied these damaged brain regions. Fisher, fascinated by this problem, during his years in Montreal and later in Boston, strove to perfect a way to study these lesions. He devised a novel way to cut the brain so as to show these small cavities but at the same time to leave undisturbed the major large arteries and their branches that supplied these lesions. The next issue was how to view under the microscope the vessels feeding the lacunes. The prevailing technique at that time was to embed cut brain sections into celloidin. These sections took time to stain. Often, the celloidin sections would not be available until 3 months after Fisher had viewed a fresh brain. He decided to experiment with paraffin embedding. After many trials using different methods of serial sectioning and staining, he concluded that to study lacunar infarcts adequately, it would be necessary to prepare continuous, uninterrupted serial sections of large blocks of brain tissue.[31] All sections would have to be stained with one stain so as to not lose the order of the slides created. To study the vascular supply of each lacune, several thousand sections had to be stained and reviewed. This project was begun in earnest in Montreal and was continued when Fisher set up his laboratory in Boston in 1954.

Brain Embolism

Fisher had begun work on the topic of the neuropathology of brain embolism while in Boston with Raymond Adams before moving to Montreal. Their early observations were described in Chapter 6. Fisher had been struck by how many brain infarcts were caused by embolism, how often the artery causing the damage did not contain a clot that could fully explain the damage, and how often there was bleeding as well as infarction (death of tissue due to inadequate supply of blood). Infarcts were commonly characterized as bland in appearance when the dead tissue was soft and white or yellow, while bleeding was quite obvious when the brain was sectioned.

When Fisher came to Montreal, he experimented with the best way to cut the whole brain so as to show the regions of damage and, at the same time, show the arteries that supplied the area of damage and the veins that drained blood from the region. While studying lacunes, he could also study brain infarcts larger than lacunes.[32]

He began to search for examples of brain embolism and especially cases in which there was hemorrhage among the 300–400 brains that he cut each year. The report on these findings was initially prepared in 1950 and was presented at the Annual Meeting of the American Association of Neuropathologists on June 11, 1950. An abstract of the presentation was published in the *Journal of Neuropathology and Experimental Neurology* in 1951.[33] The full paper was not published. Thirty-six years later, Fisher and Adams were invited to have the edited original paper included in a book on the heart and stroke.[34] In that book, Fisher also included a long chapter that reviewed the history of brain embolism.[35] In 1969, Fisher told me that he suspected that the journal editors had not behaved honorably and had refused to publish the originally submitted paper, holding on to it so that they could perform studies on the topic prior to publication of the Fisher and Adams paper. Fisher and Adams decided not to resubmit the original paper. They changed their mind when Dr. Anthony Furlan ardently requested that it be included as the first, longest, most authoritative report in his collections that comprised the book. In his memoirs, Fisher included further illustrative cases.[36]

The abstract of the original report to the American Association of Neuropathologists states clearly and elegantly the stimulus for the study:

> *The embolic process, i.e., the morbid changes which develop in an organ whose blood supply has been impoverished by the embolic occlusion of nutrient arteries, constitutes an important chapter in neuropathology and one to which little thought appears to have been given in recent years. The belief is widely held that this subject was fully elucidated by the pioneers of pathology and that further investigation of it would yield little additional information. Our recent Neuropathological experience has convinced us that such a view is by no means justified. . . . The paradoxical phenomenon of an occluded artery causing not only ischemic necrosis, but also vascular engorgement and hemorrhage in the region of its distribution, has been a controversial topic for at least a century, and many aspects of it are still disputed. Based on the casual observation that often in cases of hemorrhagic infarction of the brain at autopsy no arterial obstruction could be found at the appropriate site although the clinical setting suggested embolism (e.g., atrial fibrillation), we undertook a systematic assessment of our neuropathological material to investigate the relation of hemorrhagic infarction to embolism and the mechanism of hemorrhagic infarction.*[33]

The diagrams included in their study and in Fisher's memoirs explain the main findings. In Figure 7.4, the carotid artery branches that

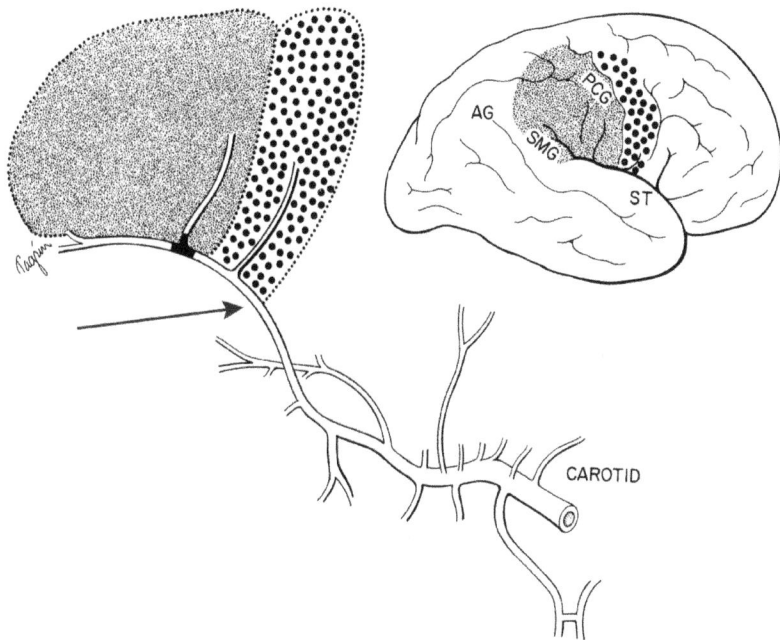

Figure 7.4 (Right) A lateral view of the right side of the brain. The stippled dotted area represents hemorrhagic transformation, and the more solid gray area represents bland nonhemorrhagic infarction at necropsy. (Left) An embolus found within a branch of the middle cerebral artery. The region beyond the embolus shows a bland infarct, while the area reperfused is hemorrhagic. AG, angular gyrus; PCG, postcentral gyrus; SMG, supramarginal gyrus; ST, superior temporal gyrus.
Source: Drawn by Edith Tagrin, medical illustrator. Reproduced with permission from Fisher CM, Adams RD. Observations on brain embolism with special reference to hemorrhagic infarction. In AJ Furlan (Ed.), *The Heart and Stroke*. London: Springer, 1987, p. 24, Figure 2.1b.

supplied a portion of the brain that became infarcted are drawn at the bottom. The location of a clot found postmortem is shown in black, the brain region containing hemorrhage is indicated by black dots, and the region of bland infarction is shown in gray. The clot must have originally stopped at a point shown by the arrow in the figure in order to deprive the supplied brain tissue of blood. When that happened, the brain cells (neurons) were injured, but also damaged were the blood vessels within the region. The clot moved on to where it was located postmortem. When the clot moved, blood flow returned to the brain region shown by black dots in the figure. The injured blood vessels were leaky and so hemorrhage developed.

Figure 7.5 is an artist's drawing of the bottom of the brain. An embolus has entered the vertebral artery—the artery at the bottom with black

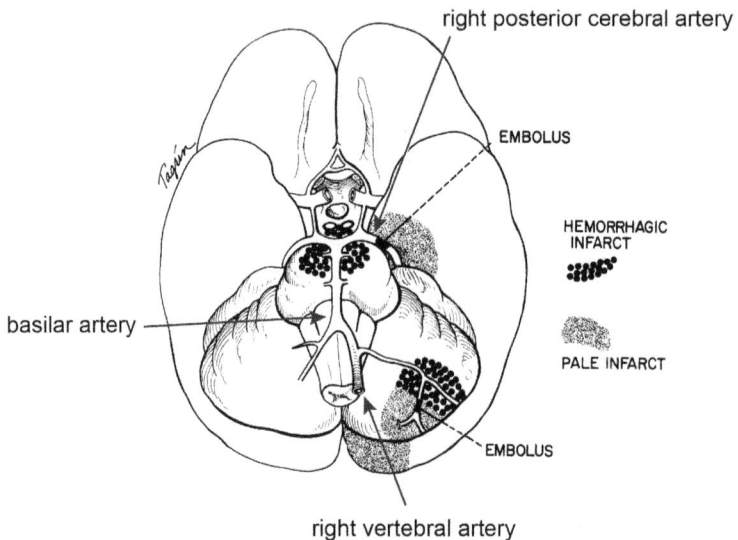

Figure 7.5 Diagram of the base of the brain showing the location of bland and hemorrhagic infarction and the clots found at necropsy. The arteries and types of infarcts are shown.
Source: Drawn by Edith Tagrin, medical illustrator. Reproduced with permission from Fisher CM, Adams RD. Observations on brain embolism with special reference to hemorrhagic infarction. In AJ Furlan (Ed.), *The Heart and Stroke*. London: Springer, 1987, p. 26, Figure 2.3 a.

circling showing where the embolus first stopped. The embolus then traveled up the vertebral artery into the basilar artery and then into the posterior cerebral artery, where it was found at autopsy. The black regions within the arteries (marked "embolus") show the location of clots found at the autopsy examination. The black dots located within brain tissue represent areas of bleeding. These are regions in which previously blocked blood flow was restored. Gray bland infarcts are located in regions in which the blood supply remained blocked.

The study by Fisher and Adams advanced information for clinicians concerning brain infarction: (1) Most brain infarcts were caused by emboli, not by localized atherosclerosis within the arteries within the cranium; (2) emboli by nature tended to move along the recipient brain-supplying arteries; and (3) bleeding into regions of brain infarction was common. The mechanism was restoration of blood flow into tissue in which the blood vessels had been injured during the time of poor perfusion. This information would prove of great practical importance when brain and vascular imaging became available in the 1970s and 1980s because areas of bleeding could be shown during life, identifying the process as embolism, and the location of emboli could be shown by vascular imaging.

Atrial Fibrillation and the Fisher Variant of Guillain–Barré Syndrome

Another observation made in Montreal formed the basis of Fisher's later research. He noted that many of the patients whose brains at autopsy showed infarcts clearly due to embolism had atrial fibrillation during life. Although he could not find thrombi that were the source of the emboli in the left atrium of the heart, he made serial sections of the left atrial appendage and found clots not evident to the naked eye within the interstices of the appendage. Atrial fibrillation as a cause of brain embolism was a topic he decided to pursue.

Fisher was a collector. He collected cases, ideas, clinical signs, information on syndromes, and pathological findings. He kept many of these collections in Manila folders, awaiting more information or clarification of the findings. An example of this behavior is that, while in Montreal, he encountered several patients who had a triad of abnormalities: They had lost their reflexes, could not move their eyes normally, and were very uncoordinated in walking and using their limbs (ataxia). After collecting more patients with these findings, he reported his findings in the *New England Journal of Medicine*. This syndrome has since been referred to as Miller Fisher syndrome.[37]

Locations of Atherosclerotic Plaques and Narrowings in the Arteries to the Head

Another major project was to attempt to define the usual locations and severities of plaques and atherosclerotic disease and narrowings found in the arteries in the neck and head that supplied the brain. While in Montreal, Fisher collected 1,100 pairs of carotid arteries at autopsies. The removal often extended to the aorta, and all of the atrial branches were dissected and preserved in formalin. The arteries within the cranium were also analyzed and preserved. Years later, I asked Fisher how he had been able to collect these specimens. He laughingly said that he gave the pathology assistants ("dieners") who worked in the pathology laboratory $5 for each specimen. Two dedicated dieners, under Fisher's guidance, broke tradition and removed the carotid arteries at autopsy, often retrieving them intact from the aorta to the place where they divided into branches within the head. Inspired by Fisher, these two dieners returned to high school and then went on to medical school. One became a university professor of surgery and president of the Royal College of Surgeons, and the other became a general practitioner.

In 1954, a group of international researchers visited Montreal to witness progress that was occurring there. A neurosurgeon who worked with Fisher brought the visiting researchers to the autopsy area to view Fisher's specimens of the blood vessels. Fisher laid his specimens out on the tables in the pathology laboratory. His exhibit was the last stop on the research tour. The researchers told him that "this was the best thing they had seen in Canada."[38] He was justifiably very proud and was determined to complete his work on disease of these brain-supplying arteries. Soon thereafter, he had a conversation with Dr. Edward Mills, the chief of the Medical Department at MGH. Mills was one of the highest ranking and most influential physician at McGill University at that time. He was a practical physician who had little or no interest in research. He told Fisher, "Why are you studying these stroke patients. They are already paralyzed. All that carotid work is a bunch of crap."[39] Fisher wryly commented in his memoirs that "to hear the unpleasant viewpoint of a figure important to my future was very unsettling."[40]

THE CALL FROM BOSTON AND LEAVING MONTREAL

Approximately 1 month after the harsh remarks of Mills that portended a difficult future for Fisher in Montreal, Raymond Adams invited Fisher to come to Boston to join the neurology service at Massachusetts General Hospital. The invitation was proffered while Adams and Fisher were walking on the boardwalk in Atlantic City, New Jersey, where they were attending a meeting. It only took four or five steps for Fisher to accept the invitation.

In 1952, Penfield had announced his intent to step down as the director of the Montreal Neurological Institute. He posited that his neurosurgical era was coming to an end and, in the future, knowledge of the functions of the nervous system would be in the hands of neurology. Penfield recommended that the directorship be transferred to a neurologist, and his choice for the leading candidate was Adams. Adams weighed the offer to come to Montreal and finally declined. Soon thereafter, Adams was appointed the Bullard Professor of Neuropathology and Chief of Neurology at Massachusetts General Hospital (MGH), positions recently relinquished by Dr. Stanley Cobb. Adams was very familiar with Fisher and his work, and he wanted Fisher to move to Boston to continue his research on cerebrovascular disease and stroke both in the neuropathology laboratory and in the wards and clinics of MGH.

Fisher commented in his memoirs that "in less than one minute, I had reached the decision to accept."[41] By then, he was determined to pursue a career centered on stroke, and he knew that he could not accomplish his goals in Montreal. He had great respect for Adams, and the opportunity to help create a new department and a stroke service was a great attraction for him.

While in Montreal, Fisher had become a productive researcher. His work on carotid artery disease and temporary episodes of eye and brain ischemia had gained him widespread recognition. Neurology leaders at the Montreal Neurological Institute (MNI) and the Royal Victoria Hospital—Preston Robb and Frances McNaughton—had developed high regard for Fisher and his contributions. They and Penfield urged Fisher to remain in Montreal.[42] Fisher recognized that epilepsy and brain tumor research and care dominated at the MNI and he had no support for stroke care and research at Montreal General Hospital. At the time Penfield was urging Fisher to stay in Montreal and at the MNI, talk of Penfield's impending retirement was rampant.[42] The situation in Montreal would be unpredictable if and when Penfield retired and a successor was chosen. The uncertainty about the future, the prior lack of interest in stroke in Montreal, and his familiarity with Boston, Adams, and Boston City Hospital (BCH) all contributed to Fisher's decision to accept the Harvard–MGH appointment. He knew Adams well and correctly decided that the future for his stroke work was far brighter in Boston than in Montreal.

NOTES

1. Fisher CM. *Memoirs of a Neurologist*. Rutland, VT: Sharp, 2006, Vol. 1, p. 51.
2. Fisher CM. *Memoirs of a Neurologist*. Rutland, VT: Sharp, 2006, Vol. 1, p. 53.
3. Louis Pasteur, Lecture, University of Lille, December 7, 1854.
4. Fisher CM. *Memoirs of a Neurologist*. Rutland, VT: Sharp, 2006, Vol. 1, p. 53.
5. Fisher CM. *Memoirs of a Neurologist*. Rutland, VT: Sharp, 2006, Vol. 1, p. 54.
6. Fisher CM. Transient monocular blindness associated with hemiplegia. *Transactions of the American Neurological Association* 1951;76:154–158.
7. Fisher CM. Occlusion of the internal carotid artery. *American Medical Association Archives of Neurology and Psychiatry* 1951;65:346–377.
8. The story of the complaints of the undertakers about Fisher's study of the carotid artery at necropsy is contained in Feindel W, Leblanc R. *The Wounded Brain Healed: The Golden Age of the Montreal Neurological Institute, 1934–1984*. Montreal, Ontario, Canada: McGill–Queen's University Press, 2016.
9. On July 7, 1927, Moniz described cerebral angiography to the medical community at a session of the Societé Neurologique in Paris. His publications on this topic include the following: Moniz E. L'encephalographie arterielle, son importance dans la localisation des tumeurs cerebrales. *Revue Neurologique (Paris)* 1927;2:72–89; and Moniz E. *L'angiographie cérébrale, ses applications et*

résultats en anatomic, physiologie et clinique [Cerebral Angiography, Its Applications and Results in Anatomy, Physiology, and Clinic]. Paris, 1934.

The contrast agent, thorium dioxide, a radioactive radiopaque substance, had a half-life of 400 years. It was never excreted and remained lodged in the liver, spleen, and bone marrow. Some of the patients he had injected later died of radiation toxicity.

10. These cases of carotid occlusion were called to my attention by Dr. Victor Oliveira of Lisbon, Portugal, and later described in a review of Moniz's carotid artery studies: Oliveira V. History of carotid occlusions: The contribution of Egas Moniz. *Journal of Stroke and Cerebrovascular Diseases* 2018;27:362–369.
11. Moniz E, Lima A, Lacerda R. Trombose da carótida interna. *Imprensa Médica* 1936;6:93–98; Moniz E, Lima A, Lacerda R. Hemiplégies par thrombose de la carotide interne. *Presse Médicale* 1937;52; Moniz E, Lima A, de Lacerda R. Par thrombose de la carotid interne. *Presse Médical* 1937:45:977. Moniz's original angiograms are still displayed in a museum within Santa Maria Hospital in Lisbon, Spain.
12. Following World War II, because of the antipathy of the British and French for Germany after two world wars, few of the German-language books and reports were translated into English or French and so were not readily available in England, Canada, or the United States.
13. Chiari Hans. Über das Verhalten des Teilungswinkels der Carotis communis bei der Endarteritis chronica deformans. *Verhandlungen Deutschen Pathologischen Gesellschaft* 1905(9);9:326–332.
14. Hultquist GT. *Über Thrombose und Embolie der Arteria carotis communis und hierbei vorkommende Gehirnstörungen*. Jena, Germany: Gustav Fischer, 1942.
15. Willis T. Instructions and prescripts for curing the apoplexy. In Portage S (Ed.), *The London Practice of Physic*. 1679.
16. Gowers WR. *A Manual of Diseases of the Nervous System*. Philadelphia: Blakiston, 1888, p. 817.
17. Osler W: *The Principles and Practice of Medicine*. New York: Appleton, 1903, p. 775.
18. Osler W: Transient attacks of aphasia and paralysis in states of high blood pressure and arteriosclerosis. *Canadian Medical Association Journal* 1911;1:919–926.
19. Caplan LR. Transient ischemic attack: Definition and natural history. *Current Atherosclerosis Reports* 2006;8:276–280.
20. Fisher CM. *Memoirs of a Neurologist*. Rutland, VT: Sharp, 2006, Vol. 1, p. 55.
21. Fisher CM. Disease of carotid arteries: A clinico-pathological correlation. Report of the Annual Meeting and Proceedings of the Royal College of Physicians and Surgeons of Canada, October 3–4, 1952, pp. 60–67.
22. Fisher CM. Transient monocular blindness associated with hemiplegia. *American Medical Association Archives of Ophthalmology* 1952;47:167–203.
23. Fisher CM. Occlusion of the carotid arteries: Further experiences. *American Medical Association Archives of Neurology and Psychiatry* 1954;72:187–204.
24. Personal communication to me from Dr. Fisher.
25. Estol CJ. Dr. C. Miller Fisher and the history of carotid artery disease. *Stroke* 1996;27:559–566.
26. Carrea R, Molins M, Murphy G. Surgical treatment of spontaneous thrombosis of the internal carotid artery in the neck: Carotid carotideal anastomosis. *Acta Neurolica Latinoamericana* 1955;1:71–78.

27. Eastcott HH, Pickering GW, Robb CG. Reconstruction of internal carotid artery in a patient with intermittent attacks of hemiplegia. *Lancet* 1954;2:994–996.
28. The first carotid endarterectomies were performed in Texas by Drs. Michael DeBakey and Denton Cooley during the 1950s (DeBakey ME. Successful carotid endarterectomy for cerebrovascular insufficiency: Nineteen-year follow-up. *Journal of the American Medical Association* 1975;233:1083–1085; Cooley DA, Al-Naaman YD, Carton CA. Surgical treatment of arteriosclerotic occlusion of common carotid artery. *Journal of Neurosurgery* 1956;13:500–506). There were 15,000 carotid endarterectomies performed in the United States in 1971; by 1985, that number had increased to 107,000. (Barnett HJM, Meldrum H. *Carotid endarterectomy: A neurotherapeutic advance. Archives of Neurology* 2000;57:40–45).

    During the 1980s, influenced by progress in treating disease of the coronary arteries in the heart, doctors began to treat carotid artery lesions by using the vascular system to reach the arteries rather than by cutting into the neck. A catheter was introduced into the femoral artery in the thigh and guided using X-ray through the aorta and into the common carotid artery. The balloon catheter could be guided into the region of the narrowing of the carotid artery and then expanded, crushing the plaque and so dilating the narrowed channel in which blood flowed. This procedure was termed angioplasty. Stents could be introduced in a similar manner to keep the artery open (carotid artery stenting). By the end of the 20th century, carotid surgery and carotid artery stenting were among the most common surgical procedures performed, and many millions of patients had undergone these treatments.
29. Durand-Fardel M. *Traite des ramollisements du cerveau.* Paris: Bailliere, 1843; Ferrand J. Essai sur l'hemiplegie des vieillards: les lacunes de desintegration cerebrale. Thesis, Paris, 1902. The historical background of lacunar infarction is reviewed in Hauw J-J. The history of lacunes. In G Donnan, B Norrving, J Bamford, J Bogousslavsky (Eds.), *Lacunar and Other Subcortical Infarcts.* Oxford: Oxford University Press, 1995, pp. 3–15.
30. Marie P. Des foyers lacunaires de désintégration et des diffeérents autres états cavitaires du cerveau. *Revue de Médeciné (Paris)* 1901;21:281–298.
31. Fisher CM. *Memoirs of a Neurologist.* Rutland, VT: Sharp, 2006, Vol. 1, pp. 121–122.
32. Fisher CM. *Memoirs of a Neurologist.* Rutland, VT: Sharp, 2006, Vol. 1, pp. 121–128.
33. Fisher CM, Adams RD. Observations on brain embolism. *Journal of Neuropathology and Experimental Neurology* 1951;10:92–94.
34. Fisher CM, Adams RD. Observations on brain embolism with special reference to hemorrhagic infarction. In Furlan AJ (Ed.), *The Heart and Stroke.* Berlin: Springer-Verlag, 1987, pp. 17–36.
35. Fisher CM. The history of cerebral embolism and hemorrhagic infarction. In Furlan AJ (Ed.), *The Heart and Stroke.* Berlin: Springer-Verlag, 1987, pp. 2–16.
36. Fisher CM. *Memoirs of a Neurologist.* Rutland, VT: Sharp, 2006, Vol. 1, pp. 74–86.
37. Fisher CM. An unusual variant of acute idiopathic polyneuritis (syndrome of ophthalmoplegia, ataxia, and areflexia). *New England Journal of Medicine* 1956;255:57–65.
38. Personal communication to me from Dr. Fisher.
39. Fisher CM. *Memoirs of a Neurologist.* Rutland, VT: Sharp, 2006, Vol. 1, p. 60.

40. Fisher CM. *Memoirs of a Neurologist*. Rutland, VT: Sharp, 2006, Vol. 1, p. 60; the account of the encounter with Dr. Mills was shared with Dr. Joseph Hanaway and me, and the identity of the "important figure" is not mentioned in the memoirs or other Fisher writings.
41. Fisher CM. *Memoirs of a Neurologist*. Rutland, VT: Sharp, 2006, Vol. 1, p. 60.
42. Penfield's urging that Fisher stay in Montreal is discussed in Feindel W, Leblanc R. *The Wounded Brain Healed: The Golden Age of the Montreal Neurological Institute, 1934–1984*. Montreal, Ontario, Canada: McGill–Queen's University Press, 2016.

PART V

Boston and Massachusetts General Hospital

Fisher's Personal Characteristics, Methods, and Major Contributions

Fisher spent the second half of the 20th century and beyond as a neuropathologist and neurological clinician at the Massachusetts General Hospital in Boston. The chapters in Part V describe his activities and modus operandi during his long career as a clinician, researcher, and teacher and his major contributions to knowledge and clinical care. Chapters 8 and 9 describe his activities, personal characteristics, and rules. Chapters 10–13 describe his contributions to the fields of medicine, neurology, and stroke.

CHAPTER 8

Boston and Massachusetts General Hospital

Fisher's Activities and Methods

MASSACHUSETTS GENERAL HOSPITAL

Raymond Adams had recruited Fisher to return to Boston to work at the Massachusetts General Hospital (MGH). MGH was founded in 1811 originally to care for the poor people of Boston.[1] At the time of its founding, it was the third oldest general hospital in the United States, preceded only by the Pennsylvania Hospital in Philadelphia and the New York–Presbyterian Hospital. MGH remains the largest hospital in New England.

When Fisher arrived in 1954, he found that MGH was in many ways quite different from Boston City Hospital (BCH), where he had had his neuropathology fellowship in 1949 and 1950, and there were some similarities. Both had a very strong tradition of medical research. The Thorndike Memorial Laboratory at BCH, established in 1923, was the first clinical research laboratory in a municipal hospital in the United States. Drs. George Minot and William Castle were pioneer clinical investigators of the highest caliber who created an atmosphere at the Thorndike Laboratory that fostered patient-centered research and attracted the best physician–scientists to work and train there.[2] Similarly, Ward 4 in the Bullfinch Building at MGH had been created in the 1920s by Dr. James Howard Means as a central region for medical research at the hospital.[3] Both hospitals were affiliated with Harvard University but differently. BCH contained units and wards affiliated with the three major medical schools in Boston—Boston University, Tufts University, and Harvard University. Only some units (including neurology) were solely aligned with Harvard University. The Peter Bent Brigham Hospital was also an important Harvard academic hospital. Dr. H. Richard Tyler (one of Dr. Derek Denny-Brown's trainees) was the neurologist at the Brigham, and the neurology residents at BCH rotated through the Brigham under Tyler's direction. MGH at the time was the major teaching hospital of Harvard Medical School. All of the medical students, house staff, and full-time faculty had Harvard University attachments or appointments.

The patients and facilities at the two hospitals were quite different. BCH was in the South End of Boston, surrounded mainly by poor, predominantly Irish neighborhoods. Patients were housed at BCH in large, open wards. They were cared for by interns and residents who were loosely supervised by full-time staff physicians. Private patients were rare. Private physicians had to have approval to teach at BCH and were not paid for their services. They could direct patients to the hospital for care by senior full-time staff physicians.

MGH was in the West End of Boston quite near the Charles River that separates Boston from Cambridge. The hospital lay at the foot of Beacon Hill. Boston Brahmins such as the Kennedys and many literati and politicians resided in Louisberg Square and on other streets within Beacon Hill. The Massachusetts State House, the Boston Common, and downtown Boston were within a short walking distance of MGH. The hospital had extensive facilities for general public patients and for private patients of staff physicians. At MGH, patients were housed in wards on three floors in the Bullfinch Building (the original building at MGH designed by the famous American architect, Charles Bullfinch; Figure 8.1). The top floor of the Bullfinch Building housed the famous Ether Dome, where ether had first been administered as an anesthetic for a general surgical procedure.[4] The conference area within the Ether Dome was the site of many grand rounds and also the place where the famous Cabot clinic–pathological cases published in the *New England Journal of Medicine* were held (Figure 8.2). When the George Robert White building opened in 1939, it also housed some general patients and included neurology beds on White 11. Two buildings, the Baker Building and Phillips House, housed private patients. Many general physicians, internists, surgeons, and obstetricians mostly in private practice were affiliated with MGH, cared for their patients at the hospital, or referred their patients to the hospital for care by full-time staff. It was generally agreed that all public and private patients anywhere in the hospital were eligible for teaching and could be seen by training

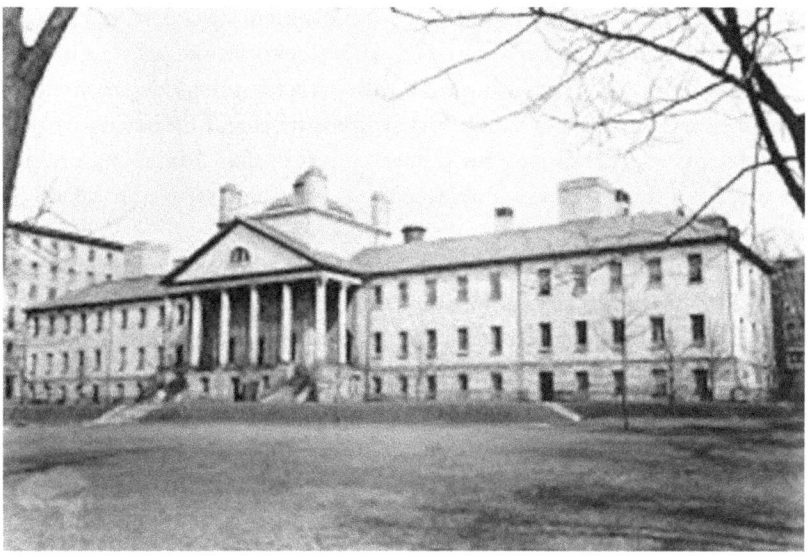

Figure 8.1 The Bullfinch Building at Massachusetts General Hospital.

and teaching staff physicians. Private practice physicians often asked for consultations by the full-time staff.

Another major difference that Fisher sensed was interest in cerebrovascular diseases and stroke. Denny-Brown, the Chair of Neurology at BCH,

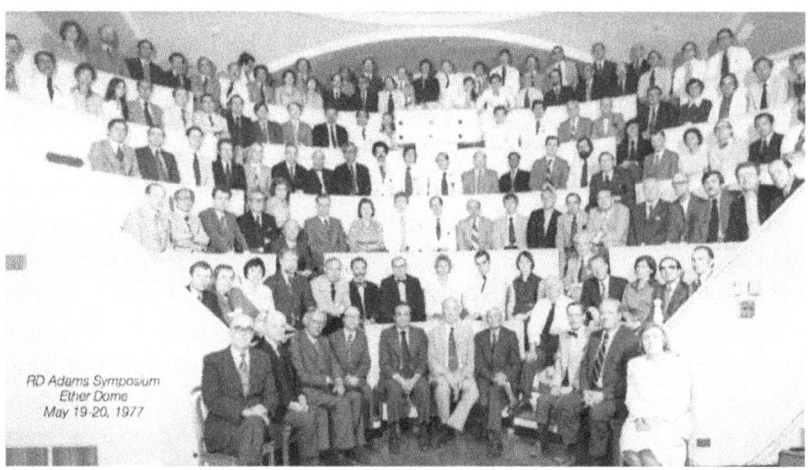

Figure 8.2 The Ether Dome at Massachusetts General Hospital on the occasion of a symposium for Raymond Adams. Fisher is seated in the first seat at the far left in the front row. Adams is in the light-colored suit seated in the middle of the first row.
Source: Submitted and reproduced with permission from Dr. Ron Kobayashi.

had studied and written elegantly about movement disorders and muscle diseases but had shown no major interest in stroke. Stroke patients at BCH were cared for on the medical wards, with little neurology department involvement. On the other hand, Fisher knew firsthand by having worked with Adams at BCH during his fellowship there that Adams maintained an intense interest in cerebrovascular disease and stroke in all of its dimensions.

Adams had been Chief of Neurology at MGH for approximately 2 years when Fisher arrived at the hospital. At the time of the Adams appointment, the Harvard Neurological Unit at BCH was the predominant neurology training program in Boston and arguably in the United States. Before Adams' arrival, the unit at MGH was small and unexceptional.[5] It was overshadowed by psychiatry, where Stanley Cobb, the Bullard Professor of Neuropathology, was in charge of the psychiatry service. Adams' charge by the MGH administration was "the maintenance of an outstanding clinical service to which the most difficult neurological problems would be referred and young physicians indoctrinated in the principles of medical neurology."[5] He sought to develop a very strong "neuromedical service" that would deliver excellent clinical care as well as perform extensive basic, pathological, and clinical research and also to create a training program equal to or exceeding that at BCH.

Adams recruited a number of scientists and budding clinicians to join the neuromedical service. Dr. Maurice Victor, a Canadian native like Fisher, was given full reign to pursue research on alcohol-related neurological conditions as well as other metabolic disorders. Dr. Robert Schwab created the first electroencephalographic laboratory in a US hospital and developed a program to manage patients with Parkinson's disease and other movement disorders. Dr. Edwin Cole directed a speech and reading clinic, one of the first in the United States. Drs. Paul Yakovlev, Jay Angevine, Phillip Dodge, Byron Waksman, Elliott Mancall, and Barry Arnason became active researchers and clinicians. Myasthenia gravis, muscle and peripheral nerve diseases, and multiple sclerosis were targets for research and patient care. Dr. David Cogan, who was later joined by Dr. Shirley Wray from Britain, was a world authority on neuro-ophthalmology and eye movement disorders. His office was in the Massachusetts Eye and Ear Infirmary adjacent to MGH. Eye movements and visual perception were major areas of interest for Fisher. Fisher, Cogan, and Wray worked very closely together.

Adams' neurology unit was one of the first to divide the department into various subunits according to disciplines and neurological conditions studied. Adams showed great intuition in choosing very capable individuals

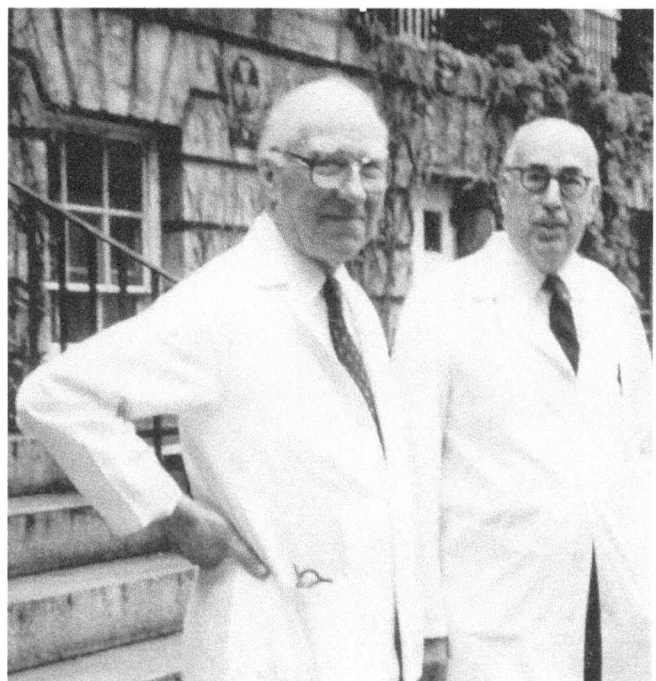

Figure 8.3 Adams and Fisher.

and then supporting them in their development of first-rate research and clinical services.[5] Figure 8.3 shows Adams and Fisher outside MGH, and Figure 8.4 shows the MGH staff during the 1960s.

FISHER'S ACTIVITIES AT MASSACHUSETTS GENERAL HOSPITAL

Soon after deciding to move to Boston, Fisher was able to purchase a large house in Winchester, a small town approximately 8 miles north of downtown Boston. The house was owned by Dr. Jost Michelsen, a neurosurgeon who worked at MGH. Michelson had become aware of the upcoming recruitment at MGH. Fisher noted in his memoirs, "The moving van from Montreal arrived early in the day after an overnight trip. Under Doris Mary's guidance we were comfortably settled in our new home by 5 p.m. ready for supper."[6] The Winchester residence remained the Fisher home for the entire time that he remained in Boston.

The assignment that Adams gave Fisher was to continue his study of cerebrovascular disease that had begun originally at BCH and flowered in Montreal. Adams gave Fisher full reign to accomplish this goal and

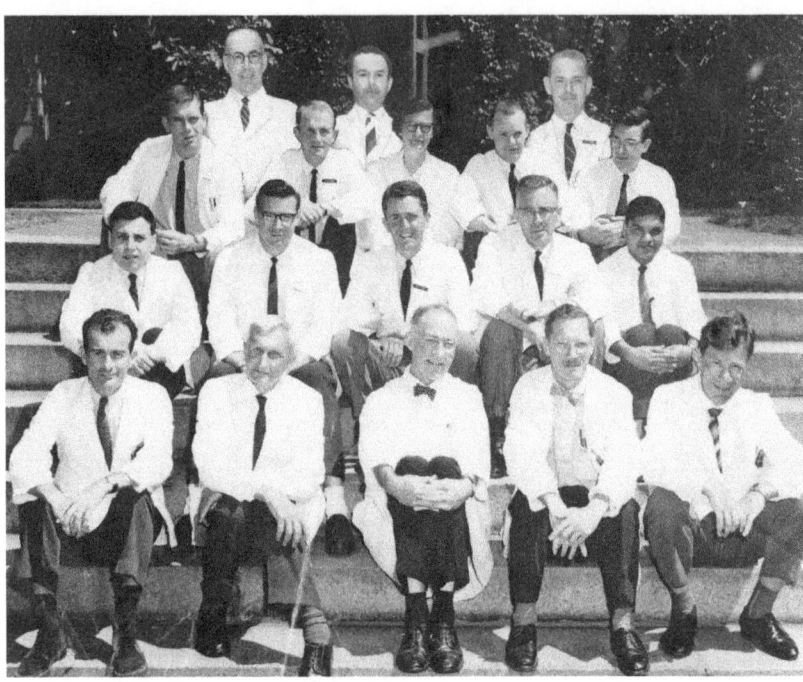

Figure 8.4 The Massachusetts General Hospital neurology staff in 1963. (From left to right) First row: Henry deF. Webster, Charles Kubik, Raymond Adams, E. P. Richardson, and Karl Astrom; second row: Shyam Pant, Alex McPhedron, Robert Young, McGee, and Joshua Hollander; third row: Peter Huttenlocher, Bennett Derby, Gwndolyn Hogan, Hallgrimson, and Joseph Foley; back row: Fisher, Otto Appenzeller, and Arthur Asbury.

never tried to manage or micromanage his work, only to provide support and guidance (but very little salary). The neurology department was small. The department's main offices and laboratories were located on the eighth and ninth floors of the Vincent Burnham Building. Fisher was given an office next to Adams, and one secretary worked for both of them.

Fisher considered his clinical and laboratory work a full-time job, meaning early in the morning until late at night at least 6 days a week and often all 7 days. During his time in Montreal and also his career at MGH, he considered that his main work in life was neurology and stroke.

Fisher commented in his memoirs, "Devotion of the activities of the Stroke Service was full-time. Hobbies, music, art, literature, sporting activities and travel were eschewed or limited. Domestic duties were minimal. Fiscal soundness was never a consideration."[7]

He gave considerable credit to his wife Doris for managing all nonmedical aspects of his existence. He noted that Doris was in charge of everything else, including the family. Fisher poignantly described her role in his memoirs:

> The practice of Neurology allowed no distractions. In the subsequent 50 years of our marriage Doris Mary (D-M) directed our ménage on her own perhaps consulting C Miller (C-M) inobviously, never plainly. D-M asked for naught and gave all. In Winchester, financial matters were D-M's bailiwick—deposits, expenses, withdrawals, investments, income tax preparation etc. C-M wrote no checks and was not known to the bank personally for the first 40 years in Winchester. The Fisher family prospered. Naturally D-M attended to the many aspects of maintenance of the property . . . painters, plumbers, electricians, heating experts and repairmen were hired without discussing the matter with C-M. The jobs were well done under D-M's trained eye. My time was devoted to the practice of neurology . . . D-M undertook all shopping. . . . Family life was happy and calm. The children required almost no disciplining. D-M attended almost all the children's high school sports games.[8]

Fisher set up a neuropathology laboratory soon after his arrival. Drs. E. P. Richardson, Charles Kubik, and Adams had also been performing major neuropathological clinical activities and research and became very trusted colleagues of Fisher in his neuropathological work. Figure 8.5 shows Fisher with Richardson, Adams, and Maurice Victor later during their careers. Fisher specified how he wanted the brains removed at

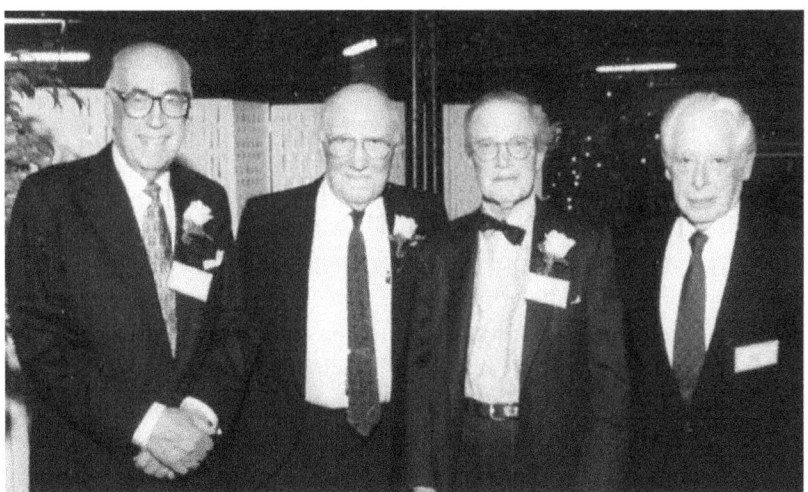

Figure 8.5 Four major leaders of Massachusetts General Hospital Neurology. (From left to right) Fisher, Raymond Adams, E. P. Richardson, and Maurice Victor.
Source: Provided by and reproduced with permission from Dr. Ron Kobayashi.

necropsy to be handled. Each brain to be studied was removed and placed in formalin in a particular way related to the blood vessels at the base of the brain. He insisted that each brain be suspended with a string around the basilar artery so that the brain floated upside down and would not become distorted, and the feeding blood vessels would not be torn. After the brain was removed from formalin, technicians cut serial sections and stained them under Fisher's directions. He spent many hours viewing the many sections and sought to learn the pathology of the blood vessels. He traced the path of the blood supply, tediously and meticulously following arteries and their branches until they reached the region of infarction. Margaret Carroll was the chief technician in Neuropathology at MGH for more than 40 years. She supervised all of the many microscopic serial section studies performed in the laboratories. Lili Bucis worked directly with Fisher. He noted that Bucis provided indispensable technical help turning out faultlessly thousands upon thousands of sections: "So devoted was Miss Bucis that if one slide in a thousand was faulty she came to my office in tears to apologize."[9] During that time (the 1950s through the 1970s), there was no apparent limit to the number of slides that were prepared in the laboratory. At the time, the expense was no problem, although later in the century the cost of providing serial sections of tissues became prohibitive.

Fisher commented in his memoirs on the clinical aspects of his assigned task to continue the study of cerebrovascular disease that had begun during his 1949–1950 fellowship in Boston and had continued in Montreal:

How does one go about a practical useful study in a broad and nebulous field where the goals are difficult to discern. It was decided to methodically consult on stroke patients throughout the hospital to determine if promising avenues of approach would not open up. One or two or three neurological Fellows at a time joined me in the project and we called it the Stroke Service.[10]

During the early 1950s, the National Institutes of Health (NIH) decided to appropriate funds to support training programs in neurology in order to overcome deficiencies in the number of clinical neurologists in the United States. NIH sought to increase the number of fully trained neurologists with academic qualifications who would teach in American medical schools. The grants covered funding for 3 years of residency training in neurology and neuropathology. Foreign medical graduates were also eligible for these grants, and many Canadians took advantage of this and trained in American neurology departments. Dr. Joseph Martin, who followed Adams as chair of neurology at MGH, was a Canadian whose American training was fully funded by NIH. Denny-Brown at BCH regularly trained Canadian-born neurologists funded under this NIH program. At that time, 2 years of training in internal medicine was required before neurology residency. NIH stipends for fellowship training in special areas of neurology, such as stroke, were also available to qualified applicants. MGH was the recipient of one of the first residency training grants. This allowed five (and later seven) physicians to be trained in neurology at MGH yearly. Before 1950, because there were very few medical school-based training programs, most budding neurologists sought training by following and shadowing clinical neurologists in private practice who consulted at several hospitals.

At that time, most neurologists in clinical practice treated both neurology and psychiatry patients.[11] The presence of residents and fellows allowed Fisher to create the first formal training in stroke and cerebrovascular disease in the United States during the 1950s. Fisher recognized that in order to examine the large number of stroke patients hospitalized at MGH, full-time stroke fellows were needed. One of the other main stroke training programs, the Mayo Clinic Stroke Service, started in July 1965 and the stroke fellowship there started at approximately the same time with one fellow per year.[12]

FISHER'S ACTIVITIES AND METHODOLOGY (MODUS OPERANDI)

Fisher awakened early, ate a meager breakfast with Doris, and then drove to the hospital, hoping to beat the traffic headed into the city. Doris made sandwiches for him to take with him to work. These he usually ate at his desk or in his laboratory. He came to the hospital every day and usually stayed until 11 p.m. or so. At times, on his way home in the evenings, he would see consultations at the Winchester Hospital near his home, in which case he would leave MGH earlier. Most days, he would call Doris at approximately 7 p.m. to talk. He enjoyed listening to sports and would have her put a game on the radio so that he could listen. On Saturdays, it was his custom to come home earlier and have dinner with Doris and the children if they were home. Afterwards, he would listen to music on the radio. He was especially fond of dance music; Lawrence Welk was his favorite. On Sunday mornings, he often slept late while the rest of the family went to church. Each summer, the family would go to the Waterloo, Canada, region for a 1-week vacation.

In his later years at MGH, Fisher would tarry a bit at home in the morning and eat breakfast with Doris. She then would drive him to the hospital usually after the traffic rush in the morning. At night, he would call her ("Car 54 Where Are you?") when he was ready to be picked up, usually around

11 p.m. She drove a large green Cadillac with giant fins. Her head could barely be seen above the steering wheel. When he arrived home, Doris and he would usually have a late snack together.

At MGH, he would spend considerable time each day in his neuropathology laboratory examining brains and microscopic sections. He taught himself vascular pathology. He was the attending physician for neurology ward patients usually approximately 2 months during each year. During those months, he would make daily rounds, examining each patient in detail with the house staff. Sometimes he had a few private patients under his care in the hospital, and he saw consultations in the private buildings of the hospital (the Baker Building and Phillips House) directed to him by full-time staff and by private practice physicians and other neurologists. He held outpatient sessions 2 days a week, during which time he saw patients referred to him. He regularly attended neurology grand rounds, which were held on Thursday mornings, and brain cutting teaching sessions, which were always at 4 p.m. on Tuesday afternoons. He played a central role in providing salient comments at these brain cutting sessions. Figure 8.6 shows him amid others at one of these conferences, and Figure 8.7 shows Fisher with Adams and Richardson at another brain cutting conference.

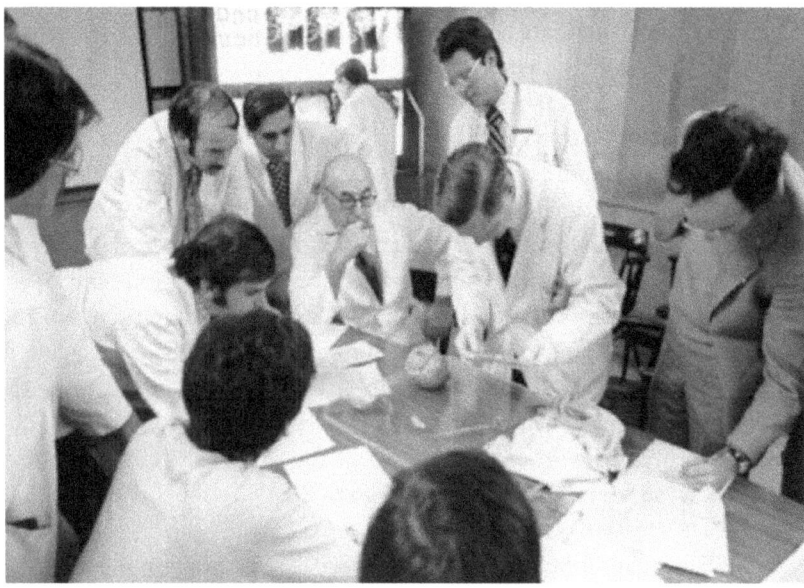

Figure 8.6 A brain cutting conference, 1978. Fisher is seated amid house staff; E. P. Richardson is to his right, bending over the brain to be cut.
Source: Provided by and reproduced with permission from Dr. Ron Kobayashi.

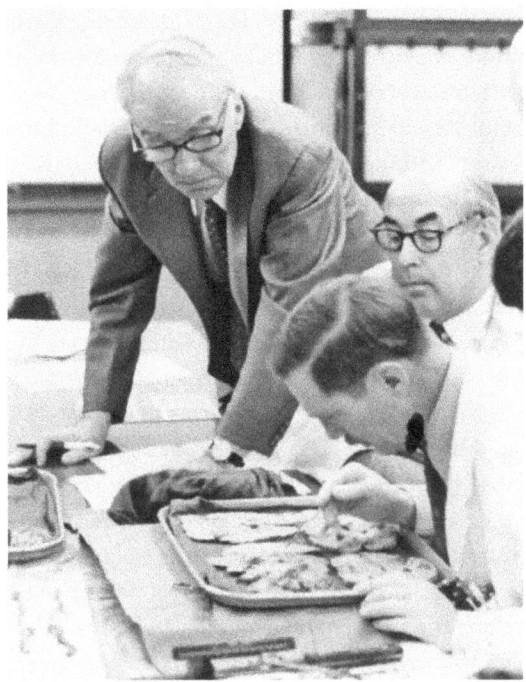

Figure 8.7 Looking at a brain after sectioning. Raymond Adams is standing, E. P. Richardson is seated and viewing the brain slices, and Fisher is peering over Richardson's head.
Source: Reproduced with permission from Loreno R. *Raymond Adams: A life of Brain and Muscle*. New York: Oxford University Press, 2009, Figure 47.

Fisher's main emphasis was learning about stroke and cerebrovascular disease. He had no master plan for that endeavor. He made himself available to see patients with the stroke fellows or residents. He could be interrupted almost any time of day except if he was already examining a patient or performing a consultation. Any and all patients in the hospital who were thought to have had strokes or transient attacks caused by vascular disease were targets for learning. Stuporous and comatose patients were of special interest because many had developed decreased consciousness due to strokes.

Until the mid-1970s, there were no imaging tests that could show the brain.[13] Diagnosis depended entirely on the history and detailed thorough general, cardiac, vascular, and neurological examinations. Recognition of the location of the problem within the brain and the likely vascular cause was solely by using the physician's eyes, ears, hands, and thinking apparatus. Those capabilities Fisher strove to understand and maximize.

Stroke fellows would often begin the day by visiting Fisher's office to learn of any new cases that would be valuable to see. Often, residents, other neurologists, and colleagues, especially cardiologists, would stop by Fisher's office to tell him about a puzzling or very challenging patient. Residents would also contact the stroke fellow to mention new stroke admissions. Many stroke patients were first seen in the emergency department of the hospital. Neurology residents and stroke fellows would be contacted, and they would see and examine the patient in the emergency department.

When urgent, after being examined, some stroke patients were brought directly to a room in the radiology department (called the Picker suite) for angiography. Until the mid- to late 1950s, angiograms at MGH were performed by the stroke fellows or by neurosurgeons. Entry into the neck arteries was by directly puncturing the carotid and vertebral arteries in the neck. The patient would lie supine with the neck extended. A needle would then be directed through the artery until the bone was met behind the artery. Then pulling the needle back, a red gush of blood aimed at the ceiling indicated that the artery had been entered. This part of the procedure was often quite frightening to the patient. Contrast dye would then be injected by hand into the artery. The stroke fellow would then rush to hold and pull the radiology films as the blood circulated through the neck and brain arteries and veins. The speed of pulling the films would depend on whether a fast or slow circulation was likely. Only one view [frontal or anteroposterior or side (sagittal)] could be filmed after an injection. Depending on the results of viewing the films after the first injection, a second frontal view or a side view would be obtained after a second dye injection. In some patients, both carotid arteries or a vertebral artery were injected depending on the suspected localization of the process in the brain. Fisher would sometimes be available to watch the procedure and to view the films as they were printed.

Routinely, Fisher would see patients with the stroke fellow at the end of the day. Fisher and the fellow would usually meet in the cafeteria while Fisher ate dinner. The fellow would describe the case, try to answer Fisher's queries, and then, after dinner, Fisher and the fellow would see the patient. Usually, each night one or two patients would be seen in great detail. After seeing the patient, Fisher would return to his office and record the details of the patient and place the material in a Manilla folder. He kept a small notebook in his pocket in which he would jot down words that the patient uttered or other information that he believed was worth noting.

HOW BEST TO DESCRIBE FISHER'S MAIN ATTRIBUTES AND ROLES?

Fisher was an extraordinary individual. Herein, I describe his attributes as a person, physician, researcher, writer, teacher, and colleague.[14]

Learner–Student

Fisher was a lifelong student, and perhaps this was his most important attribute. One of Fisher's mentors early in his career told him, "You've got a question mark stamped on your forehead."[15] His inquisitiveness and studies were not limited to stroke or neurology or medicine. He studied almost everything and in depth. He studied people—his fellows, colleagues, patients, and family. He characterized his learning method as follows:

> *Through the years I have been asked repeatedly how I go about doing what I do, what goals I set myself, and how the research is organized. . . . My work has not, for the most part, lent itself to a research protocol or research aim. Each day has been a small odyssey of discovery: of what, one never knew. Hardly a day passed without some, new for me, observation. Each day I became a more knowledgeable clinician, a better neurologist. It is my impression that thinking is a matter of keeping one's personal think tank pleasantly stocked with questions—what, when, where, who, which.*[16]

He examined every patient in detail hoping to find a new observation or to clarify questions in his mind. He was extremely interested in how both normal brains and brains of patients with stroke or any other medical or neurological condition worked. Stroke was of special interest because nearly all brain infarcts and hemorrhages involved only a part of the brain. Localizing the damage to a particular brain region gave clues to how that part of the brain worked: "In the neurological sick room every symptom, every sign, every word, every fragment of behavior, every event is grist for the neurologist's mill."[17]

He reflected on his approach to learning and studying patients:

> *Making a diagnosis and providing a service are, to be sure, the heart of medical practice. In 30 years, I was never too busy to see another patient. For the scientific clinician, however, there must be more. There is the task of extending the observations and increasing their precision. Does the case ring a familiar bell? Does it bear out former experience or not? Is a clinical shoe-horn being used to ease the case into a convenient but erroneous category? Are there any atypical, unusual, or novel features? Have there been similar cases? Are any new rules emerging? Does the clinical picture fit any special pattern, arrangement, or relationship? Does the case illustrate or illuminate any neurological principle? Is an informative experiment of nature being witnessed? Does a generalization concerning nervous system function suggest itself? What points may require attention in future cases? All of this might well be abridged into I wonder whether . . . and one wonder begetteth another and another.*[18]

He studied topics by collecting materials:

> *The details of every stroke case seen by the Stroke Service were written or typed, often briefly, on a sheet or two, and roughly and simply piled in broad categories—hemorrhage, aneurysm, embolism, thrombosis, unknown etc. Later, they might be filed according to carotid disease, lacunar syndromes, TIAs, migraine etc. All filing was done in Manila folders, placed in the open and no records were filed by drawers. In a day or two on some weekend we could roughly review every significant stroke case of the previous five years, constantly keeping before us in this way the interesting, puzzling, and the unusual. Experience is not experience unless it is retrievable. A hundred cases may mean little unless they are brought forward for review. The system must not be complex, else it will bog down.*[19]

Fisher practiced before personal computers became available, and he was skeptical that they would facilitate collecting. In studying a problem or answering a query, he would often wait until he had collected sufficient cases and materials and had reviewed the literature on a topic before writing a report for publication. Naming was an important part of collecting. Fisher commented,

> *An important custom was assigning every new finding an identifying designation or name, when it was first noted: for example, wrong-way eyes, normal pressure hydrocephalus, the string sign, the cord sign, the one and a half syndrome etc. A descriptive name is easily remembered compared with an unnamed complex phenomenon.*[20]

Fisher also studied his residents and fellows and colleagues. Typically, if he was in his office, a doctor might come by and ask, "Dr. Fisher, have you heard about this patient—Mr. or Mrs. X." Fisher would invariably reply, "No, tell me about him or her." Then that physician would describe the case, peppered intermittently by Fisher asking for points of clarification. Then Fisher would ask, "What do you think was wrong?" Later, a second physician might come to the office and inquire whether Fisher had heard about the same patient. Again, Fisher would reply, "No, please do tell me about the case." Fisher would later in the day go to see that patient. He would keep in mind what each physician had told him about the patient. This evaluation of the thoroughness, clarity, and analysis of the case descriptions and diagnosis would give him information about the reliability and expertise of the physicians who had told him initially about the case. He had a low tolerance for misbehavior. Although he did not talk about others' foibles and misdeeds, he clearly was aware of them and used them as the measure of the person. He was never mean to a trainee, a colleague, or a patient or a patient's family.

Fisher was very interested in individual attributes of patients and colleagues. One patient described lifting small cars as part of his work. Fisher inquired at length on how this was done and how he had trained to be able to accomplish this feat. Another very obese patient in his 70s was in the hospital for a minor ailment. Fisher saw that the breakfast plate in front of him contained scrambled eggs, milk, cream, and butter. On inquiry, this patient had had no vascular events. Fisher inquired in depth about his diet and activities, trying to understand how this individual had escaped vascular disease despite his obesity, inactivity, and high intake of fats. He was very interested in his patients' various occupations and would query patients in depth about their training, activities, and how they were able to fulfill and even excel at their work. He was particularly fascinated by odd habits and unusual abilities. He liked people.

Unfortunately, his wife Doris developed a progressive decline in cognitive functions and ultimately was clinically diagnosed with Alzheimer disease. When she began to display difficulty with memory, Fisher studied her decline in detail, hoping to gain insight about the condition. Being in very close daily contact with her, he was well positioned to make lengthy observations about the nature and course of the disease. Doris died in 2008 after a lengthy decline in function.

Fisher also studied himself when he had an ailment or symptom. One weekend, he was at work and developed back pain. He tried to make a diagnosis:

> *After an hour of restlessly moving about, it was decided to carry out what I call a pain-o-gram, a methodical detailed analysis of all aspects of the pain. It was an ache of 6/10 intensity. Constant, not cramping or throbbing. It was deep, posterior in the spine or close to it, in the midline 8½ inches below the vertebra prominens. . . . Bending, tilting, twisting, and jarring did not aggravate the pain.*[21]

Later jaw pain, tenderness in the mouth, and deep aching appeared in both arms. He concluded it was not likely to be a mechanical back problem. He went back to work but became fidgety and had difficulty concentrating. He called Doris and asked her to pick him up. Doris responded, "Miller you must be very ill. This has never happened before. Go immediately to the emergency department." He heeded her advice. The diagnosis turned out to be an acute myocardial infarction with a very slow pulse and reduced blood pressure. Doris proved to be a better diagnostician than Fisher on that occasion. In later years, after retirement he became very interested in his visual problem and its variability. Before his death, he wrote directions for an autopsy to be performed on himself soon after death, to include a dissection of the eyes.

Fisher often learned by listening to others at meetings. He seemed to have great patience in meetings and encounters in listening carefully to what others said and thought without the necessity of announcing his own ideas. He did not want others to parrot back or be unduly influenced by his own pronouncements. He preferred to listen and potentially be swayed by their uninfluenced discussions.

He was an avid reader of the literature. He often could be found in the library in the evenings looking up *Virchow's Archives* in German and investigating any journal (English, French, or German) that had articles and reports on a topic he was researching. He assiduously read and analyzed past contributions and ideas about topics. His writings were most often very carefully and thoroughly referenced.

Physician

More than any other descriptor, Fisher thought of himself primarily as a doctor—a medical practitioner. He loved what he did. Once, he said that he was "amazed that you could get paid for doing neurology" because figuring out the neurologic puzzle was so rewarding. He always kept the patient in mind and aimed to translate his observations into treatment of individual patients.

He responded quickly to medical students, residents, and colleagues who wanted him to see a relative or friend or a perplexing patient. He saw the prospective patient as soon as required, fitting them in to his busy schedule as a high priority. Often, the patient was seen on weekends, which were not as heavily scheduled. Fisher thought the best of his patients and tried to think of them as he would himself or his family:

> In reflecting on 50 years of medical practice there comes to mind first and foremost the virtuous personal qualities exhibited by almost all patients.... I have been impressed by the essential right-mindedness of patients, their eagerness to be helped, their forbearance and optimism, and their slowness to animadversion. In the long run their courage, resolve, loyalty and gratitude make medicine a most rewarding pleasure. For this physician, the practice of medicine at a highly skilled level must be one of the most satisfying endeavors of human existence.[22]

He was very patient and understanding with his patients, and he clearly tried to convey empathy:

> It was my endeavor to develop a friendship with each patient. In a consulting practice there is not always time for the basics of ministering to the ill, but generally I lingered attempting to place the patient's ailment in correct perspective.[23]

Fisher was a tall man. He presented an imposing figure in his white coat (Figure 8.8). He was soft-spoken and considerate with patients. They knew that he would spend as much time as needed with them and would be available if they encountered problems. Most patients and their families came to love and worship him.

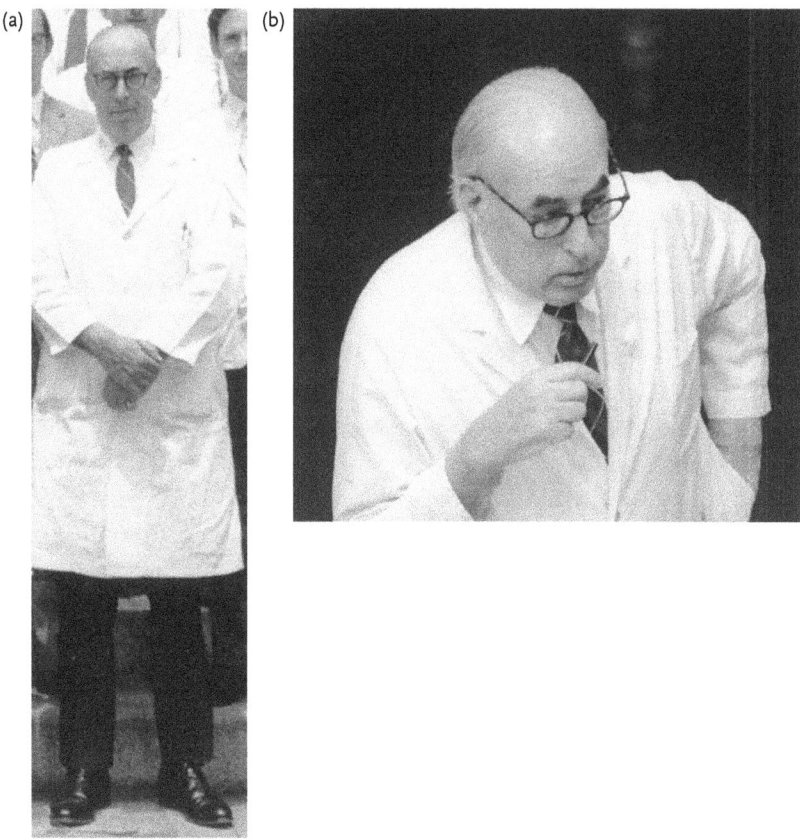

Figure 8.8 Photographs of Fisher standing (A) and lecturing (B).
Sources: A, provided by and reproduced with permission from Dr. Ron Kobayashi; B, reproduced with permission from Caplan LR. *Caplan's Stroke* (5th ed.). Cambridge, UK: Cambridge University Press, 2016.

Teacher and Mentor

Fisher was a superb teacher and mentor. He did not, however, teach by didactic transmission of information. He taught in three main ways: as a role model, using the Socratic method of questioning, and by his written publications.

My own experiences during daily rounds serve as examples of his teaching methodology. Discussions with other residents and fellows assured me that my experiences were not unique and were clear examples of his usual modus operandi.

We would usually meet at approximately 6 p.m. in his office or at a table in the cafeteria for patient rounds. I use the example of a 60-year-old man who had come to the hospital the day before because of headache and weakness of his left limbs. The patient had been seen by me that morning. It was early in my stroke fellowship, perhaps after only a few weeks of mentoring. Fisher would ask me to tell him about the patient I had seen. I would begin with the history. Fisher would interrupt and ask for clarification or further information. If I noted that the patient had been hypertensive, Fisher might inquire, "For how long, at what levels, and how was the hypertension managed?" If a stroke had developed after a day that the patient considered normal, Fisher would ask for more details as to exactly what the patient had done that day. If I had not characterized the headache in detail, Fisher would ask about prior headaches: "How was this headache different from past ones?" "How abrupt was the onset of the headache?" "Where was it located?" "How long did it last?"

After relating the history, Fisher would ask me to describe my examination. Again, Fisher would require more details. If the patient had a left hemianopia (inability to see objects to the left with either eye), Fisher might inquire, "Did the patient's vision change depending on the amount of ambient light?" "Did detection of a moving object brought from the left side differ depending on the size of the object stimulus [hand, finger, or head of a pin]?" "Could the patient identify colors?" "Could the patient read?" I would try to answer the best that I could but would admit when I had not performed the testing mentioned in his inquiries. If I told Fisher that the patient had a left hemiparesis (weakness of the limbs on the left side of the body), he would ask about quantification of the weakness: "Was the weakness equal in the left face, arm, and leg?" "In the left upper limb, was there a difference in the weakness in the shoulder, arm, forearm, and hand?" "How long could the patient hold his arm outstretched?" He then might ask a question about a part of the potential examination that I had not performed: "Could the patient draw a clock, a house, a bicycle?"

"Could the patient copy objects that you drew?" "How did the patient fare in describing the Poppelreuter figure [a drawing of overlapping objects]?"[24] At that time, I knew nothing about the Poppelreuter figure. Invariably, my examination was incomplete in relation to Fisher's inquiries. I would seldom be able to answer many of the queries in a satisfactory manner. His questioning taught me what I should be looking for. As the stroke fellowship progressed, I became more facile at producing the desired detailed history and examination information that Fisher required.

In his queries, Fisher had been generating hypotheses about where in the brain the stroke abnormality was located and what was the cause. The technique of localization of a given lesion in the brain can be likened to finding a son or daughter whose vehicle has broken down. A telephone call informs the father that the car is non-operative. "Come and get me," the driver states. The parent responds, "Where is it?" "Somewhere on Route 9" is the reply. Route 9 extends for many miles. The parent, knowing various landmarks and intersections on Route 9, then proceeds to interrogate the driver: "Where on Route 9? Before the Route 128 turnoff? Near Route 16?" etc. Similarly, when trying to identify a location within the brain, knowing one finding, the clinician asks about other findings known to be in the near vicinity or pathway of a symptom. If weakness of the left limbs was accompanied by a visual abnormality, that would indicate involvement of visual fibers near the occipital lobe. Drawing and copying abnormalities, depending on their nature, might indicate a parietal lobe location, as would loss of feeling in the left limbs.

During my early training, I had not sufficiently mastered the technique of hypothesis generation and sequential testing, but this improved with time as a result of Fishers questioning. After my description of the history and examination, Fisher would ask me, "What did you make of the case? What is your diagnosis?" I would proffer my analysis. He would then ask, for example, "Then how did you fit in this observation that you made?" "How do you explain the lack of lethargy?" "Why is his speech normal?" After my bumbling responses, he would say, "Now let's go to see the patient."

We would then go together to the patient's bedside, and Fisher would elicit a very thorough history. I had missed several points of importance. Then he would conduct a meticulous examination. He might spend an hour exploring the patient's visual capabilities and the patient's ability to describe objects and people from memory and then from pictures. Could the patient describe directions to and from various regions? Could the patient visualize a map and tell directions for traveling to and from one location to another place? If one traveled from Boston to Miami what directions would they be going? If the patient answered correctly south, Fisher might ask,

"On what side of the car would the Atlantic Ocean be located?" He would study the patient's ability to draw objects such as a clock, house, and bicycle and to copy a complex diagram. He might have the patient look at a figure and describe what they saw after the picture was removed from view. He might ask the patient to copy a specific figure while looking directly at it and then, after a 5- or 10-minute interval, to redraw the image to test visual memory. Of course, my examination had been quite incomplete.

After the patient encounter, he would ask again about my formulation of the case: "What do you think now?" "What type of stroke did the patient have?" "Where was the abnormality in the brain located?" "What further testing would you suggest?" "What treatments are available and which would you choose?" Depending on my replies, he would often then suggest, "Why don't you have a look at . . ." and then mention three or four references that would amplify or question my formulation of the case. He had shown me how to get the maximal information from the patient encounter and how to study and learn. During the first 6 months of my fellowship, he never told me anything directly. His technique was entirely Socratic. He did not want me to parrot back his own thoughts, ideas, statements, or formulations. He wanted me to think on my own and to learn how logically and thoroughly to assess and describe a patient encounter. He also wanted to learn and gain from my formulations—maybe I could teach him something he had not considered. During the fellowship, I became much more adept and thorough, but the patient encounter with him always resulted in my learning something new or questioning a tenet that I previously held.

During the years after my fellowship, I continued to use Fisher as my oracle. I would call him about cases that puzzled me. He would ask about the details. He believed that the details were what distinguished the expert from the novice, the men from the boys, the women from the girls. After my description, he would ask questions. When I could not answer his queries, he seemed always able to pinpoint the key unanswered question. If you can answer that question, he would say, the cause will become clear.

Fisher was not a polished speaker. He was slow and at times rambling. He seemed not to be on top of the topic. It often seemed as if he had not sufficiently prepared beforehand for the formal exposition of the topic. He did like to show pictures, particularly of pathological specimens. He kept hundreds of slides on his desk scattered about. Before a presentation, he would dive into the pile and select the ones he wanted to show. It seemed uncanny that he somehow knew where the key slides were located in the large pile. He disliked making didactic speeches. He was quite good at commenting on cases at grand rounds or during brain cutting sessions, but formal lecturing was not his forte.

Fisher was a very careful and compulsive author. He opined that it was the clinician's duty to write and share observation, ideas, and formulations. He often waited until the ideas and concepts were clear in his own mind before making reports: "It is essential that the progressive clinician write for publication. Persuasive imagination is disarmingly deceptive and requires a sobering thorough methodical written exposition."[25]

Fisher had a very broad vocabulary and loved to apply many descriptors, sometimes presented as a list of nouns, adjectives, or adverbs. For example, when trying to define the word "emotional," he wrote in his memoirs,

> The term "emotional" is used in its broadest connotation to cover an array of emotions, some of which are difficult to define or identify. Included are: anxiety, tension, worry, fear, alarm, anger, desperation, frustration, depression, grief, fatigue, exhaustion, quandary, disbelief, disappointment, defeat, emotional crisis, arrest of action and thought and others.[26]

In describing personality characteristics, Fisher wrote,

> Crackpots, windbags, lazy people, eccentric persons and even fools do not realize their quirks and foibles. The person who is domineering or demanding or impatient or bad tempered is often incapable of seeing it himself. What is obvious to everyone else is not so obvious to him. Our idiosyncrasies, our bad habits, our short comings are more evident to others. Occasionally, we are made aware of them by our wives! The thief, the psychopath, and the anarchist are not fully aware of their aberrations.[27]

Fisher described people, objects, findings, activities, and events quite well. His published reports were often very long and extensively referenced. He did not like anyone to tinker with his wording. An example is the first publication that bore both his and my name.[28] He did not show a draft of the report to me until after it was published. He did not want me to change one word. Two of his very long studies were published in the *Acta Neurologica Scandinavica Supplements*.[29,30] This was definitely not a journal that was routinely read in the United States or Europe. At that time, as well as now, most general and neurological journals did not accept for publication very long original observations and reviews. Many reviewers and editors suggested cutting portions of the paper and altering the wording. Fisher and Adams insisted that all of the case materials and discussion be included in their publications. They did not want to shorten the reports and, in doing so, weaken the message. They also did not want anyone to tinker with the language. Considering these two issues, shortening and editing, Fisher and Adams had three alternatives: publish with book companies, publish on their own, or allow their material to be published as a supplement in *Acta Neurologica Scandinavica*. Book publishers were unlikely to publish single long reports as books; self-publishing long reports or chapters was quite expensive. The authors could publish a supplement in *Acta Neurologica Scandinavica* without any editorial changes; they would only have to pay a meager publishing charge—much less than it would cost to self-publish.

NOTES

1. Kowalczyk L. Massachusetts General Hospital at 200: A great institution rises and with it the healing arts. *Boston Globe*, February 26, 2011. An account of the history of the hospital is also available from Wikipedia.
2. Elrod JM, Karnad AB. Boston City Hospital and the Thorndike Memorial Laboratory: The birth of modern haematology. *British Journal of Haematology* 2003;121(3):383–389; Tishler PV. The sociology of the deceased Harvard Medical Unit at Boston City Hospital. *Yale Journal of Biology and Medicine* 2015;88(4):423–426.
3. Means JH. *Ward 4: The Mallinckrodt Research Ward of the Massachusetts General Hospital*. Cambridge, MA: Harvard University Press, 1958; Stanbury JB, Chapman EM. James Howard Means. In Castleman B, Crockett DC, Sutton SB (Eds.), *The Massachusetts General Hospital, 1955–1980*. Boston: Little, Brown, 1983, pp. 63–68.
4. Ether anesthesia was first administered in 1842 by Crawford Long under a tree in Jefferson, Georgia, but Long did not publish his use until 1849. The credit for making ether known to the public goes to William T. G. Morton, a dentist, who in 1846 held his famous public demonstration of ether in the dome of the Bullfinch in the presence of Drs. J. C. Warren and Henry Bigelow. The "Ether Dome" at MGH commemorates this event.
5. The early history of the neurological service at MGH and Adam's career are described in depth in Adams R. Neurology service. In Castleman B, Crockett DC, Sutton SB (Eds.), *The Massachusetts General Hospital, 1955–1980*. Boston: Little, Brown, 1983, pp. 158–1164; and in Laureno R. *Raymond Adams: A Life of Brain and Muscle*. New York: Oxford University Press, 2009.
6. Fisher CM. *Memoirs of a Neurologist*. Rutland, VT: Sharp, 2006, Vol. 5, p. 138.
7. Fisher CM. *Memoirs of a Neurologist*. Rutland, VT: Sharp, 2006, Vol. 4, p 84.
8. Fisher CM. *Memoirs of a Neurologist*. Rutland, VT: Sharp, 2006, Vol. 5, pp. 138–140.
9. Fisher CM. *Memoirs of a Neurologist*. Rutland, VT: Sharp, 2006, Vol. 1, p. 143.
10. Fisher CM. *Memoirs of a Neurologist*. Rutland, VT: Sharp, 2006, Vol. 1, p. 132.
11. When I began my neurology training during the early 1960s, I was advised by several practicing physicians that I would need to do mostly psychiatry in order to earn a living.
12. Personal communication from Dr. Robert Brown of the Mayo Clinic Neurology Department.

13. Computed tomography scanning became available in most large US hospitals during the late 1970s. Magnetic resonance imaging was introduced into neurological practice during the 1980s.
14. I attempt to portray Fisher's main attributes from the viewpoint of a former trainee and long-term colleague. In 1969–1970, during slightly more than 1 year as his only stroke fellow, I spent 4–6 hours each day, 6 days a week with him as a private tutorial. I have also consulted many of his residents, fellows, and colleagues to be able to attempt to characterize his attributes. I continued to have very frequent contact with Fisher after my training up to the time of his death.
15. Fisher CM. *Memoirs of a Neurologist*. Rutland, VT: Sharp, 2006, Vol. 1, p. 7.
16. Fisher CM. *Memoirs of a Neurologist*. Rutland, VT: Sharp, 2006, Vol. 1, p. 162.
17. Fisher CM. *Memoirs of a Neurologist*. Rutland, VT: Sharp, 2006, Vol. 1, p. 133.
18. Fisher CM. *Memoirs of a Neurologist*. Rutland, VT: Sharp, 2006, Vol. 1, p. 162.
19. Fisher CM. *Memoirs of a Neurologist*. Rutland, VT: Sharp, 2006, Vol. 1, p. 162.
20. Fisher CM. *Memoirs of a Neurologist*. Rutland, VT: Sharp, 2006, Vol. 4, p. 84.
21. Fisher CM. *Memoirs of a Neurologist*. Rutland, VT: Sharp, 2006, Vol. 1, p. 229.
22. Fisher CM. *Memoirs of a Neurologist*. Rutland, VT: Sharp, 2006, Vol. 1, p. 166.
23. Fisher CM. *Memoirs of a Neurologist*. Rutland, VT: Sharp, 2006, Vol. 1, p. 166.
24. See Sells R, Larner A. The Poppelreuter figure visual perceptual function test for dementia diagnosis. *Progress in Neurology and Psychiatry* 2011;15(2):18–21. The original descriptions of the Poppelreuter figure are in Poppelreuter W. Zür Psychologie und Pathologie der Optischen Wahrnehmung. *Zeitschrift für Gesamte Neurologie und Psychiatrie* 1923;83:26–152; and Poppelreuter W. *Die psychischen Schädigungen durch Kopfschuss im Kriege 1914/17: Mit besonderer Berücksichtigung der pathopsychologischen, pädagogischen, gewerblichen und sozialen Beziehungen* (2 vols.). Leipzig, Germany: Voss, 1917–1918.
25. Fisher CM. *Memoirs of a Neurologist*. Rutland, VT: Sharp, 2006, Vol. 1, p. 167.
26. Fisher CM. *Memoirs of a Neurologist*. Rutland, VT: Sharp, 2006, Vol. 3, p. 354.
27. Fisher CM. *Memoirs of a Neurologist*. Rutland, VT: Sharp, 2006, Vol. 1, p. 234.
28. Fisher CM, Caplan LR. Basilar artery branch occlusion: A cause of pontine infarction. *Neurology* 1971;21:900–905.
29. Fisher CM. The neurological examination of the comatose patient. *Acta Neurologica Scandinavica* 1969;45(Suppl. 36):5–56.
30. Fisher CM, Adams RD. Transient global amnesia. *Acta Neurologica Scandinavica* 1964:40(Suppl. 9):1–83.

CHAPTER 9

Fisher's Collegiality, Personality Traits and Idiosyncrasies, and "Rules"

FISHER—A MODEL COLLEAGUE

Fisher was always a team player. He never publicly uttered an unkind word about his colleagues and would readily come to their defense if they were unfairly criticized. He chose particular consultants and colleagues with whom to work. Dr. Robert Ojemann, a trusted and skilled neurosurgeon, worked closely with him in treating patients with cerebrovascular conditions that required surgery—for example, brain aneurysms, brain vascular malformations, and carotid artery disease. A number of the cardiologists at Massachusetts General Hospital (MGH) were often asked to consult on his patients—Drs. Roman DeSanctis, Allan Friedlich, Paul Dudley White, among others. He developed a very close relationship with them and would often meet at a lunch table to discuss vascular disease. E. P. Richardson, Jr., a neuropathologist and clinical neurologist, and Fisher collaborated on many neuropathological projects and had a very close relationship.

After 1972, Fisher handed the direction and management of the stroke fellows over to Dr. J. P. Mohr. This gave Fisher more time to spend in his neuropathology laboratory. Mohr had been Fisher's stroke fellow in 1968–1969. After his fellowship, in order to fulfill his required military commitment during the Vietnam War, Mohr was assigned to the neurology and neuropathology departments of the Walter Reed Army Hospital in Washington, DC. He returned to MGH in 1972 at Fisher's request to assume directorship of the Stroke Service. In 1978, Mohr left Boston to chair the neurology department at the University of South Alabama. He later moved to Columbia University as the first Daniel Sciarra Professor of Neurology. He developed the first stroke service and training program at Columbia's New York–Presbyterian Hospital and has remained at Columbia ever since, but he maintained close contact with Fisher until Fisher's death in 2012.

When Mohr returned to MGH, he asked Dr. J. Phillip Kistler to be the first of many subsequent stroke fellows. Mohr had been Kistler's supervising medical resident when he was a medical intern at Columbia's Mary Imogene Bassett Hospital in Cooperstown, New York. Kistler was a board-certified internal medicine physician. He had spent his military service from 1968 to 1970 as Chief of Medicine at a large US Air Force hospital. During his stroke fellowship year, Raymond Adams, Fisher, and Mohr urged Kistler to stay and take the neurology residency program at MGH. Kistler joined the MGH Stroke Service in 1976 to work with Mohr. After Mohr left MGH in 1978, Adams and Fisher encouraged Kistler to take on the leadership of the Stroke Service, which he did for 26 years until 2004. During these years, Mohr and Fisher remained very close advisers and colleagues of Kistler.

During the 1970s and thereafter, Dr. Robert Ackerman, created a laboratory to investigate stroke risk factors and ultrasound exploration of the arteries supplying the brain. Ackerman had been trained in medicine and neurology at North Carolina and at MGH; he then further trained in Boston and London to become a qualified neuroradiologist. He also performed some of the early work on positron emission tomography analysis of brain infarction at MGH. Fisher worked very closely with Mohr, Kistler, and Ackerman and was always available to help steer the MGH Stroke Service in the right direction. In 1984, Ackerman began to arrange and schedule meetings of stroke-oriented physicians in the Boston area. These occurred three or four times a year and were reliably attended by Fisher.

In 1977, Adams decided to step down from the directorship of the Neurology Service at MGH. Adams decided to devote more time to pediatric neurology. In 1978, Dr. Joseph Martin succeeded Adams as the Neurology Chair at MGH and led the department through the 1980s.[1] Figure 9.1 shows Fisher with Adams, Richardson, and Martin. In the mid-1970s, the Kennedy family funded renovation of the top two floors of the Vincent Burnham Building, which housed the offices of the MGH Neurology Department. After Martin became the chair, he shared an examining room with and had the same secretary as Fisher and often would consult with Fisher on patients seen in their adjoining offices. Dr. Verne Caviness, Jr., a former MGH neurology trainee, became the director of the MGH pediatric neurology program, and he had offices adjacent to Martin and Fisher. Figure 9.2 shows Caviness with the other leaders

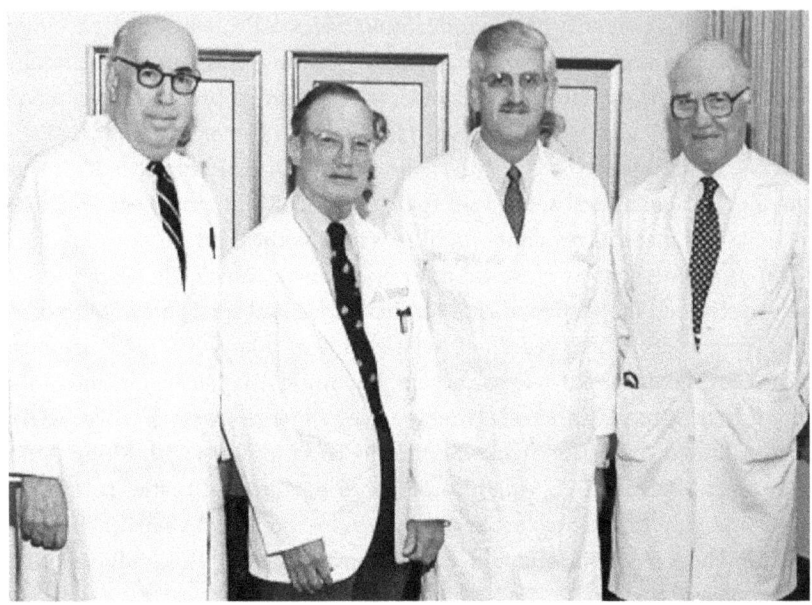

Figure 9.1 (From left to right) Drs. Fisher, E. P. Richardson, Joseph Martin, and Raymond Adams.
Source: This Photograph was kindly provided by Dr. Joseph Martin and was published in Martin JB. *Alfalfa to Ivy: Memoir of a Harvard Medical School Dean.* Edmonton, Alberta, Canada: University of Alberta Press, 2011.

of MGH Neurology during Martin's regime as chief. After a sojourn at the University of California at San Francisco, Martin became the dean of the Harvard Medical School. Dr. Anne Young assumed the leadership of the MGH Neurology Department in 1991. Fisher served as a key member of the teaching faculty during the chairmanships of Martin and Young and was an important adviser to both chairs.

Adams and Fisher encouraged their residents and stroke fellows to be well trained in caring for both neurology and neurosurgery patients. The first neurology/neurosurgery critical care unit was set up by Robert Ojemann in a room containing four beds on the floor of the neuroscience department on White 12. During the mid-1970s, Ojemann and Mohr advised the MGH architects on the design of a new larger intensive care unit (ICU) in the adjacent Gray Bigelow Building. A few years later, Drs. Alan Ropper and Brooke Swearingen (a neurosurgeon) became the first co-directors of the larger Neuro-critical Care Unit. After Ropper left to chair the neurology department of St. Elizabeth Hospital in Boston, Drs. Daryl Gress and Walter Koroshetz followed as co-directors of neurocritical care at MGH. Fisher and Kistler were very supportive of the neurocritical care ICU, which contained many patients with acute strokes as well as postoperative

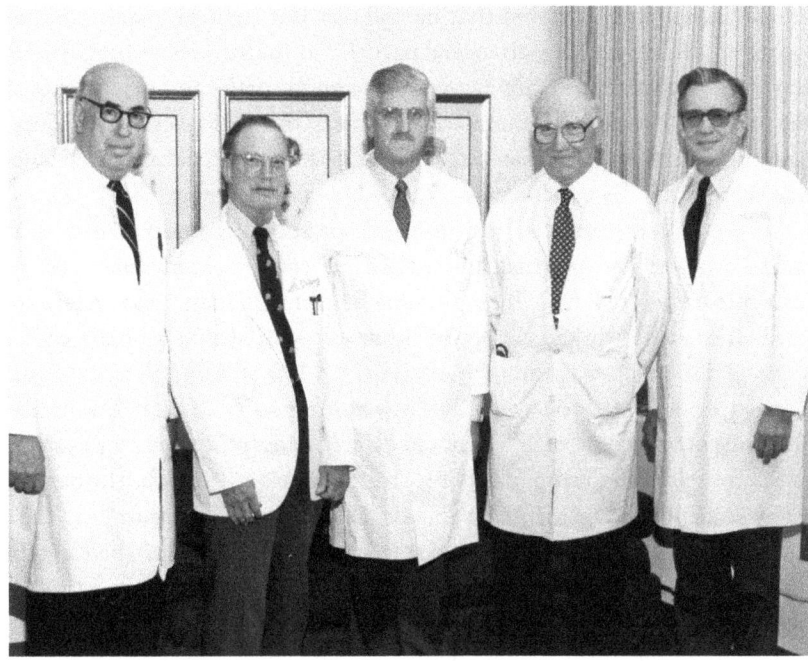

Figure 9.2 Senior staff during Martin's Chairmanship of Neurology at MGH. (From left to right) Drs. Fisher, E. P. Richardson, Joseph Martin, Raymond Adams, and Verne Caveness. *Source*: This photograph was kindly provided by Dr. Joseph Martin and was published in Martin JB. *Alfalfa to Ivy: Memoir of a Harvard Medical School Dean*. Edmonton, Alberta, Canada: University of Alberta Press, 2011.

cases. Stroke fellows often saw patients and spent time training in the ICU. Later, neurointensive care of hemorrhagic and ischemic stroke was integrated into the stroke fellowships.

FISHER'S PERSONALITY TRAITS AND IDIOSYNCRASIES
Lack of Concern About Time

Fisher never seemed in a hurry and was completely oblivious to the time of day or night. He never rushed. He spent as much time as he needed to thoroughly analyze neuropathology specimens, to review literature in the library, and at the bedside until he satisfied himself that he had milked the case of all salient details. When asked "Where do you get the time?" he responded, "Not wearing a watch may help. At night I was always the last to retire. A night hawk propensity was an innate endowment."[2] On many occasions, he would spend hours at the bedside of an "important case" unconcerned that patients in the clinic might be waiting or that he had other obligations. For example, in one case, a patient stated that he had just lost sight in one eye. Fisher looked in the eye and saw abnormal particles in the arteries in that eye. He stayed with the patient many hours, following the paths and movements of the particles. He drew diagrammatic pictures of the eye vessels and the location of the particles.[3] All other activities had to be delayed or canceled. Fisher was heard to say, "History is here. We need to take advantage of it."

This very slow, protracted pace was the despair of many students, residents, and fellows who were in a rush or wanted a quick answer. Many characterized his approach as "tedious." The nickname "shifting dullness" was widely applied. Those who worked closely with him recognized that a phone call or a casual discussion was rarely brief and could last an hour or more. Some would duck out of the way when they saw him and so avoid a long encounter. This trait of very slow pace was noted even in Montreal, where a physician preceptor told him to stop "dawdling." His disregard of time was the bane of many students and residents on rounds. Patients in his office waiting their turn to be seen by him often had to stay long after his secretary had left for the day. Patients did understand that Fisher would spend as much time as needed with them, so they rarely complained about waiting.

Fisher arrived at the hospital early in the morning and stayed until late at night. Telephone calls to his office or home for advice were very common, even late at night. A clinician remarked that "his own wife doesn't know where he is. When I called one morning around 2:00 a.m. she said she'd check to see if he has come in."[4] During the later years of his career at MGH, his wife Doris would drive to the hospital from Winchester, collect him, and take him home. He would call her when he was ready to leave. Once she had been called, he disliked keeping her waiting. If he was called to the emergency room while she was on her way, he could proceed with haste and not dawdle. At all other times, he chose not to hurry.

Perhaps the years that he spent in the prisoner-of-war camp in Germany with not much to do and no time constraints fueled this innate tendency to ignore time.

Unconcern About Money and Other Practical Matters

Fisher wrote,

> *Financial matters relating to practice can bring their share of quirky behavior. . . . None of my secretaries was permitted to send a second bill. Keeping track of fiscal transactions was deemed unworthy of my attention or time. Making money was incidental.*[5]

He clearly focused entirely on medical activities. His disregard and unconcern about practical and financial matters were legendary. A personal example of this occurred early in my experience with him. He interviewed me in the fall of 1968 after I had applied to become a stroke fellow during the 1969–1970 period. Soon after that interview, I received a very brief note in the mail informing me that I was accepted for the fellowship and that I should report to his office at MGH on July 1, 1969. I dutifully appeared on that date, and he proceeded to briefly describe where I could get a white coat and where I was to work. Then he said, "I hope that you have arranged your salary." I was stunned. Neither he nor anyone else had remotely mentioned salary during the initial interview or thereafter. I naively assumed that I would be paid. At that time in my life, I was over 30 years old and had a wife and five young children at home. I dreaded going home and telling my wife that there was one small problem: I was to work for more than a year without pay. Fisher saw the dismay and alarm in my face, and he said, "Do not worry, we will take care of it." He called Raymond Adams and had me placed on the house staff list so that I would get some meager pay, the same as his neurology residents. He then said that I should apply to the National Institutes of Health (NIH) for funding. He reached in a drawer, pulled out papers, and handed me a multipage application. He said, "Fill this out. I also have to fill out forms." I went home and spent that night writing and typing in the lengthy detailed information requested. The next morning, I showed my completed application to him and asked if he had had time to fill out his portion of the application. He pulled out of the desk another multipage packet. He wrote on the top, "I guarantee that his time will be well spent—C. Miller Fisher." He then handed the entire packet to me and said "send it in." In a month or so, I received word from NIH that indeed my fellowship would be supported fully and I would receive a reasonable stipend.

Fisher rarely carried any money. Doris would on occasion give him some dollars and coins to carry if he had an expense coming up. On one occasion, he went to a meeting in New York. He became bored by the proceedings and tried to locate his wife. He had no money in his pockets. Failing to reach her (cell phones were completely unknown at that time), he decided impulsively to return home to his work and somehow got to Boston and his office without funds.

I doubt that he ever shopped with his wife for food or other necessities.

Compulsiveness

Fisher was a very compulsive note taker and collector. His memoirs are packed with copies of talks and speeches that he once delivered. His comments at tributes to others (Mohr, Kistler, Ojemann, Zervas, and myself) at various occasions are printed in full in his memoirs. Also included are the speeches that he gave at the annual MGH dinners. The minute details that he included in his memoirs more than 30 years later about events that occurred during his early years and surrounding his prisoner-of-war period indicate that he must have been taking notes at that time. He also included in his memoirs many unpublished drafts that must have been meticulously thought out but never submitted. He always kept a small notebook in his pocket. He scribbled in that book often, particularly noting verbatim descriptions by patients. He kept the previously used notebooks in his desk and referred to them later.

Before he died, he bequeathed all of his patient notes and his files of journal articles that he had collected and organized during life to the Harvard Countway Library, where they can be reviewed upon request. The collection includes many boxes of material.[6]

Forward Looking and Flexible

Fisher was always future-oriented. He was delighted with new technology and new ideas. When computed tomography (CT) scanning and, later, magnetic resonance imaging (MRI) appeared and were integrated into the diagnostic evaluation of patients, Fisher was very enthusiastic about their ability to help in the care of patients. He even mused that were he to begin training again, he might have become a neuroradiologist. He gave advise to the committee that was in charge of the development of MRI at MGH, and one of his own patients was the first patient studied using the new machine. He was enthusiastic that these newer imaging techniques would shed important new information about the stroke subtypes that he had carefully studied in his neuropathology laboratory and in the clinic. He adapted quickly to the new technology and used both CT and MRI in investigating brain infarcts, hydrocephalus, and hemorrhages inside and outside the brain.

Acting

Fisher loved to pretend and act. He often presented a persona different from his true self. He often played possum. For example, with patients, after an individual had shared their history of events, he would say, "Let me review with you what I have heard you tell me." Then he would proceed to relate the history but would misquote many details and sometimes add to the story. He wanted to find out if the patient would correct him. How consistent was the story the patient provided? How forthright was the patient that he would challenge the errors related to him? Dr. Steve Cramer listed among the 25 things that Fisher taught him the following Fisher quote: "If you want to know the truth, lead the patient with the wrong question."[7]

In dealing with patients whose problem was considered to be psychogenic, Fisher would often play games that miraculously sometimes worked. For example, there was the apocryphal story of a 12-year-old boy who had a terrible balance problem referred to Fisher by a pediatric neurologist who had failed to help the adolescent.[8] The boy was homebound and could not attend school because he could not walk safely. He had already been seen by multiple physicians in Montreal, New York, and Baltimore to no avail. After the history and examination, Fisher told the boy, his parents, and the pediatric neurologist who was witnessing the encounter that it was a simple weight problem that was causing the imbalance. He was weighed to one side. Fisher then proceeded to put objects first in the boy's left front pocket and then in the right front pocket. With new weights the boy tilted to that side. Finally, when the weights were equal, the lad was able to walk well. The problem was fixed.

Similarly, with doctors, as previously noted, Fisher would pretend he had not heard previously about a patient in order to gain insight into the acumen of the doctor who told Fisher the story he had already heard from others.

When he was invited to lecture at other hospitals and meetings, Fisher would play the bumbling novitiate. He would fumble with his notes and forget to show one or more slides and then show them later. His lectures were poorly organized and were not remotely indicative of his knowledge of a topic. He disliked didactic talks and often wanted to keep his observations and thoughts close to the vest before putting them to words in print.

After retirement, Fisher's son, Dr. Hugh Fisher, was amazed at witnessing Fisher playing with his grandchildren and their trains. Fisher pretended to be the conductor and tried to make the train excursions as close to real life as possible for his grandchildren. Hugh had never had this type of light play with his father while Hugh was growing up.

Patriot

Fisher was very proud of being an American. He kept a cube with an American flag on his desk. He reveled in July 4th celebrations and liked to attend patriotic parades. He watched congressional hearings on CNN. He also revered his country of birth, Canada. He was very proud of serving in the Canadian Navy during World War II. He was very moved by his native country installing him in the Canadian Medical Hall of Fame in 1998.

FISHER'S "RULES"

The neurology department at MGH honored Fisher on September 7, 1980, with a Festschrift celebration of his career at the hospital. Former residents, fellows, and colleagues were invited and urged to give presentations.[9] I made a brief presentation that I titled "Fisher's Rules." Dr. Solomon Hakim, who attended the celebration, urged me to submit my talk for publication in a neurological journal. I edited the material, and it was published a year later.[10] These rules were never told to me directly. I surmised these precepts from Fisher's words, his procedures and methods, and by his personal example as a role model. He has read them and never disapproved. They have been cited in a number of subsequent publications that discussed his life and works. Herein they have been amplified:

1. The bedside can be your laboratory. Study the patient seriously.

    Many physicians employ vigorous scientific principles when performing laboratory experiments but take care of patients in a haphazard fashion. Fisher always urged an equally systematic scientific approach at the bedside. Clinical observation requires time and patience. The method of clinical observation should be just as rigorous and systematic as that of an experiment in the laboratory. During the history taking, make hypotheses about the nature of the disease process and its location in the brain and in the blood vessels supplying the brain. Test these hypotheses by thorough questioning. Next, think of tests that can be performed at the bedside during the general and neurological examinations that will either corroborate your hypotheses or argue against them. Then think of imaging and laboratory testing that will further clarify the diagnosis.
2. Settle an issue as it arises at the bedside.

    Whenever possible, do not leave a strong "maybe" after the history and physical examinations of the patient. An accurate complete diagnosis is the key to effective patient management. A wonderful quote from Miguel de Cervantes, the author of *Don Quixote*, is "For when the cause of the complaint is unsure, twould be a miracle to find a cure."

It is commonplace now for physicians to carry out brief slipshod histories and examinations and then order many imaging, electrophysiological, and laboratory tests; this method is often referred to as a shotgun approach. This approach should be vehemently discouraged in this time of cost containment. A loose, imprecise, indefinite formulation of a clinical problem at the bedside is seldom improved or clarified by laboratory testing.

3. Make a hypothesis and then try as hard as you can to disprove it or find the exception before accepting it as valid.

   This rule is similar to that taught to students in elementary geometry, reductio ad absurdum—disprove a theorem by showing it leads to a ridiculous, absurd, or impractical conclusion. Fisher's formal statement of a concept and its publication often appeared years after the observations and ideas were originally generated. During that interval, he would test and retest his ideas to uncover weaknesses and pitfalls, always trying to "trip it up." He would try them out on fellows and colleagues for additional input. He was wary of stating ideas that had not stood the test of time and inquiry.

4. Always be working on one or more projects: It will make the daily routine more meaningful.

   Once you make an observation or a hypothesis, you can begin collecting data at the bedside and in the clinic. Patients can also serve as normal controls. For example, if a physician is interested in visual exploration and perception, he or she can select scenes to show to all patients, even those who have no cognitive or behavioral issues. The responses of patients with none of these issues serve as normal controls to be contrasted with those of patients who have brain lesions that impact on visual behavior. A physician can gain in this way from any clinical encounter. Active exploration of projects allows the clinical encounters to be more meaningful and more productive.

5. In arriving at a clinical diagnosis, think of the five most common findings (historical, physical examination, or laboratory) found in a given disorder. If at least three of these five are absent in a given patient, the diagnosis is likely to be wrong.

   This is a practical rule of thumb that helps focus thinking. For example, concerning a patient who is a brain tumor suspect, the five most common features are headache, symptoms that suggest a localized neurological lesion, findings on examination that point to a localized place in the brain, seizures, and a localized mass on imaging (CT and/or MRI). This precept stimulated Fisher to determine and file mentally the *rules* concerning each condition and diagnosis.

6. Describe quantitatively and precisely.

    Medical students, trainees, and even seasoned physicians often have occasion to present a patient's physical and neurological findings to other doctors individually or at conferences and meetings. Ideally, those who hear the presentation should be able to visually picture the findings. This is facilitated if the findings are described quantitatively—for example, by terms such as mild or slight weakness. Better would be a description that listeners could visualize or repeat if they subsequently examined the patient. For example, one could state, "The patient could hold their leg 3 feet above the bed for a period of 20 seconds" or "On looking to the left side, the patient had 5 beats of rapid nystagmus consisting of 2 mm excursions." These quantifications also are helpful in writing a note so that the same or another physician could compare the new examination with the old.

7. The details of the case are important: Their analysis distinguishes the expert from the journeyman.

    The history and physical and neurological examinations can provide subtle clues to the correct diagnosis. These clues will be missed by a superficial or casual approach.

8. Collect and categorize phenomena: Their mechanism and meaning may become clearer later if enough cases are gathered.

    I have already commented extensively about Fisher's method of collecting cases, data, and references in Manila folders. His desk and work area contained many Manila folders that contained collections of unusual signs, historical accounts, or observations that defied understanding. Headings on these folders included "Patients Who Write off the Edge of the Paper," "Intermittent Interruption of Behavior," "Nonsense Speech," and "Oval Pupils."

    He would often wait until he had sufficient observations to be able to characterize a finding, a diagnosis, or a treatment. Especially in patients with unknown diagnoses or puzzling unusual findings, an observation or a case or imaging might appear months or even years later that shed light on the previous conundrum.[11]

9. Fully accept what you have heard or read only when you have verified it yourself.

    Be a doubter. Test the ideas, statements, and publications of others before embracing them as valid. The literature and dogma of medicine and neurology are loaded with hearsay, half-truths, and imaginings. Misinformation and poorly tested "facts" are often passed on from generation to generation.

10. Learn from your own past experiences and those of others (literature and experienced and respected colleagues)

    Explore the literature. Learn how ideas and concepts were generated and evolved. Each generation cannot relive the history of neurology. Fisher often visited the stacks of the MGH and Harvard libraries day and night.

    He listened avidly to others whose opinions he respected. He often bounced new ideas off of his fellows and colleagues to obtain their reactions and thoughts.

11. Didactic talks benefit most the lecturer. We teach others best by listening, questioning, and demonstrating.

    Fisher liked to query attendees at a didactic talk days later to determine how much they retained and how accurate was their understanding. He concluded that they retained very little. His teaching forte was at the bedside. He was a master of the Socratic technique.

12. Write often and carefully. Let others gain from your work and ideas.

    Fisher set a goal of producing at least one major and two minor reports each year. This gave him a timeline. He invariably surpassed and seldom lagged behind that aim. Many observations and ideas are lost if not recorded and published. These observations can then be amplified and clarified by readers, investigators, and clinicians.

13. Pay particular attention to the specifics of the patient with a known condition and diagnosis; it will help later when similar phenomena occur in an unknown case.

    Many doctors stop acquiring information when the diagnosis becomes clear. For them, the goal of the clinical encounter is to make a diagnosis. For example, listening to detailed descriptions of the visual phenomena in a patient with a known migraine aura may prove very valuable when confronted by a patient who has an undiagnosed unusual visual experience. Compare the unknown case with the 100 or more migrainous visual accompaniments that have been carefully collected. Neurological diagnoses are often made by pattern matching. Does the new case fit the patterns encountered previously? Fisher was a compulsive collector of patterns.

14. Be a good listener; even from the mouths of beginners may come wisdom.

    In the writings of Shakespeare and Mark Twain, it was often the least likely character who uttered the most important wisdom—Polonius in *Hamlet* by Shakespeare and Huck Finn in *Adventures of Huckleberry Finn* by Twain. Students and novitiates often have good ideas worth hearing.

15. Resist the temptation to prematurely place a case into a diagnostic cubbyhole that fits poorly.

    Allowing material to remain unknown and imprecisely categorized stimulates continuing activity and thought. Fisher had an uncanny ability for recognizing the unusual patient or a facet of a case that did not quite conform to the rules. He was also keenly aware of the limitations of present-day medical knowledge. Identifying the unique case or finding led to further analysis, seeking information that would clarify the observation or diagnosis. Ultimately, further clarification often led to a report of a newly identified sign or condition or variant.

16. The patient is always doing the best that he or she can do.

    Be supportive. Never become short or angry with patients or their families. Take time to hear their stories, their problems, and their concerns. Empathy is a very important part of patient encounters.

17. Maintain a lively interest in patients as people.

    Fisher was always interested in what his patients did and what their life was like. He showed a special interest in unusual hobbies, interests, and attributes and would question patients at length about these features. His interest in people also extended to his students, residents, fellows, and colleagues. He was never too busy to discuss a vexing clinical problem or conundrum, share ideas about a new report or new medical advance, or simply chat about the recent news of the day. His success as a clinician in interacting with patients can be at least partially attributed to his more general interest in humanity and its trials, tribulations, successes, and sufferings.

NOTES

1. A description of neurology at MGH during Dr. Martin's chairmanship is provided in Martin JB. *Alfafa to Ivy: Memoir of a Harvard Medical School Dean.* Edmonton, Alberta, Canada: University of Alberta Press, 2011.
2. Fisher CM. *Memoirs of a Neurologist.* Rutland, VT: Sharp, 2006, Vol. 1, p. 147.
3. The description and drawings of the findings in the eye are contained in Fisher CM. Observations in the fundus oculi in transient monocular blindness *Neurology* 1959;9:337–347.
4. This remark is cited in Mohr JP, Caplan LR, Kistler JP. C. Miller Fisher: An appreciation. *Stroke* 2012;43:1739–1740.
5. Fisher CM. *Memoirs of a Neurologist.* Rutland, VT: Sharp, 2006, Vol. l, p. 170.
6. The C. Miller Fisher collection is housed in the Harvard Countway Library, 10 Shattuck Street, Boston, MA 02215, within the History of Medicine department.
7. Fisher CM. *Memoirs of a Neurologist.* Rutland, VT: Sharp, 2006, Vol. 2, p. 57.

8. The story of this boy's treatment is told in Fisher CM. *Memoirs of a Neurologist.* Rutland, VT: Sharp, 2006, Vol. I, pp. 168–169.
9. Adams and Richardson published a brief note describing the event: Adams RD, Richardson EP Jr. Salute to C. Miller Fisher. *Archives of Neurology* 1981;38:137–139.
10. Caplan LR. Fisher's rules. *Archives of Neurology* 1982;39:389–390.
11. I discuss this issue of collecting in Caplan LR. "Caplan's syndrome"—Revisited and lessons learned. *Practical Neurology* 2005;5(5):304–307.

CHAPTER 10

Neurological Examination of the Stuporous Patient, Lacunar Infarction, Intracerebral Hemorrhage, and Aneurysmal Subarachnoid Hemorrhage

Once Fisher had identified an area of interest, he often continued to contribute to knowledge regarding that topic throughout his long career. When new technology or new observations that would advance research on that topic became available, he would redirect his attention to further understanding that area of interest. For these reasons, his work is not presented chronologically but instead is discussed under major topic headings. Contributions were often made over time. Fisher often worked on different areas of interest concurrently. When Fisher prepared a list in 1998 of his own contributions for a Canadian Medical Hall of Fame biographer, he listed 101 separate contributions.[1] Here, it is not possible to describe each. Discussions are limited to his major contributions and are grouped under broad topics.

STUPOR AND COMA AND FINDINGS DURING NEUROLOGICAL EXAMINATIONS

Soon after arriving at Massachusetts General Hospital (MGH) in 1954, Fisher turned his attention to a vexing clinical problem: patients who arrived at the hospital unconscious or nearly so or became unconscious after entry into the hospital. Little had been written about diagnosis in patients with stupor and coma, and the potential causes were many: bleeding into and around the brain, serious infections such as meningitis and encephalitis, head injuries, intoxications, chemical imbalances within the body such as liver or kidney failure, low blood sugar, diabetic acidosis coma, cardiac arrest with low blood flow to the brain, strokes, and others. Fisher recognized that stuporous or frankly comatose patients could not give an account of their symptoms, and often the family or others could not clarify the preceding events. The history of how the symptoms began and progressed, long acknowledged to be the cornerstone of neurological diagnosis, was not as helpful in patients with reduced consciousness as it was in those with other neurological conditions. Fisher had to focus on the physical and neurological examination to attempt to render diagnoses.

During the 1950s and 1960s, there were no tests available that could image the brain: Computed tomography (CT) scanning was not available until the mid-1970s, and magnetic resonance imaging (MRI) was introduced a decade after CT. The only test available, skull X-rays, could show fractures but gave no image of the brain inside the skull. Blood tests and analysis of the spinal fluid that circulated around the brain could help diagnose some cases, and electrical activity as measured from the scalp [electroencephalography(EEG)] was helpful in showing a patient's state of alertness; however, these were the only tests available to Fisher and colleagues at that time. Doctors had to depend on their eyes, ears, hands, and brain to try to uncover the cause of the reduced consciousness.

Fisher had read available reports of animal studies that had shed light on the physiology of consciousness.[2] He knew that consciousness resided in the cerebral hemispheres and that abnormalities that affected both cerebral hemispheres—for example, intoxications and lack of blood flow—could cause coma. The cerebral hemispheres were constantly stimulated by structures in the brainstem (the reticular activating system). The brainstem was a critical region for survival that connected the cerebral hemispheres above with the spinal cord below. The cerebellum was attached to the brainstem. The other mechanism that caused coma was dysfunction of the brainstem. Coma could ensue if the reticular activating system within the brainstem was damaged by a process within the brainstem (e.g., a stroke) or by pressure on the brainstem caused by space-taking lesions in one cerebral hemisphere or the cerebellum (e.g., large bleeds or brain infarcts).

These various mechanisms of coma involved different locations in the brain. Fisher hypothesized that if clinicians could localize the problem to various regions within the brain, that would help identify the likely cause. Fisher opened his subsequently published article, "The Neurological Examination of the Comatose Patient," as follows:

> An accurate assessment of the comatose patient can be of great practical importance. A detailed neurological examination will usually establish the principal site of the intracranial pathology, provide important clues to the etiological diagnosis and not infrequently indicate the proper approach to therapy.[3]

Characteristic of his approach to unsolved problems, Fisher went to the literature and to the bedside for answers. From his reading, he recognized the importance of various reflex responses that involved the pupils, eye movements, and the response of the limbs to stimuli. He wrote in his memoirs,

> The history of neurology contained no record of the methodical examination of the comatose patient. Starting with the important observations of Klingon on eye movements in brain stem lesions, over a period of five years, little by little, probing here and probing there, the Stroke Service painstakingly and haltingly evolved the concept of utilizing each and every reflex response to determine the localization of the process and estimate its severity.[4]

Fisher and his stroke fellows set out to examine consecutive hospitalized patients who had stupor or coma. They noticed the spontaneous presence and absence of movements and activities such as coughing, sneezing, swallowing, tongue protrusion, lip licking, sighing, and yawning. The patterns of breathing were also very important to note. They examined the eyes in detail: They categorized the size of the pupils, their position within the iris, and their response to light and painful stimuli. They carefully noted the position of the eyes at rest and tested eye movements to each side and up and down after various stimuli were given.[5] Horizontal, vertical, and oblique eye movements are controlled at different levels of the brainstem. Yoking of the eyes together so that both eyes work optimally together is controlled by a different cell group within the brainstem. The position of the arms and legs at rest and their response to passive movement and to painful stimuli were studied, ultimately describing various automatic reflex movements of the arms and legs. Irregular, rapid, deep, intermittent, and other abnormalities of respiration seemed to indicate dysfunction at various levels of the brainstem.

Fisher and his fellows were able, after methodically examining hundreds of patients with reduced levels of consciousness, to describe in the literature the significance of various abnormalities of the pupils and eye movements.

Fisher strove to give these abnormalities names that were easy to recall and would aptly characterize the abnormality: Oval pupils, wrong-way eyes, 1 and ½ syndrome, pseudo-sixth nerve palsy, and ocular bobbing are some of these designations.[6] Identifying the abnormality helped localize the pathology within the brainstem.

The previous discussion relates to diagnosis of the cause and localization of the condition responsible for the stuporous and comatose states. The two other very important values of the systematic examination of the unconscious patient are its utility for prognosis and for recognizing changes—worsening of the level of consciousness or improvement. The best example of the prognostic value of the examination is in patients who arrive at the hospital unconscious after a cardiac arrest. Will the patient survive? If the patient survives, what will their function be like? Vegetative, demented, disabled, dependent, homebound, or relatively normal and able to return to work and be a productive family member? Brain electrical activity monitoring had not proven helpful in rendering a prognosis unless electrical activity was absent (a "flat" EEG). Even when CT scanning and MRI became available later, these tests were not definitive. The neurological examination performed each day proved to be more accurate in suggesting the likely duration of the coma and the final outcome than any of the imaging and other technology.

Because the comatose patients cannot say how they are now compared to in the past, without detailed neurological examination it was difficult for doctors to determine whether they were better, the same, or worse. Repeated imaging or other technology studies were impractical and not often definitive. Fisher believed that it was the neurological examination performed by a trained and experienced neurologist that had the most value (and was the least expensive).

Fisher made other important contributions to the physical and neurological examination of patients. Careful feeling of the pulses of the arteries supplying the face proved helpful in recognizing occlusion of the carotid arteries in the neck[7] and in diagnosing temporal arteritis,[8] a serious inflammatory condition of the arteries supplying the eyes and brain. Simple tests of repetitive tapping of the fingers[9] and feet[10] proved helpful in identifying disorders of coordination of the limbs, often caused by disease of the cerebellum. Fisher also studied and described abnormalities of gait that were helpful in separating various neurological conditions.[11]

He had added to the daily armamentarium of neurologists in evaluating patients. His clinical observations and identification of important abnormalities detected during neurological examinations are very important for clinical neurologists who examine patients in the hospital and in the clinic even today.

LACUNAR INFARCTION AND DISEASE OF THE SMALL BRANCH ARTERIES THAT PENETRATE INTO THE BRAIN

While performing neuropathology in Montreal, Fisher had become interested in the frequent occurrence of small holes (lacunes) located deep within the brain in elderly patients. His initial studies on the topic in Montreal were discussed in Chapter 8. He had read the French literature concerning the topic,[12] and at MGH he turned his attention to studying and analyzing the usual characteristics, locations, and dimensions of these small infarcts; the causative abnormality in the arteries and arterioles that supplied the infarcts; and the clinical symptoms and signs noted during life.

In his neuropathology laboratory, Fisher meticulously dissected the brains of patients that contained lacunar infarcts, and he laboriously studied innumerable microscopic sections. Dr. Martin Samuels told of his experience of examining the brain of a patient with Fisher when Samuels was a neurology resident at MGH.[13] The patient had had a stroke that Fisher believed was due clinically to a lacune in the thalamus, a region that lay deep within the cerebral hemisphere. Fisher followed the patient clinically during the 5 years after the stroke until his death and then undertook a postmortem examination. Fisher spent at least 5 hours carefully dissecting the brain, cutting it in such a way as to not interrupt the blood supply to the suspected region that he posited harbored the lacune. When he approached the thalamus, Samuels, who was watching attentively, noted that Fisher switched to a razor for cutting to make very thin cuts. After many hours, lo and behold, there was a tiny lacunar infarct where Fisher predicted it should be located. He cut a block of tissue that contained the infarct and its vascular supply and made serial sections to be examined under the microscope.

It took years for Fisher to arrive at the best method to analyze the nature of the causative vascular process. At first, he made two separate blocks of the tissue containing the lacune. Then he had a technician stain every 10th section with one stain and every 11th and 12th section with different stains. This process was very time-consuming and costly, and it also proved ineffective in clarifying the vascular process because it was difficult to follow the sequences of sections. Fisher later switched strategies to making a much larger block that he thought would contain the lacune and then directed his technician to stain every section with one stain—a phosphotungstic acid–hematoxylin combination. Each block of tissue could yield up to 3,000 stained sections. Trays of slides from a single case were often stacked in a pile that stretched up to the ceiling in his office. It took Fisher many hours to review the slides and to reconstruct the location and cause of the vascular process responsible for the lacunar infarct.

In total, it was 10 years before Fisher was able to satisfactorily identify and define the nature of the condition within the tiny arteries that caused the infarcts and to correlate the pathology with the clinical findings during life. Lacunar infarcts were virtually never fatal; many patients lived for decades after their stroke, and by the time of autopsy, they often had accumulated many other lesions and sometimes the location of the initial infarct studied clinically had been obliterated by a hemorrhage that had developed later.

Among 1,042 brains that Fisher studied at autopsy, 114 (11%) had lacunar infarcts, often multiple.[14] The most common locations were deep within the brain: the internal capsule, basal ganglia, thalamus, and the pons. These were the same locations that Fisher found were the most frequent locations for hypertensive brain hemorrhages. The appearance of the lacunar infarcts varied depending on the time elapsed since their occurrence. The recent infarcts represented small regions of brain softening. Older lesions were cavities ranging from 1 to 17 mm in size. Often, strands of fibrillary connective tissue traversed the cavities. A typical lacune photographed by Fisher is shown as Figure 10.1.

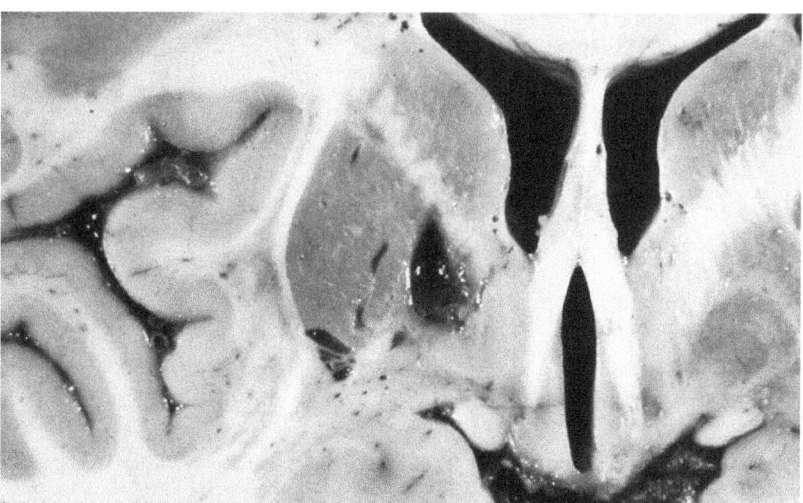

Figure 10.1 A necropsy specimen showing a cavity due to an old lacunar infarct located in the medial basal ganglia (mostly the globus pallidus) and extending through the internal capsule in a patient with a pure motor hemiplegia during life.
Source: Provided by Dr. C. Miller Fisher.

Fisher studied the small penetrating arteries and arterioles that supplied these small deep infarcts.[15] An artist's drawing of these arteries is shown in Figure 10.2. He had Edith Tagrin, his trusted medical illustrator, make a drawing that showed the method used to analyze the pathology within penetrating arteries that supplied these lacunes. Figure 10.3 is her diagram of the tissue studied. In the figure, the line pointing to segmental occlusion shows the site of the blocked artery. The artery before (retrograde occlusion) and after (antegrade occlusion) this blockage was also occluded because of lack of blood flow. Fisher showed that an area labeled in the figure "segmental occlusion" contained severe abnormalities located within the walls of these small arteries. He called this pathology "segmental arterial disorganization," indicating that the pathology was localized to a segment of the artery and that the pathology resulted in severe reduction of blood flow beyond the area of

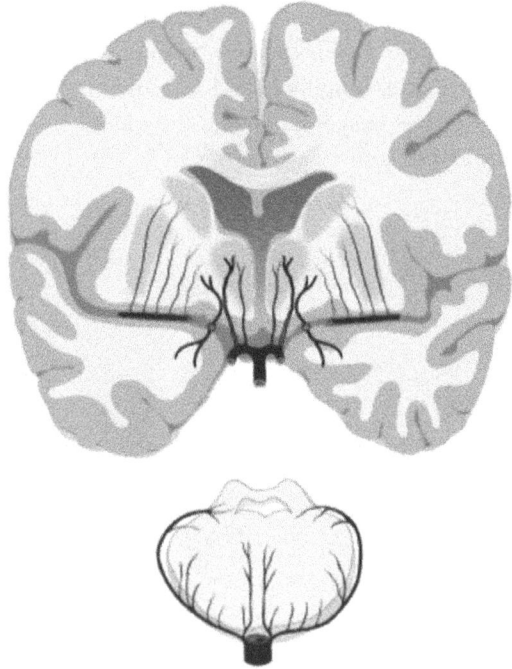

Figure 10.2 Artist's drawing showing penetrating arteries that supply the basal ganglia and thalamus.
Source: Reprinted with permission from Caplan LR. *Caplan's Stroke: A Clinical Approach* (4th ed.) Philadelphia: Elsevier, 2009.

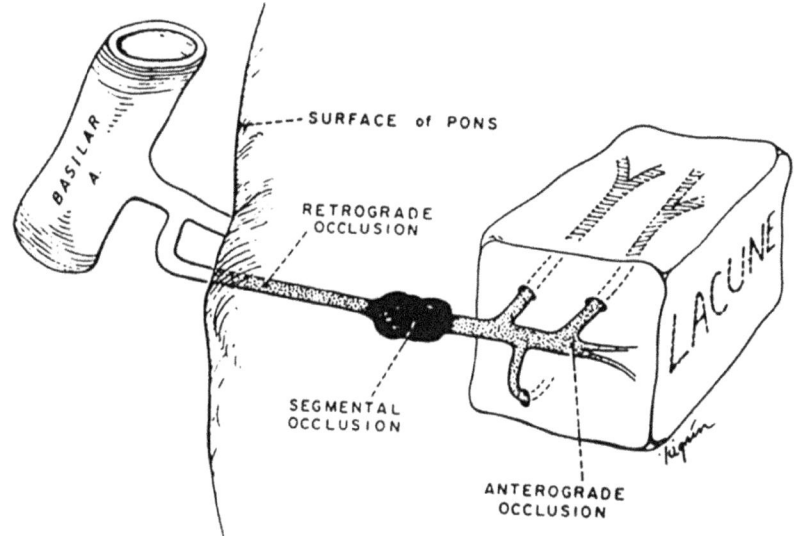

Figure 10.3 Diagram showing the relationship of a lacune in the pons to the causative penetrating artery vascular lesion. The artery beyond the region of arterial disorganization is thrombosed (anterograde occlusion), and thrombus has also formed in a retrograde manner extending toward the parent basilar artery.
Source: From Fisher CM: The arterial lesion underlying lacunes. *Acta Neuropathologica* 1969;12:1–15, with permission. Reprinted from Caplan LR. *Caplan's Stroke: A Clinical Approach* (5th ed.). Cambridge, UK: Cambridge University Press, 2016.

abnormality. He also applied the term "lipohyalinosis" to the segmental abnormality, indicating that fatty material (lipid) was present within the arterial wall and that the wall took on a glassy (hyaline) appearance. Lipid material and connective tissue called fibrinoid thickened the wall of the small arteries, causing encroachment on the lumen where blood flowed. Figure 10.4 is a photograph that Fisher took of one of these diseased arterial segments. The wall of the artery is grossly thickened. Only a very small lumen (the white area shown by the black arrow) remains. The dark area of abnormality within the arterial wall (shown by the white arrow) represents fibrinoid necrosis.

Some regions within the penetrating arteries studied showed focal enlargements, dilatation of the vessels. Fisher suggested that these dilated regions represented the formation of microaneurysms explained by weakening of the arterial wall. Some of these vessel-expanded regions were located just beyond regions of luminal blockage, a phenomenon characterized as post-stenotic dilatations.

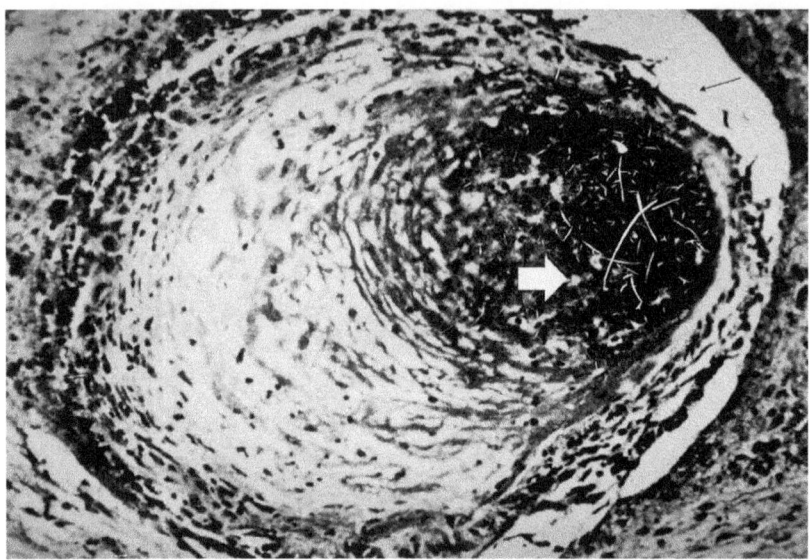

Figure 10.4 Small penetrating artery showing lipohyalinosis and fibrinoid necrosis. The large white arrow shows the fibrinoid material which stains black. The small thin black arrow is inside of the lumen. The lumen is considerably compromised. The large white arrow shows the fibrinoid material which stains black. The small thin black arrow is inside of the lumen.
Source: Provided by Dr. C. Miller Fisher.

Fisher noted the frequency of the various abnormalities in his major detailed report on the nature of the arterial lesions that caused lacunar infarction:

> *In 45 of 50 consecutive lacunes there was a total occlusion of the artery supplying the territory of the infarct. The associated vascular lesions were: segmental arterial disorganization 40 (with enlargement 31, with hemorrhage 26, with fibrinoid deposit 14); thrombosis of a fusiform asymmetric microaneurysm, 2; plaque of foam cells (atherosclerosis) 3.*[15]

He emphasized that this pathology was quite different from what he found in the large arteries in the neck and in the head that supplied the brain. He searched through the records of the patients in whom lacunes were found and noted that nearly all had either high blood pressure at the time of the stroke or had been treated for high blood pressure in the past.[16] Fisher posited that hypertension had a severe effect predominantly on small penetrating arteries; the wear and tear of being pounded by higher than normal pressure led to lipohyalinosis and blockage that caused lacunar infarcts and also explained rupture of these diseased arteries that led to hemorrhages within the brain.

Later studies of deep infarcts during the 1970s led to another explanation for small deep infarcts.[17] The initial designation for this alternate pathology was "basilar branch infarcts" because the pathology was found in studying branches of the basilar artery. This pathology could also involve branches of the main arteries supplying the cerebral hemispheres and was labeled "intracranial branch atheromatous disease."[18] Figure 10.5 is an artist's drawing that shows this pathology. A small plaque in the parent artery blocks flow into the penetrating artery branch (Figure 10.5A); or the

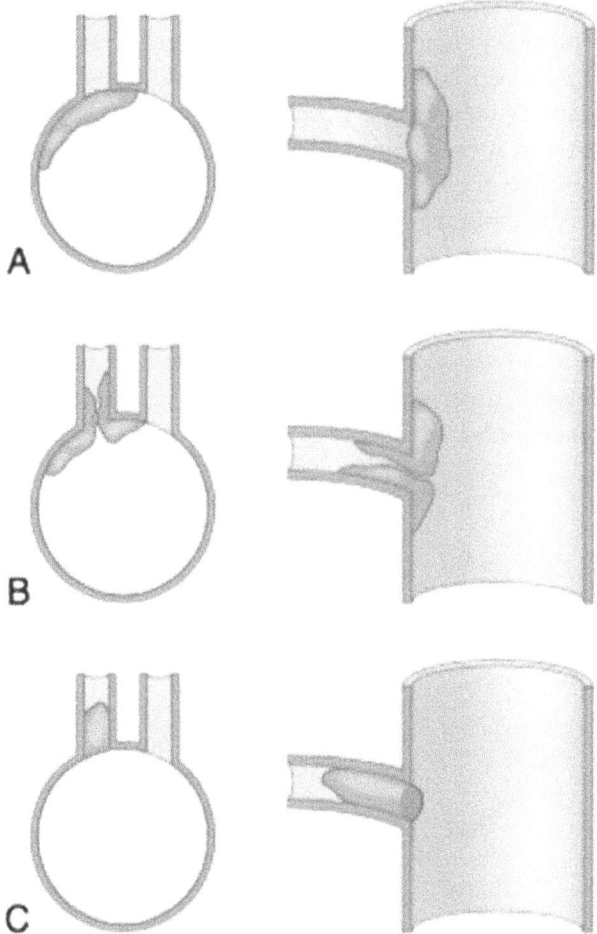

Figure 10.5 Drawing showing the arterial pathology in atheromatous branch disease. (A) Plaque in parent artery obstructing a branch. (B) Junctional plaque extending into the branch. (C) Microatheroma formed at the orifice of a branch.
Source: Reprinted with permission from Caplan LR. *Caplan's Stroke: A Clinical Approach* (5th ed.). Cambridge, UK: Cambridge University Press, 2016.

plaque extends into the branch and blocks flow (Figure 10.5B); or a tiny lipid collection, a "microatheroma," forms at the orifice of the branch and blocks it (Figure 10.5C).

These pathologies (lipohyalinosis and atheromatous branch disease) caused brain infarcts explained by reduction of blood flow. The locations deep within the brain and the size, shape, and morphology of the resultant brain infarcts were quite different from those that were explained by disease referable to the heart and aorta and to the large arteries in the neck and head that supplied the brain with blood. The heart, aortic, and large artery pathology caused release into the circulation of particles (emboli) that traveled within the supply arteries to branches within the head. The size of the emboli determined what sized arteries were blocked. The emboli traveled in the direction of superficial branches and were unlikely to suddenly redirect into penetrating arteries that branched off of the main arteries at right angles (90°). The resultant infarcts were usually located more near the surface of the cerebrum and the cerebellum than solely in deeper brain regions. Figure 10.6 is an artist's depiction of one such superficial infarct.

Fisher taught that noting the location and size of brain infarcts, at first during postmortem examinations and later by brain imaging (CT and MRI scanning), should direct physicians to search for different causes and potentially different treatments for the two classes of infarcts—lacunes and superficial embolic brain infarcts.

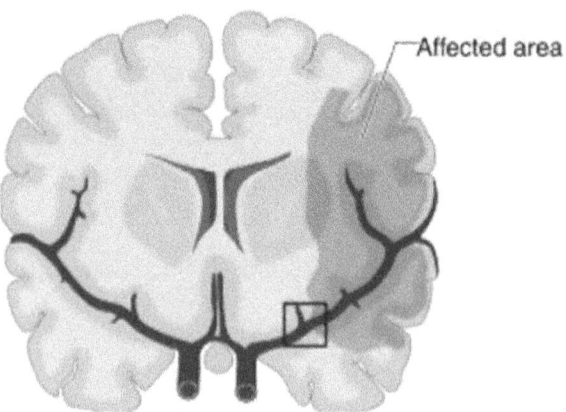

Figure 10.6 Artist's drawing of a superficial brain infarct caused by embolism. A thrombus that originated in the heart embolized to the middle cerebral artery (the site shown in the box), causing an embolic brain infarct.
Source: Reprinted with permission from Caplan LR. *Caplan's Stroke: A Clinical Approach* (5th ed.). Cambridge, UK: Cambridge University Press, 2016.

Concurrent with his examination of brains in the neuropathology laboratory, Fisher also explored the clinical findings in patients with lacunar infarcts. Could certain symptoms and signs found clinically reliably predict the presence of lacunar infarction? The first two clinical syndromes that he identified were pure motor and pure sensory strokes.[19] He examined patients who had important weakness of the face, arm, and leg on one side of the body in isolation—that is, no cognitive, behavioral, sensory, or other abnormalities. They all had lacunar infarcts in the internal capsule or pons. Other patients whose symptoms were purely sensory and included numbness or abnormal sensations limited to the face, body, arm, and leg on one side of the body without weakness, motor, cognitive, behavioral, or other abnormalities often had lacunar-type infarcts in the ventral lateral thalamus. In patients who were examined thoroughly and found to have either pure motor hemiparesis or pure sensory stroke syndromes, none had superficial infarcts at autopsy or by brain imaging when it became available. Later, Fisher added other syndromes—slurred speech with accompanying clumsiness of one hand (the "dysarthria clumsy hand syndrome")[20] and the combination of weakness and incoordination on one side of the body (ataxic hemiparesis)[21]—as entities for which clinicians could reliably predict that the cause was a lacunar stroke. In later years, Fisher authored reviews of the lacunar syndromes and their importance.[22]

HEMORRHAGES WITHIN AND OUTSIDE OF THE BRAIN

Fisher relied on studies that he performed in his neuropathological laboratory, the prior literature, and clinical observations to tackle the topic of hemorrhage within (intracerebral) and outside of the brain but inside the skull. Bleeding is the polar opposite of ischemia: In hemorrhage, there is too much blood in the head, whereas in ischemia, not enough blood is delivered to brain cells. The first major presentation of his findings concerning hemorrhage was at a March 1959 meeting at the Texas Medical Center that was organized by Dr. William Fields (Figure 10.7).[23] Fields had been a trainee with Fisher at Henry Ford Hospital, and they had remained close friends and esteemed colleagues.[24]

Fisher's presentation about the pathology of intracerebral hemorrhage began with a description of his own series of cases.[23] He had examined 134 brains that contained brain hemorrhages during a period of 3½ years. Most of the hemorrhages in patients with hypertension occurred at four sites: the basal ganglia, thalamus, pons, and cerebellum. (These were the

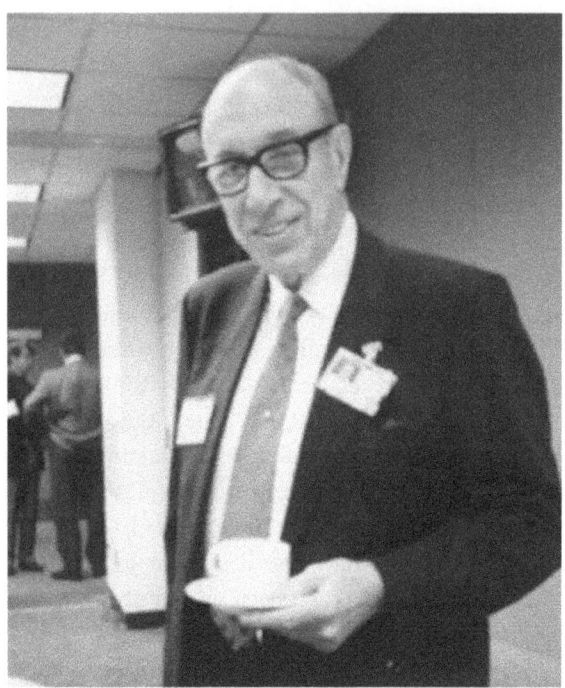

Figure 10.7 William S. Fields.
Source: Reprinted with permission from Caplan LR. *Caplan's Stroke: A Clinical Approach* (5th ed.). Cambridge, UK: Cambridge University Press, 2016.

same regions in which lacunar infarcts were found.) Some hemorrhages occurred in the cerebral lobes near the junction of the gray and white matter. Fisher noted, "In most of the 61 cases with a recent large hemorrhage, the hemorrhage was the cause of death and was usually massive, forming a clot 5, 8, or even 10 cm in extent."[25] The mass effect of the hemorrhage caused death by pressure on vital centers within the brainstem. Old smaller hemorrhages tended to spread and dissect along white matter tracts, often forming a slit-like cavity after the blood was absorbed. Although these small hematomas were not "harmless," clearly patients often made good recoveries. Before his time, most clinicians thought a brain hemorrhage was a uniformly fatal or devastating condition. Fisher attempted to define the bleeding site by injecting a neoprene solution into the intracranial artery that fed the hematoma region. In several specimens, the neoprene could be traced back to a leaking penetrating artery site. The hemorrhage had obliterated the rupture site within the artery that bled and so no definitive pathology that led to the leakage was discoverable.

Fisher commented,

> It is remarkable that hemorrhages arise from deep penetrating arteries and yet vessels of comparable size lying on the surface of the brain in the subarachnoid space rarely if ever rupture. The large arteries of the Circle of Willi (at the base of the brain) rupture only when saccular aneurysms are present. Some fundamentally important fact must underlie the difference between the behavior of penetrating and superficial arteries. A parallel might be drawn with the occurrence of occlusive atherosclerosis in the penetrating vessels with lacunar formation while similar lesions are rarely found in the superficial territories. It has been suggested that the small penetrating arteries are subjected to especially high pressures by virtue of their origins at right angles from the major arterial trunks at the base of the brain.[26]

Fisher continued his autopsy studies of brain hemorrhages and in 1971 published a seminal paper on his findings.[27] Studying hematomas in serial section, he noted that small globoid caps were often situated around the circumference of the hematoma. These caps represented bleeding capillaries or small arterioles. Figure 10.8 shows a diagram that he made of the bleeding globes in a patient who died of a hemorrhage in the brainstem. Fisher interpreted the circumferential bleeding sites as evidence that the hematomas developed gradually, with pressure effects beginning and maximal at the center of the hematomas. Pressure-related damage developed sequentially to vessels on the periphery of the expanding hematoma.

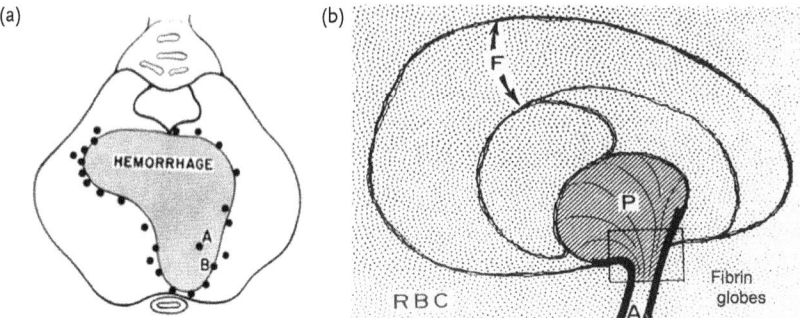

Figure 10.8 Fisher's drawings of a necropsy specimen of a patient who died of a pontine hemorrhage. (A) Along the circumference of the hemorrhage, dots mark the presence of fibrin globes that represent recently ruptured capillaries. (B) View of the fibrin globes that represent enlarged capillaries or arterioles; platelets (P) are in the center, and fibrin (F) is on the periphery. A, artery; RBC, red blood cells.
Source: From Fisher CM. Pathological observations in hypertensive cerebral hemorrhages. *Journal of Neuropathology and Experimental Neurology* 1971;30:536–550. Reprinted with permission from Caplan LR. *Caplan's Stroke: A Clinical Approach* (5th ed.). Cambridge, UK: Cambridge University Press, 2016.

Hypertension caused a penetrating artery to rupture. Often, this occurred when the hypertension first developed. Hemorrhages would begin small. Pressure in the center due to the high pressure within the leaking artery exerted force on vessels at the periphery, causing them in turn to bleed. The hematoma grew on its outer circumference much like a snowball rolling downhill. This process of growth of the hematoma would stop if and when the hematoma drained onto the brain or ventricular surface, and in so doing partially decompressed itself. Alternatively, tissue pressure and intracranial pressure external to the hematoma would increase until pressures inside and outside the hematoma equalized. The clinical course of patients with brain hematomas corresponded to what would be expected from gradual enlargement of the lesions.

Fisher commented,

> *When hemorrhage occurs when the patient is under observation, it will be found that the deficit comes not instantaneously but gradually and steadily over an appreciable length of time, possibly 10 minutes or a few hours or even a few days (rarely 7 to 14 days). This is to be contrasted with the fluctuating intermittency of signs in cerebral thrombosis and the lightning like development of signs in cerebral embolism.*[28]

Before Fisher, most authors described sudden-onset, maximal at onset symptoms and signs. Fisher analyzed the clinical findings in patients with hematomas found at the common sites for hypertensive intracerebral hemorrhage: putamen, thalamus, pons, and cerebellum.[29] He systematically noted the positioning and movement of the eyes; pupillary responses; abnormalities of movement and sensation; any accompanying reflex abnormalities; and alteration of alertness and speech and cognitive functions. Clearly, his experience in meticulously and thoroughly examining patients with stupor and coma had prepared him to make these important and novel clinical observations that contrasted the finding in patients with hematomas at various sites. These observations were also generally applicable to conditions other than hemorrhages (e.g., brain infarcts, tumors, and abscesses) and became key patterns that taught brain localization to young neurologists.

These descriptions of the clinical findings found in patients with hematomas at the various sites occurred B.C. (i.e., before CT scans). Hematomas during that time could only be diagnosed if corroborated at autopsy or if they caused blood in the spinal fluid or mass effect on cerebral angiography. Only the larger hematomas were diagnosed so that the clinical findings described at that time by Fisher applied only to larger hematomas.

When CT and, later, MRI became available, Fisher and colleagues were able to add descriptions of smaller hematomas, some within the subdivisions of the pons, thalamus, and basal ganglia.

Fisher and colleagues, in a very important benchmark paper published in 1965, described the clinical findings that they thought would improve clinical recognition of cerebellar hemorrhage.[30] Before this report, there was no consensus on how to diagnose hemorrhages or infarcts in the cerebellum. The authors of a 1942 report that described 15 new patients who had cerebellar hemorrhages and reviewed the 109 cases previously reported concluded that there was no consistent pattern of symptoms and signs in patients with cerebellar hemorrhages (most of whom died).[31] In 1960, an esteemed London neurosurgeon, Wylie McKissock, reviewed his experience with cerebellar hemorrhage and concluded,

> *The neurological signs presented by these patients were in the main singularly unhelpful. Localizing signs could not be elicited in those patients who were unconscious except that most of them had constricted and non-reactive pupils and periodic respirations. In the conscious patients, signs of cerebellar dysfunction were present in less than half.*[32]

Fisher and colleagues' report described in detail the findings in 3 patients who had cerebellar hemorrhages.[30] After the paper had been accepted, the authors mentioned in an addendum that they had since seen 8 additional patients in whom the rules derived from the original 3 patients had allowed the diagnosis of cerebellar hemorrhages that were confirmed at surgery.[30] Fisher and colleagues emphasized the importance of several clinical findings. All patients vomited and lost the ability to stand unsupported or walk unaided. Another very important abnormality, previously not emphasized, was noted when observing the position and movement of the eyes. Cerebellar hemorrhage patients developed an inability to gaze with both eyes or an abducting eye to one side.[33] Fisher had previously emphasized that patients who had hemorrhages in the deep portion of one cerebral hemisphere often had deviation of both eyes to the side of the hemorrhage and had difficulty looking to the other side. All had paralysis of the limbs on the side of the body opposite to the region of bleeding. But in the cerebellar hemorrhage patients with eye deviation, none had weakness or paralysis of the limbs on one side of the body. So eye deviation without one-sided paralysis was virtually diagnostic of cerebellar hemorrhage in the patients studied. Some patients developed bilateral increased deep tendon reflexes and Babinski signs. Headache, neck stiffness, limb incoordination, slurred speech, and dizziness were variable findings. Because at the time there was no definitive brain imaging available, Fisher and colleagues urged surgical exploration when the clinical signs were typical. In fact, it was a surgical emergency because of the mass effect on the brainstem created by the cerebellar hematoma mass. Later, several large clinical series of patients with cerebellar hemorrhages corroborated the frequency of the symptoms and signs noted in this report.[34]

Fisher had confidence in his ability to diagnose cerebellar hemorrhages at the bedside. This was illustrated in his discussion of a case he was asked to present at a conference; the discussion was published in the prestigious *New England Journal of Medicine* in 1967, 2 years after his seminal report.[35] The patient was a 48-year-old hypertensive man who one morning suddenly developed headache and vertigo. He walked to the bathroom, but when he tried to return, he fell to his knees. He was unable to walk and crawled back to his bed. He vomited twice. He later tried to walk but could not, consistently leaning and veering to the left. When seen at the hospital, examination showed a stuporous man whose eyes were deviated to the right and could not be moved to the left side. He did not have paralysis on one side of the body. A neurosurgeon made incisions in both the right and left sides of the cerebellum and found no hemorrhage or other abnormality. The patient died, and Fisher was invited to discuss the case and to predict the findings at autopsy. In his formulation of the diagnosis, the abnormality of eye movement was the most important sign. Vomiting, inability to walk, and absence of one-sided paralysis were other typical findings in Fisher's previously examined patients with cerebellar hemorrhage. Fisher concluded, "In summary, so strongly do the clinical signs in the case point to cerebellar hemorrhage that I am obliged to make that diagnosis despite the negative surgical exploration. In fact, no other diagnosis comes to mind."[35] The autopsy showed a large left cerebellar hemorrhage (Figure 10.9), as Fisher had predicted.

Fisher and colleagues also made important observations in patients whose hemorrhages involved regions outside the brain. Typically, these subarachnoid hemorrhages were caused by leakage of aneurysms or vascular malformations. Subarachnoid refers to the location of the blood; bleeding is distributed under one of the brain coverings called the arachnoid membrane that lies just outside of the brain substance. Pathologists described aneurysms located on large arteries at the base of the brain in 1814.[36] These aneurysms had, at autopsy, been shown to rupture and cause death. And yet the linkage between aneurysmal rupture and the syndrome of aneurysmal subarachnoid hemorrhage was not made until 1924. Sir Charles Symonds, a British neurologist, during his mentorship with neurosurgeon Harvey Cushing in Boston first used the term subarachnoid

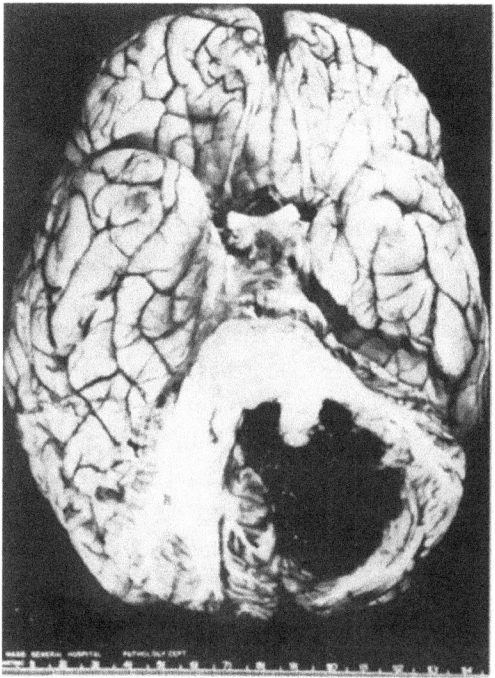

Figure 10.9 Brain at autopsy showing a very large left cerebellar hemorrhage (black region located at the bottom right of the figure).
Source: Reproduced with permission from Fisher CM, Richardson EP. Sudden headache and vertigo in a man with hypertension: Case 35-1967. *New England Journal of Medicine* 1967;277:423–428.

hemorrhage, described the clinical features, and identified aneurysmal rupture as the usual cause.[37]

Fisher maintained a long-term interest in subarachnoid bleeding, and he and Raymond Adams reviewed the then current treatment of aneurysmal subarachnoid bleeding in 1960.[38] But it was not until the advent of CT scanning during the 1970s that Fisher and colleagues were able to make further contributions to the care of patients with ruptured aneurysms. The presence and clinical features related to the initial aneurysm rupture and rerupture were widely known. Fisher observed that often during the end of the first week after aneurysmal rupture, patients would develop focal neurological deficits unrelated to rupture of an aneurysm. Sometimes, CT scans in these patients would show a localized brain infarct. At autopsy, infarcts were found within the brain substance. Fisher and colleagues Glenn Roberson, a neuroradiologist, and Bob Ojemann, a neurosurgeon, called this condition delayed ischemic deficit (DID) and studied the relationship of the ischemic lesions to constriction of intracranial arteries ("vasospasm") shown by angiography.[39] They reported in 1977 on the results of a study of 50 patients who had verified intracranial ruptured saccular aneurysms among whom half developed a DID, most often on day 8 after the initial bleed.[39] All of the DID patients had severe vasospasm shown by cerebral angiography. In their study, vasospasm accounted for all DIDs; in the absence of vasospasm, DID did not occur. Before this report, others had concluded that there was no clinical picture consistently present coincident with cerebral vasospasm.[40] With the aid of Phil Kistler, a former MGH Stroke Fellow, Fisher and colleagues analyzed the relation of the amount and localization of the blood to the development of vasospasm. They grouped patients according to the CT findings: Group 1, No detectable blood on CT; Group 2, Diffuse blood that was not dense enough to represent a large, thick homogenous clot; Group 3, Dense collection of blood that represented a clot greater than 1 mm thick in the vertical plane or greater than 5 × 3 mm in longitudinal and transverse dimension in the horizontal plane; and Group 4, Intracerebral or intraventricular clots but with only diffuse blood or no blood in the basal cisterns.[41] This method of grading blood on CT scan in patients with subarachnoid hemorrhage became widely known as the "Fisher scale," which is used even today.

In his memoirs, Fisher noted,

> *The site of vasospasm in the angiogram could be accurately correlated with the location and amount of subarachnoid blood seen in the CT scan. This has probably been confirmed as a reliable finding and strongly suggests that a chemical constituent within the blood clot is the agent responsible for the spasm.*[42]

Fisher's studies on subarachnoid hemorrhage stimulated later research on the nature of the substances that trigger vasospasm and its management.

NOTES

1. Fisher CM. *Memoirs of a Neurologist*. Rutland, VT: Sharp, 2006, Vol. 2, pp. 501–504.
2. Fisher was aware of animal studies reported in Bremer F. *Some Problems in Neurophysiology*. London: Athlone Press, 1953; Moruzzi G, Magoun HW. Brain stem reticular formation and stimulation of the EEG. *Electroencephalography and Clinical Neurophysiology* 1949;1:455–473; and Starzl TE, Taylor CW, Magoun HW. Ascending conduction in reticular activating system with special reference to the diencephalon. *Journal of Neurophysiology* 1951;14:461–477.
3. Fisher CM. The neurological examination of the comatose patient. *Acta Neurologica Scandinavica* 1969;49(Suppl. 6):4–57.

4. Fisher CM. *Memoirs of a Neurologist.* Rutland, VT: Sharp, 2006, Vol. l, p. 133.
5. One important study of reflex eye movements cited by Fisher was Klingon GH. Caloric stimulation in localization of brainstem lesions in a comatose patient. *Archives of Neurology and Psychiatry* 1952;68:233–235.
6. Descriptions of abnormalities of the pupil and eye movements are contained in Fisher CM. Oval pupils. *Archives of Neurology* 1980;37:502–503; Fisher CM. Some neuro-ophthalmologic observations. *Journal of Neurology, Neurosurgery, and Psychiatry* 1967;30:383–392; Fisher CM. Ocular bobbing. *Archives of Neurology* 1964;11:543–546; Fisher CM. Dilated pupil in carotid occlusion. *Transactions of the American Neurological Association* 1966; 91:230–231; and Fisher CM. Ocular flutter. *Journal of Clinical Neuro-Ophthalmology* 1990;10:155–156.
7. Fisher CM. Facial pulses in internal carotid artery occlusion. *Neurology* 1970;20:476–478.
8. Fisher CM. Palpation of arteries in temporal arteritis. *Journal of the American Medical Association* 1961;11:335–336; Fisher CM. Ocular palsy in temporal arteritis. *Minnesota Medicine* 1959;42:1258–1268, 1430–1437, 1617–1630.
9. Fisher CM. A simple test of coordination of the fingers. *Neurology* 1960;10:745–746.
10. Fisher CM. An improved test of motor coordination in the lower limbs. *Neurology* 1961;11:335–336.
11. Fisher CM. The clinical picture in occult hydrocephalus. *Clinical Neurosurgery* 1977;24:270–284. Fisher CM. Hydrocephalus as a cause of disturbance of gait in the elderly. *Neurology* 1982;32:1358–1363.
12. Durand-Fardel M. *Traite des ramollisements du cerveau.* Paris: Bailliere, 1843; Ferrand J. Essai sur l'hemiplegie des vieillards: les lacunes de desintegration cerebrale. Thesis, Paris, 1902; Marie P. Des foyers lacunaires de désintégration et des difféerents autres états cavitaires du cerveau. *Revue de Médeciné (Paris)* 1901;21:281–298.
13. Samuels later became the first full-time chief of the Department of Neurology at the Brigham and Women's Hospital and the Miriam Sydney Joseph Professor of Neurology, Harvard Medicine School.
14. Fisher CM. Lacunes, small deep cerebral infarcts. *Neurology* 1965;15:774–784.
15. Fisher CM. The vascular lesion in lacunae. *Transactions of the American Neurological Association* 1965;90:243–245; Fisher CM. The arterial lesions underlying lacunes. *Acta Neuropathologica* 1969;12:1–15.
16. During the time of these studies (1960s), there was not a very effective treatment for hypertension, and many individuals had uncontrolled high blood pressure.
17. Fisher CM, Caplan LR. Basilar artery branch occlusion: A cause of pontine infarction. *Neurology* 1971;21:900–905; Fisher CM. Bilateral occlusion of basilar artery branches. *Journal of Neurology, Neurosurgery, and Psychiatry* 1977;40:1182–1189.
18. Caplan LR. Intracranial branch atheromatous disease: A neglected, understudied and underused concept. *Neurology* 1989;39:1246–1250.
19. Fisher CM. Pure motor hemiplegia of vascular origin. *Archives of Neurology* 1965;13:30–44; Fisher CM. Pure sensory stroke involving face, arm, and leg. *Neurology* 1965;15:76–80; Fisher CM. Thalamic pure sensory stroke: A pathologic study. *Neurology* 1978;28:1141–1144; Fisher CM. Pure sensory stroke and allied conditions. *Stroke* 1982;13:434–447.
20. Fisher CM. A lacunar stroke, the dysarthria–clumsy hand syndrome. *Neurology* 1967;17:614–617.

21. Fisher CM, Cole M. Homolateral ataxia and crural paresis, a vascular syndrome. *Journal of Neurology, Neurosurgery, and Psychiatry* 1965;28:48–55; Fisher CM. Ataxic hemiparesis. *Archives of Neurology* 1978;35:126–128.
22. Fisher FM. Capsular infarcts. *Archives of Neurology* 1979;36:65–73; Fisher CM. Lacunar strokes and infarcts: A review. *Neurology* 1982;32:871–876.
23. Fisher CM. Pathology and pathogenesis of intracerebral hemorrhage in pathogenesis and treatment of cerebrovascular disease. In W Fields (Ed.), *Proceedings of the Annual Meeting of the Houston Neurological Society*. Springfield, IL: Charles C Thomas, 1961, pp. 295–317.
24. Fields devoted his entire career to advancing knowledge about cerebrovascular disease and stroke and caring for stroke patients.
25. Fisher CM. Pathology and pathogenesis of intracerebral hemorrhage in pathogenesis and treatment of cerebrovascular disease. In W Fields (Ed.), *Proceedings of the Annual Meeting of the Houston Neurological Society*. Springfield, IL: Charles C Thomas, 1961, p. 302.
26. Fisher CM. Pathology and pathogenesis of intracerebral hemorrhage in pathogenesis and treatment of cerebrovascular disease. In W Fields (Ed.), *Proceedings of the Annual Meeting of the Houston Neurological Society*. Springfield, IL: Charles C Thomas, 1961, p. 308.
27. Fisher CM. Pathological observations in hypertensive cerebral hemorrhages. *Journal of Neuropathology and Experimental Neurology* 1971;30:536–550.
28. Fisher CM. Clinical syndromes in cerebral hemorrhage in pathogenesis and treatment of cerebrovascular disease. In W Fields (Ed.), *Proceedings of the Annual Meeting of the Houston Neurological Society*. Springfield, IL: Charles C Thomas, 1961, p. 319.
29. Fisher CM. Clinical syndromes in cerebral hemorrhage in pathogenesis and treatment of cerebrovascular disease. In W Fields (Ed.), *Proceedings of the Annual Meeting of the Houston Neurological Society*. Springfield, IL: Charles C Thomas, 1961, pp. 318–342; Fisher CM. The pathological and clinical aspects of thalamic hemorrhage. *Transactions of the American Neurological Association* 1959;84:56–59; Walshe T, Davis K, Fisher CM. Thalamic hemorrhage, a computed tomographic–clinical correlation. *Neurology* 1977;29:217–222.
30. Fisher CM, Picard E, Polak A, Dalal P, Ojemann R. Acute hypertensive cerebellar hemorrhage: Diagnosis and surgical treatment. *Journal of Nervous and Mental Diseases* 1965;140:38–57.
31. Mitchell N, Angrist A. Spontaneous cerebellar hemorrhage: Report of fifteen cases. *American Journal of Pathology* 1942;18:935–953.
32. McKissock W, Richardson A, Walsh L. Spontaneous cerebellar hemorrhage. *Brain* 1960;83:1–9.
33. Fisher credited Dr. Herb Karp, his stroke fellow at that time, with calling his attention to the eye movement abnormality in the cerebellar hemorrhage patients. Karp was puzzled over this abnormality. Fisher CM. *Memoirs of a Neurologist*. Rutland, VT: Sharp, 2006, Vol. 1, pp. 134–135.
34. Brennan R, Berglund R. Acute cerebellar hemorrhage: Analysis of clinical findings and outcome in 12 cases. *Neurology* 1977;27:527–532; Ott K, Kase C, Ojemann R, et al. Cerebellar hemorrhage: Diagnosis and treatment. *Archives of Neurology* 1974;31:160–167; Kase CS. Cerebellar hemorrhage. In CS Kase, LR Caplan (Eds.), *Intracerebral Hemorrhage*. Boston: Butterworth-Heinemann, 1994, pp. 425–443.

35. A clinical–pathological discussion of a case seen at MGH. Fisher CM, Richardson EP. Sudden headache and vertigo in a man with hypertension: Case 35-1967. *New England Journal of Medicine* 1967;277:423–428.
36. The first pathological identification of aneurysms was probably made in Biumi F. Observations anatomicae, scholiis ilustratae: Observatio V. In: Sandifort E (Ed.), *Thesaurus Dissertationum*. Milan: Luchtmans, 1765 (reprinted 1778), Vol. 3, p. 373.
37. Symonds CP. Spontaneous subarachnoid haemorrhage. *Quarterly Journal of Medicine* 1924;18:93–123.
38. Fisher CM, Adams RD. Subarachnoid hemorrhage due to ruptured aneurysm. In Conn HF (Ed.), *Current Therapy*. Philadelphia: Saunders, 1960, pp. 523–524.
39. Fisher CM, Roberson GH, Ojemann RG. Cerebral vasospasm with ruptured saccular aneurysm: The clinical manifestations. *Neurosurgery* 1977;1:245–248;and later Fisher CM, Kistler JP, Davis JM. Relation of cerebral vasospasm to subarachnoid hemorrhage visualized by computerized tomographic scanning. *Neurosurgery* 1980;6(1):1–9.
40. A very influential neurologist, Dr. Clark Millikan, then the editor and the first editor of the journal *Stroke* and Professor of Neurology at the Mayo Clinic, published a study that denied that vasospasm had a role in causing DID: Millikan CH. Cerebral vasospasm and ruptured intracranial aneurysm. *Archives of Neurology* 1975;32(7):660–667.
41. Kistler JP, Crowell RM, Davis KR, Heros R, Ojemann RG, Zervas NT, Fisher CM. The relation of cerebral vasospasm to the extent and location of subarachnoid blood visualized by CT scan: A prospective study. *Neurology* 1983;33:424–437.
42. Fisher CM. *Memoirs of a Neurologist*. Rutland, VT: Sharp, 2006, Vol. 1, p. 158.

CHAPTER 11

Carotid Artery and Cerebral Atherosclerosis, Transient Ischemic Attacks, Symptoms and Signs Correlated with Lesions at Various Brain Locations, Cervical and Cranial Arterial Dissections, and Hydrocephalus and Gait Abnormalities

CAROTID ARTERY AND CEREBRAL ATHEROSCLEROSIS AND BRAIN ISCHEMIA AND INFARCTION

While in Montreal, Fisher became interested in studying the severity and location of abnormalities that involved the arteries within the neck and within the head that could serve as causes of stroke. With the help of the pathology dieners at Montreal General Hospital, he had collected specimens of the arteries that supplied the head. They were removed as continuous uninterrupted vessels that extended from the arch of the aorta, through the neck, and inside the head. These specimens showed the locations and severity of atherosclerosis and arterial narrowing within the circulatory system that fed the brain. In 1954, when an international research group visited Montreal, the group lauded Fisher on this remarkable collection. He did not publish the results of this study, but he continued his interest and activity in describing cervical and cerebral atherosclerosis after coming to Massachusetts General Hospital (MGH).

In 1965, Fisher along with Dr. Paul Dudley White, a prominent cardiologist, and two pathologists reported the results of a large series of postmortem examinations of the arterial system of patients studied at MGH.[1] They began their collection and analysis in 1960 and continued until 178 cases had been studied. The patients were predominantly Caucasian; there were 91 men and 87 women. They examined the aortas, coronary arteries, and the carotid and vertebral arteries in the neck and head and their intracranial branches. They introduced a grading system for the severity of atherosclerosis, considering the presence of flat and raised plaques, ulceration, calcification, and arterial narrowing in each area. They also studied changes over time and in reference to hypertension.[2]

In nearly all specimens, the aorta contained the most severe atherosclerosis, followed by the coronary arteries, carotid arteries in the neck, vertebral arteries in the neck, and intracranial arteries. Men showed an increase in atherosclerosis in their 40s and 50s, whereas women showed little atherosclerosis until the end of the sixth decade. Hypertension decreased the age of onset and increased the severity of atherosclerosis. In hypertensive patients, the intracranial arteries were slightly more often involved than the vertebral arteries in the neck. Within the carotid arterial system, the most severe atherosclerosis developed at the origin of the internal carotid arteries in the neck. The carotid siphon was the next most common area. Involvement of the common carotid artery was rarely severe. Occlusions of the internal carotid artery in the neck were often found. Within the vertebral arterial system, the most common site of severe atherosclerosis or occlusion was near the origin of the arteries from the subclavian arteries. Intracranial involvement was mostly at the first part of the basilar artery and at the end regions of the intracranial vertebral arteries. Thrombi were found in 42 (23%) of the cases.[1]

This published report became widely known as it corroborated Fisher's prior publications that indicated the importance of narrowing and occlusion of the carotid arteries within the neck.[3] This study also reinforced the observation that occlusive disease within the intracranial arteries (with the exception of the vertebral–basilar artery junction region) was uncommon.

Fisher understood that the availability of collateral blood flow was often important in determining the presence and extent of brain infarction after a vascular occlusion. He included in his studies of brains at autopsy a thorough analysis of the anatomy of the large arteries at the base of the brain—the circle of Willis. He studied and reported the results of the anatomical configuration of the circle of Willis among 414 unselected autopsies.[4] He noted whether the anomalous vessels were large or small. His report included diagrams of the anomalies found that were drawn by Edith Tagrin (Figure 11.1). This was the first detailed analysis of these anomalies.

Fisher also continued to study the pathology of carotid artery disease in his neuropathology laboratory. He discussed this project in his memoirs:

> *A most ambitious undertaking was the clinic–pathologic correlation of carotid endarterectomy plaques removed surgically by Dr. Robert Ojemann in the treatment of symptomatic carotid artery disease. Dr. Ojemann removed the plaque intact in one piece, placed it in formalin without incising it or disturbing the contents of the lumen. Again we turned to serial sectioning and each plaque provided hundreds of sections. . . . Some 150 specimens were processed and the piles of trays of slides literally filled a room. It was the first methodological study of such surgical specimens and the pathological findings within the artery could be correlated with the clinical symptoms the patient had been having in the days just prior to the operation.[5]*

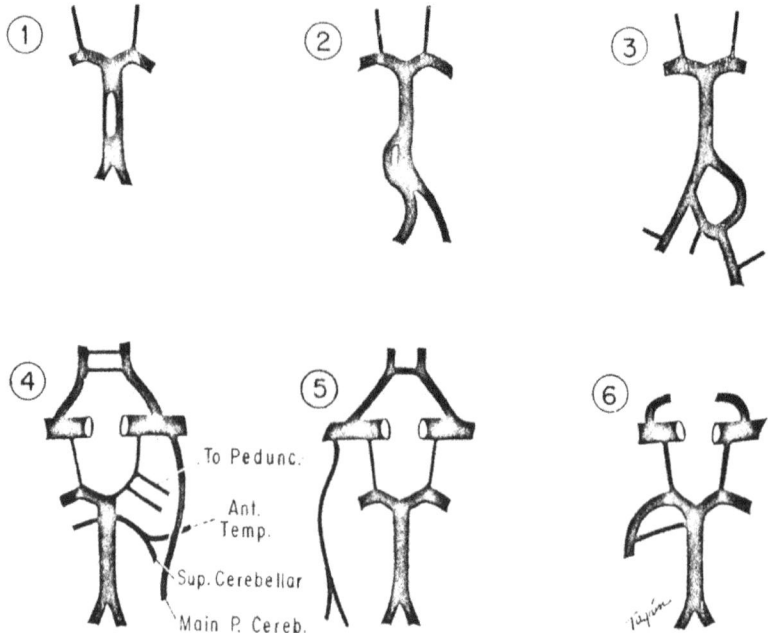

Figure 11.1 Anomalies of the circle of Willis. 1 and 2, fenestrations (windows) within the basilar artery; 3–6, unusual arteries arising from the main vertebral and basilar arteries.
Source: Reproduced with permission from Fisher CM. The circle of Willis: Anatomical variations. *Vascular Diseases* 1965;2(2):99–105. Drawings by Edith Tagrin.

The task of examining carotid artery specimens and correlating the findings with the clinical symptoms during life stretched over a period of 15 years.[6] Fisher divided the patients studied into those with temporary neurological symptoms, those with transient monocular blindness, those with strokes, and those who had no relevant symptoms. He concluded that many instances were not explained by recurrent microembolism alone.

TRANSIENT ISCHEMIC ATTACKS AND THE DIAGNOSIS OF CAROTID ARTERY DISEASE

While in Montreal, Fisher made important contributions concerning the importance of temporary neurological spells and transient and persistent eye ischemia in the diagnosis of carotid artery disease.[7] He was the first clinician to emphasize and describe the occurrence of prodromal, transient episodes that preceded and warned of an imminent stroke. He dubbed these spells transient ischemic attacks (TIAs), a designation that stuck and became popular.[8] By 1954, Fisher was a widely respected authority on brain ischemia and the carotid artery. He was invited to present material from his work and to discuss his ideas about cerebrovascular disease at the first American Conference on Cerebrovascular Disease held in Princeton, New Jersey. He commented on TIAs at that conference:

> *If a satisfactory history can be obtained ... one finds in a great many cases that there had been a warning prior to the stroke. The warnings may go back weeks or months. There may have been only one or as many as 500. Some of these very interesting cases lying in the wards are described simply as "had a stroke this morning" but in going into the details many premonitory symptoms may be elicited. I have seen a man with eight attacks a day for two months, each attack characterized by numbness around the lip, numbness of the thumb and index finger and drooping of the lip. Attacks occurred in physicians' offices. Finally the patient awakened one morning with a massive hemiplegia from which there has been practically no recovery.*[9]

Fisher emphasized the importance of recognizing the warning attacks, which gave physicians an opportunity to intervene and prevent a stroke from occurring. His work on carotid artery disease and its occurrence, pathology, symptom complex, evaluation, and treatment continued during his entire career at MGH. He reported that feeling the branches of the external carotid artery in the face could be a clinical clue in some patients that the internal carotid artery was occluded. Figure 11.2 shows these pulses, which Fisher labeled ABC for ready recall (angular, brow, and cheek).[10] He

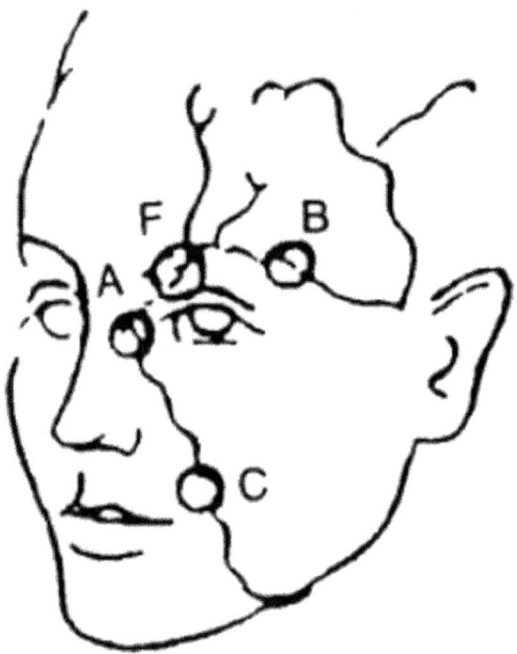

Figure 11.2 Artist's drawing of facial pulses. A, angular; B, brow; C, cheek; F, frontal.
Source: Reproduced with permission from Caplan LR. *Stroke, a clinical approach* (2nd ed.). Boston: Butterworth-Heinemann, 1993, p. 86.

also noted that carotid artery occlusion could be associated with dilation of the pupil on the side of the occlusion.[11]

A very important and often cited publication was his personal observation of the retina through an ophthalmoscope in a patient who developed blindness in one eye while hospitalized.[12] The patient was a pharmacist who had had many prior attacks of partial or total blindness in the left eye. He was sitting in a chair reading when, at 8:55 a.m. during a period of 1 minute, his vision failed in all fields of the left eye except the upper temporal quadrant. Vision remained unchanged when Fisher examined him 20 minutes after the onset of the attack. The visual loss lasted 1 hour. Fisher noted a whitish platelet embolus that blocked a main artery. The embolus moved during Fisher's examination of the eye. He included within his report his own drawings (Figure 11.3) and descriptions of the retinal arteries that changed as he watched.[12] This report emphasized the importance of careful observation of a single patient and the usefulness of looking in the eyes of individuals suspected of having carotid artery disease.

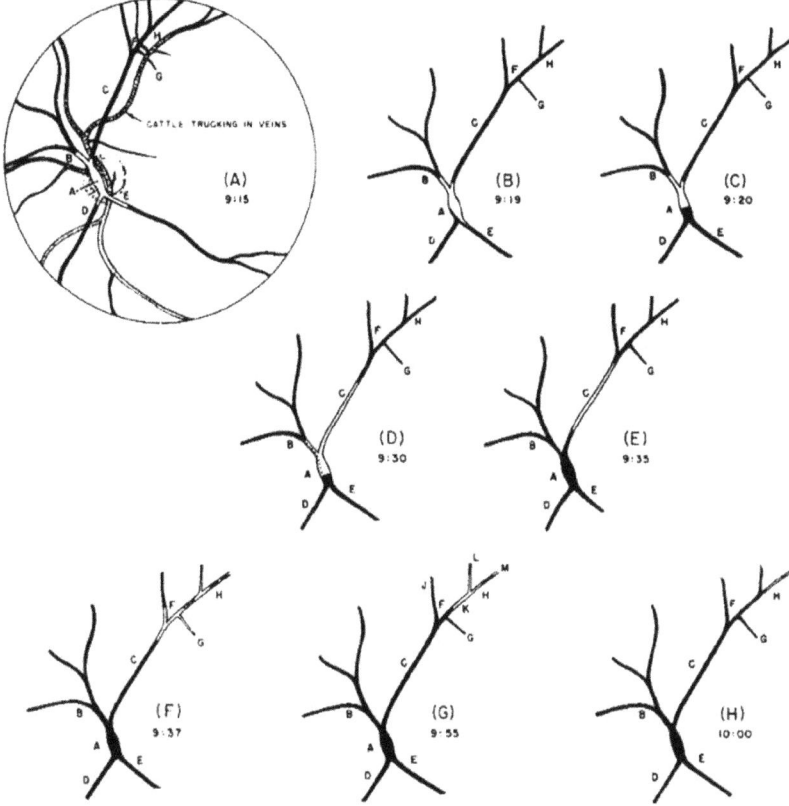

Figure 11.3 Fisher's drawings of the blood vessels of the left eye in a patient with transient left eye blindness. These drawings diagram the appearance of the retinal vessels at intervals during the period of blindness.
Source: Reproduced with permission from Fisher CM. Observations of the fundus oculi in transient monocular blindness. *Neurology* 1959;9:333–347.

Fisher worked closely with Dr. Robert Ackerman, who had developed a diagnostic laboratory at MGH that utilized ultrasound examinations of the neck and head to evaluate patients with suspected carotid and other arterial occlusive disease. Fisher and Ackerman noted that strokes seldom occurred in patients with carotid artery disease unless plaques narrowed the artery, leaving less than a 2-mm lumen for blood flow, and the patients developed symptoms. This was important because surgery on patients with carotid artery disease, even when individuals had no symptoms and the lumen of the artery was still widely open, had become widespread. Fisher noted that TIAs were due to "intermittent failure of flow in a compromised region. TIAs correlated best with severe carotid stenosis and when a stroke was imminent, the stenosis had advanced to virtual occlusion."[13]

Fisher, Ojemann, and colleagues commented extensively on the indications for carotid artery surgery in a meeting of the Congress of Neurological Surgeons held in 1975.[14] In later years, monitoring of the middle cerebral artery branch of the carotid artery by Ackerman and others showed that microembolism was common in patients with severely narrowed carotid arteries but mostly occurred without symptoms. When carotid artery blood flow became greatly diminished, the blood flow stream became inefficient at washing out these emboli and transient symptoms and strokes developed.[15]

In 1961, Fisher wrote an editorial concerning disease of the subclavian artery. He dubbed the entity described in an accompanying report the "subclavian steal syndrome."[16] In this condition, blockage of a subclavian artery—for example, the left—diminished blood flow in the left vertebral artery, the first large branch in the neck. Blood flowed from the right vertebral artery in the head and traveled down the left vertebral artery to the portion of the subclavian artery beyond the blockage to help supply blood to the left arm. In essence, blood was stolen from the brain to supply the arm. Fisher and colleagues also reported many studies of the symptoms and findings in patients who had occlusions of other blood vessels that supplied the brain. These included studies of the vertebral arteries in the neck and their branches in the head[17] and studies of the intracranial carotid artery and its branches.[18] Arguably Fisher's major contribution to the care of patients with cerebrovascular disease and brain ischemia and strokes was his lengthy descriptions and diagrams of the symptoms and signs in patients with occlusive cerebrovascular disease that appeared in textbooks of internal medicine and neurology. The first major presentation of this material was in a chapter included in a volume of the proceedings of a March 1959 meeting at the Texas Medical Center that was organized by Bill Fields.[19] The drawings and much of the text that Fisher presented at this meeting were later incorporated into chapters in very popular and widely read medical textbooks.

The involvement of Fisher in these texts illustrates the role of serendipity in explaining history: Luck and chance played a major role. During the early 1950s, Dr. Tinsley Harrison had organized a textbook of internal medicine. He and a group of renowned clinicians and internists were editors of the first edition of the *Principles of Internal Medicine*, which was published in 1950. Subsequent editions used the same title until the sixth edition published in 1971, when the work was retitled *Harrison's Principles of Internal Medicine*.[20] The editors decided to include a section on neurological function in the 1954 edition and sought an academic neurologist to write the section and, potentially, to also become an editor. They approached several individuals, including H. Houston Merritt, the Chair of Neurology at Colombia University; all declined, saying they were too busy.

Finally, they contacted Raymond Adams, the Chair of Neurology at MGH, who agreed to provide a neurology segment for the second edition of the textbook.[21] Adams submitted 15 chapters on various aspects of nervous system function, including discussions of topics usually considered psychiatric in nature, such as anxiety, depression, lassitude, sleep, and delirium. He also wrote elementary short chapters on typical neurological topics—cranial nerve, motor, sensory, speech, and equilibrium functions.[21]

Adams was made an editor of the third and subsequent editions of *Harrison's Principle of Internal Medicine*. A large section of neurology consisting of 157 pages was the largest single section devoted to organ functions in the third edition. All subsequent editions included large sections devoted to nervous system function. Harrison later joked that the textbook should have been called the *Principles of Internal Medicine and the Details of Neurology*.

Fisher, Karp (Fisher's stroke fellow), and Adams were the authors of a 46-page chapter on cerebrovascular disease and stroke in the third edition of Harrison's internal medicine textbook.[22] The text and diagrams from this chapter concerning the symptoms, signs, and management of individuals with cerebrovascular disease and stroke were included in all subsequent editions of the volume. Figures 11.4a and 11.4b are two of these diagrams. Fisher wrote the text and supervised the drawing of the diagrams; usage of virtually the same diagrams in his presentation as was published in the proceedings of the March 1959 meeting at the Texas Medical Center made it clear that the chapters were authored by him, with some editing and polishing by Adams. This tome of internal medicine became required reading for many medical students and internal medical trainees.[23]

Adams decided to incorporate much of the neurology text material published in Harrison's internal medicine volumes into a larger book aimed at neurology trainees and practicing neurologists. Co-authored with Dr. Maurice Victor, the book was titled *Principles of Neurology*.[24] This book also contained Fisher's long chapter on cerebrovascular disease with the very same diagrams that were featured in Harrison's text and Fisher's chapter in the Field's symposium. This neurology textbook became one of the most popular medical textbooks, read and referenced by nearly all trainees in neurology and owned and referred by most neurologists. Drs. Martin Samuels and Allan Ropper, trainees of Fisher and Adams, took over the editorship of Adams and Victor's text. Their edited volumes still contain an authoritative chapter on stroke and cerebrovascular disease that features many of Fisher's original diagrams (now some in color) and text, edited by his trainees (Mohr, Caplan, and Kistler). And so, perhaps, with the two previously mentioned seminal works and the contributions made by

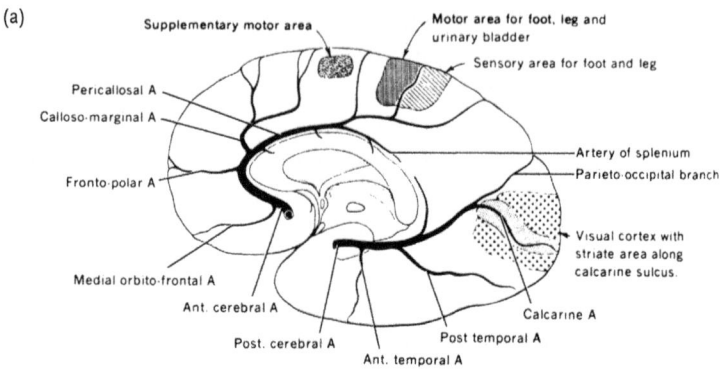

Signs and symptoms	Structures involved
Paralysis of opposite foot and leg	Motor leg area
A lesser degree of paresis of opposite arm	Involvement of arm area of cortex or fibers descending therefrom to corona radiata
Cortical sensory loss over toes, foot, and leg	Sensory area for foot and leg
Urinary incontinence	Posteromedial part of superior frontal gyrus (bilateral)
Contralateral grasp reflex, sucking reflex, gegenhalten (paratonic rigidity), "frontal tremor"	Medial surface of the posterior frontal lobe (?)
Abulia (akinetic mutism), slowness, delay, lack of spontaneity, whispering, motor inaction, reflex distraction to sights and sounds	Uncertain localization—probably superomedial lesion near subcallosum
Impairment of gait and stance (gait "apraxia")	Inferomedial frontal–striatal (?)
Mental impairment (perseveration and amnesia)	Localization unknown
Miscellaneous: dyspraxia of left limbs	Corpus callosum
	Corpus callosum
Tactile aphasia in left limbs	
Cerebral paraplegia	Motor leg area bilaterally (due to bilateral occlusion of anterior cerebral arteries)

Figure 11.4 Conttinued

Fisher, one of his major legacies was his role in educating medical students, internists, and neurologists in the fundamentals of cerebrovascular disease through his many chapters in authoritative, widely read textbooks.

DISSECTION OF BRAIN-SUPPLYING ARTERIES

Fisher and his surgical colleague Robert Ojemann were among the very first to call attention to dissection of arteries in the neck and head that supplied the brain.[25] At the time of their reports (the 1970s), arterial dissection was well known to occur in the aorta but was not often thought to involve systemic arteries in the neck, head, abdomen, and coronary circulations. Dissection refers to a mechanically or traumatically induced tear within the wall of an artery. The tear causes bleeding within the arterial wall that can spread (dissect) within the wall.[25] As had been true in many other

(b)

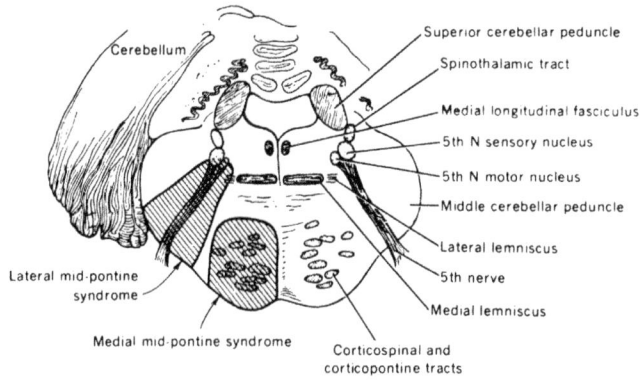

Signs and symptoms	Structures involved
1. Medial midpontine syndrome (paramedian branch of midbasilar artery)	
a. On side of lesion	
(1) Ataxia of limbs and gait (more prominent in bilateral involvement)	Middle cerebellar peduncle
b. On side opposite lesion	
(1) Paralysis of face, arm, and leg	Corticobulbar and corticospinal tract
(2) Deviation of eyes	
(3) Variably impaired touch and proprioception when lesion extends posteriorly. Usually the syndrome is purely motor.	Medial lemniscus
2. Lateral midpontine syndrome (short circumferential artery)	
a. On side of lesion	
(1) Ataxia of limbs	Middle cerebellar peduncle
(2) Paralysis of muscles of mastication	Motor fibers or nucleus of fifth nerve
(3) Impaired sensation over side of face	Sensory fibers or nucleus of fifth nerve

Figure 11.4 (A) Findings in patients with cerebral infarcts that involve the paramedian segments of the cerebral hemispheres. (B) Findings in patients with brainstem infarcts located in the pons. A, artery; Ant, anterior; N, nerve; Post, posterior.
Source: Diagrams and text reproduced with permission from Fisher CM. Clinical syndromes in cerebral arterial occlusion. In W Fields (Ed.), *Proceedings of the Annual Meeting of the Houston Neurological Society*. Springfield, IL: Charles C Thomas, 1961, pp. 151–181.

conditions that Fisher described, the first observation came from his pathology laboratory. He commented on this discovery in his memoirs:

> *It was largely a chance observation that contributed to the opening of the field of dissection of the carotid and cerebral arteries. Dr. Robert Ojemann and I had described the pathological findings in a patient with carotid obstruction whom he had operated on by removing the blocked segment. The diagnosis of dissection was established. Only 10 cases of carotid dissection had been previously described in the literature and almost all had been fatal. Our patient's angiogram had shown a thin column of dye in the carotid where the lumen was compromised by blood dissecting in the wall of the artery. Three of the cases in the literature had a somewhat similar appearance. The*

narrow column of dye was termed "the string sign" and tentatively it was suggested that it might be a sign of dissection. Not long afterwards there was admitted to the hospital another stroke patient with the string sign on angiography. . . . After the introduction of the "string sign" as a diagnostic clue, it was not long before we were consulted concerning numerous cases far and wide. The "string sign" was extended to dissection in other arteries, middle cerebral, vertebral, and posterior cerebral and the ranks of obscure strokes underwent further shrinkage.[26]

Recognition of the findings on angiography led Fisher to be able to diagnose arterial dissection clinically. He then analyzed and reported the major clinical features found in subsequent patients with arterial dissections in the neck diagnosed angiographically: neck pain, headache, Horner's syndrome, pulsatile tinnitus (in patients with carotid artery dissection), and focal neurological signs due to embolism of clot material from the region of dissection in the neck. Later, he and his colleagues reported instances of arterial dissection involving the internal carotid and other arteries within the skull and the associated clinical symptoms and signs.[27] By the later years of the 20th century, arterial dissection had become a relatively common and important diagnosis. The string sign and other details originally described by Fisher, Ojemann, and colleagues became important in rendering a diagnosis of arterial dissection.

HYDROCEPHALUS AND GAIT ABNORMALITIES, ESPECIALLY IN OLDER ADULTS

An excess of water within the ventricles of the brain (hydrocephalus, which literally means water in the head) was a well-known condition in infants and children. Before computed tomography (CT) scanning was introduced during the mid-1970s, it was not a common diagnosis in adults. The causes and neurological symptoms and signs that accompanied the development of hydrocephalus in adults had not been well studied or described. In adults, most physicians assumed that the ventricles became enlarged because of loss of brain tissue. The brain and its fluid contents are contained and restrained in a closed system surrounded by the hard skull bones. When brain substance was lost, the water content inside of the skull increased to take up the space previously occupied by the lost brain tissue. The symptoms and findings in these adults, often geriatric patients, were attributed to the loss of brain tissue (atrophy) and not to the supposed compensatory increased ventricular water content—hydrocephalus.[28]

Before Fisher's time, there was almost no information about the symptoms and signs that were attributable to hydrocephalus. These signs could not be separated from the brain conditions that caused the ventricles to enlarge: brain atrophy, tumors, traumatic injuries, and bleeding. An observation in a single patient led to further clarification of the symptoms and signs attributable to hydrocephalus. The patient was a 59-year-old woman, the wife of a businessman from Colombia, South America. Dr. Solomon Hakim, a neurosurgeon from Bogota, Colombia, referred the patient to Raymond Adams in Boston because of "mental and physical slowness."[29] She was hospitalized at MGH in 1959. She had become forgetful and had difficulty concentrating. Fisher was consulted. He noted that she had a "peculiar wobbling" gait and had become incontinent of urine. The first diagnostic lumbar pressure had shown that the fluid was under normal pressure. The major available study at that time, decades before the availability of CT scanning, was a pneumoencephalogram. This procedure was performed by injecting air into the spinal fluid through a lumbar puncture performed in the patient's back. The air ascended and went into the ventricles and surrounded the brain after exiting the ventricles. This study showed striking enlargement of the ventricles and delayed emptying of the gas that was introduced (Figure 11.5). After the pneumoencephalogram, her function worsened. Adams noted that she became stuporous: She

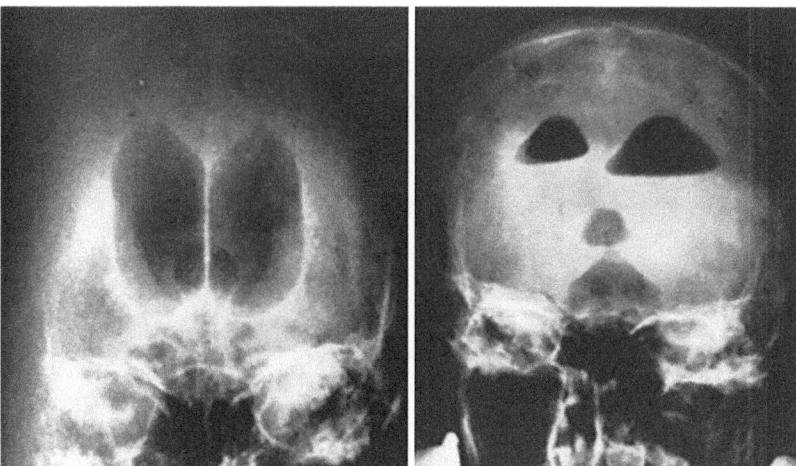

Figure 11.5 X-rays of the skull after air has been inserted into the lumbar cerebrospinal fluid. (Left) Very large lateral ventricles distended with air. (Right) A later X-ray that shows air remaining in the ventricles. The ventricles in the upper part of the image are the lateral ventricles. The round air-filled midline structure below is the third ventricle. The triangular air-filled structure below the third ventricle is the fourth ventricle. There is no air around the brain.
Source: Reproduced with permission from Adams RD, Fisher CM, Hakim S, Ojemann RG, Sweet WH. Symptomatic occult hydrocephalus with "normal" cerebrospinal fluid pressure (a treatable syndrome). *New England Journal of Medicine* 1965;273:117–126.

would not speak and was inattentive to everything going on about her. Fisher described her as "severely abulic (akinetic mute), lying awake, silent, immobile, unresponsive to all stimuli except pain, and incontinent of bladder and bowel."[30] She remained completely inactive during the ensuing 5 weeks. A repeat lumbar puncture showed that the fluid removed was under abnormally high pressure. Adams commented, "We were appalled by what had happened as was her husband. . . . Not knowing what to do I asked Dr. William Sweet to drain the ventricle."[31] A ventricular drain was placed. To her treating physicians' astonishment, during the next week

> she was back to not only the state in which she entered the hospital, but, according to her husband, she had regained her normal level of mentation. She proved to be an intelligent woman; her gait returned to normal. . . . She was buying cookies for our residents, knew them all by name and joked about their affairs.[31]

Six weeks after the ventricular shunting, the patient fell and broke her hip. Two days after the fall, she returned to the mute unresponsive state that preceded shunting. Her doctors discovered that the plastic connector of the shunt tubing that had been placed by Sweet had become disconnected as a result of the fall. Effective cerebrospinal fluid drainage was reestablished 6 days after the fall. She improved dramatically during the next 24 hours, and she continued to improve thereafter. One month later, her family reported that she had returned to her normal self with full restoration of memory, animation, and intellect, and she walked normally and was no longer incontinent. The patient was followed for the next 6 years, during which she remained in excellent health.

Fisher commented in his memoirs,

> Review of the puzzling course of events suggested that her illness was not due to cerebral atrophy and resultant ventricular enlargement, but more likely was related to the communicating hydrocephalus. Furthermore, the hydrocephalus must have caused symptoms because the shunting had caused their disappearance. The temporary exacerbation of symptoms when the shunt tubing was damaged proved that the relief of symptoms was related to the shunting.[32]

Further proof that the clinical syndrome was attributable to the hydrocephalus came when she returned to normal after shunting the fluid out of the enlarged ventricle occurred following the shunt blockage. Recognition of the symptoms and signs in this single patient led Fisher, Adams, and Hakim to seek other patients with hydrocephalus and to further analyze and describe their findings and the effect of treatment. This case and the subsequent analyses are an excellent example of the quote of Louis Pasteur: "In the field of observation chance favours only the prepared mind."[33] Fisher, Adams, and Hakim clearly had minds that were prepared to learn and profit from this single patient experience.[34] Hakim and Adams published a report in 1965 concerning two patients described in detail and others mentioned briefly who had developed hydrocephalus and had benefitted from shunting.[35] One patient was a 16-year-old boy who developed symptoms a month after head injury that had caused bleeding in the subarachnoid space around the brain; the other patient was a 52-year-old man. In another patient, significant improvement in symptoms occurred after removing fluid by lumbar puncture. Spinal fluid pressures were not elevated. The major portion of this report was devoted to discussion of cerebrospinal fluid hydrodynamics that explained how the ventricles could become quite enlarged and yet the pressure within the ventricles and fluid still remain normal.[35]

In 1965, Adams, Fisher, and Hakim wrote a landmark report published in the *New England Journal of Medicine* about their experience with adult patients with hydrocephalus who had improved after shunting of fluid.[36] This paper was widely cited and has remained one of the most frequently referenced papers even up to the present time. The first patient was the woman from Bogota described previously. The second patient was a 62-year-old pediatrician in whom a pneumoencephalogram showed a cyst in the third ventricle that blocked cerebrospinal fluid flow: "The symptomatology was unobtrusive having no assignable date of onset, and evolved over a period of weeks or a few months."[36] The major symptoms in these and the other patients included unsteadiness of gait, loss of spontaneity and initiative, poor concentration, apathy, general lack of interest, slowness, and distractibility. All had urinary incontinence, two only after the pneumoencephalogram. One patient improved temporarily after removal of a large amount of fluid by lumbar puncture. Spinal fluid pressures measured by lumbar puncture were within normal levels. The authors concluded, "An important aspect of the present study is that it has permitted for virtually the first time a clear delineation of the specific symptomatology of chronic hydrocephalus in general."[36] Prior theories had attributed the enlargement of the ventricles to high pressures. Because in their materials the measured spinal fluid pressures were often normal, the authors chose to call the syndrome normal pressure hydrocephalus (NPH). Fisher commented in his memoirs, "What was new was the conclusion that hydrocephalus with normal pressure could be symptomatic in its own right and that reducing the pressure to still lower levels could relieve the symptoms."[37]

One of Fisher's most notable behavioral characteristics during his entire career was his perseverance with projects. Once started, he continued to study and analyze in order to settle questions left unclear initially. This attribute was despite the fact that he had many continued projects, all of which he continued to juggle simultaneously. His continued pursuit of gait abnormalities and their cause and relationship to hydrocephalus is an example of this attribute.

Fisher commented after study of the initial patient from Bogota,

Subsequent cases led to the formulation of the NPH syndrome consisting of dementia, psychomotor retardation, slowness, paucity of thought and action, unsteadiness of gait and urinary incontinence. Lack of spontaneity and initiative, faulty concentration, distractability, lack of interest, apathy and inertia were other terms that were used. The onset was unobtrusive and had no assignable date.[38]

Four years after the *New England Journal of Medicine* report, Ojemann, Fisher, and colleagues published their 10-year further experience in patients with hydrocephalus.[39] They described 28 patients, 12 in detail, 2 of whom had been described in the original report. These patients all had the gradual development during weeks to months of impaired memory, physical and mental slowness, unsteadiness of gait, and urinary incontinence. Four of the patients had had subarachnoid hemorrhages in the past; 3 had had serious head trauma years before; 1 had a febrile illness, most likely meningitis years before; and 2 had obstructing lesions in the third ventricle. In 5 of the patients with hydrocephalus, the enlargement of the ventricles was attributable to brain atrophy due to probable Alzheimer disease. None of the patients with Alzheimer disease improved after shunting. All of the other patients showed improvement, some partial.[39]

Fisher continued to study patients he personally examined and treated who had hydrocephalus. In 1977, he reported an analysis of 30 of his own patients.[40] Among these patients, 16 had definite sustained improvement after shunting, 1 had only temporary improvement, 11 showed no definite improvement, and in 2 patients an effective shunt was not established. The report emphasized the nature of the symptoms and their sequential appearance. Gait abnormalities were most often the first symptom. Gait abnormalities were prominent in all the patients who improved after shunting. Patients who presented with mentation difficulties before the development of gait difficulty or at the same time as altered gait failed to improve. Urinary incontinence often developed later. Some patients had spells of falling or leg weakness.[40]

In 1982, fully two decades after the first patient was seen, Fisher reported another series of patients.[41] By this time, CT scanning had become available. All patients were older than age 60 years, and gait abnormalities were a prominent complaint. The gait abnormality often began as imbalance or falling. Navigating curbs and stairs became difficult. The patients described weakness or tiredness of the legs on walking. As the gait abnormality worsened, steps became shorter and shuffling; scuffing of the feet on the ground developed, and turning became very slow and precarious and was performed using multiple small steps. When the lower extremities were examined in bed or in a chair, no strength or reflex abnormalities were found. Fisher reviewed his notes on 60 gait abnormality patients who had been previously seen and on another 49 who were prospectively studied. Among the 109 patients, another diagnosis (neurological, orthopedic, rheumatologic, etc.) explained the walking abnormality. Fisher also analyzed 50 patients in whom gait abnormality was not explained. Most patients were older than age 70 years: 42% were aged 70–79 years, and 38% were older than 80 years.[41]

After these studies, Fisher directed his attention to a somewhat different but related question:

> Cases of unexplained gait disturbance in the elderly are not uncommon. When several patients followed for several years because of unsteadiness on their feet proved in the long run to have symptomatic NPH that was corrected or relieved to some extent by shunting, the question became, to what extent might NPH account for the large number of cases of unexplained gait disturbance in the elderly.[42]

He began to pay attention to the size of the ventricles found on imaging studies of the brain. Using an ordinary ruler, he measured the span of the ventricles on CT scans in their most frontal location using prescribed directions for acquiring the scans and for their magnification, and he identified the individual scan on which to make the measurement. An example of the measurement to be taken is displayed as Figure 11.6. Among the 50 patients with unexplained gait difficulties, 46 had ventricular spans greater than 12 mm, whereas only 5 of 80 control patients (6.3%) had spans greater than 12 mm. He concluded that there was a "strong correlation between unexplained disturbance of walking in the elderly and ventricular enlargement."[43] Seven of the patients with large ventricles were shunted and their walking improved. Walking temporarily improved in 10 others. Some of the patients walked better after lumbar punctures that removed a large volume of cerebrospinal fluid.[41,43]

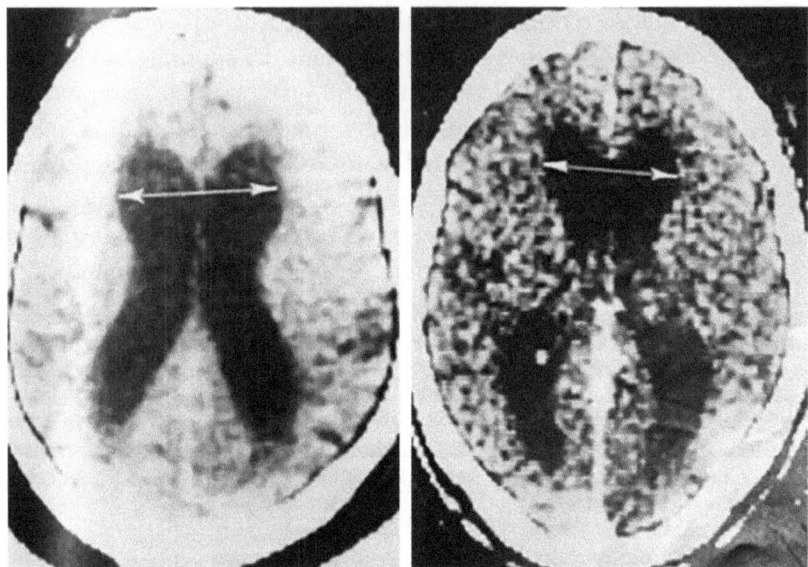

Figure 11.6 CT scans. The white arrows show the span measurement used by Fisher.
Source: Reproduced with permission from Fisher CM. Hydrocephalus as a cause of disturbances of gait in the elderly. *Neurology* 1982;32:1358–1363.

During nearly a quarter of a century, Fisher and colleagues, especially Adams, Ojemann, and Hakim, had brought hydrocephalus to the forefront of investigation. Fisher had also drawn attention to the common problem of walking difficulty and falls in the elderly—their nature, causes, and management.

NOTES

1. Fisher CM, Gore I, Okabe N, White PD. Atherosclerosis of the carotid and vertebral arteries—Extracranial and intracranial. *Journal of Neuropathology and Experimental Neurology* 1965;24:455–476.
2. The only detailed prior study of the arteries was by Dr. A. B. Baker, a Minnesota neurologist, and his colleague Dr. Iannone. These authors reported the presence and location and morphology of atherosclerosis of arteries within the head, emphasizing the presence of calcification, and did not include studies of the neck or systemic arteries. Baker AB, Iannone A. Cerebrovascular disease: I. The large arteries of the circle of Willis. *Neurology* 1959;9(5):321–332; Baker AB, Iannone A. Cerebrovascular disease: II. The smaller intracerebral arteries. *Neurology* 1959;9(6):391–396; Baker AB, Iannone A. Cerebrovascular disease: III. The intracerebral arterioles. *Neurology* 1959;9(7):441–446.
3. Fisher CM. Occlusion of the internal carotid artery. *American Medical Association Archives of Neurology and Psychiatry* 1951;65:346–377; Fisher CM. Occlusion of

the carotid arteries: Further experiences. *American Medical Association Archives of Neurology and Psychiatry* 1954;72:187–204.
4. Fisher CM. The circle of Willis: Anatomical variations. *Vascular Diseases* 1965;2(2) 99–105.
5. Fisher CM, Ojemann RG. A clinico-pathological study of carotid endarterectomy plaques. *Revue Neurologique (Paris)* 1986;39:273–299.
6. When I was Fisher's stroke fellow in 1969, stacks of trays of carotid specimens stretched to the ceiling of the room that we shared. How Fisher had the time and perseverance to examine carefully each slide mystified me at that time.
7. The prior studies on the carotid artery, transient monocular blindness, and transient ischemic attacks were cited and extensively commented on in chapter 7. Fisher CM. Occlusion of the internal carotid artery. *Archives of Neurology and Psychiatry* 1951;65:346–377; Fisher CM. Occlusion of the carotid arteries. *Archives of Neurology and Psychiatry* 1954;72:187–204; Fisher CM. Transient monocular blindness associated with hemiplegia. *Transactions of the American Neurological Association* 1951;76:154–158; Fisher CM. Disease of carotid arteries: A clinico-pathological correlation. Report of the Annual Meeting and Proceedings of the Royal College of Physicians and Surgeons of Canada, October 3–4, 1952, pp. 60–67; Fisher CM. Transient monocular blindness associated with hemiplegia. *American Medical Association Archives of Ophthalmology* 1952;47:167–203.
8. Fisher CM. Concerning recurrent transient cerebral ischemic attacks. *Canadian Medical Association Journal* 1962;86(24):1091–1099.
9. Luckey H (Ed.). *Cerebral Vascular Diseases: Transactions of a Conference Held Under the Auspices of the American Heart Association, Princeton, New Jersey, January 24– 26, 1954.* New York: Grune & Stratton, 1955, pp. 95–96.
10. Fisher CM. Facial pulses in internal carotid artery occlusion. *Neurology* 1970;20:476–478.
11. Fisher CM. Dilated pupil in carotid occlusion. *Transactions of the American Neurological Association* 1966;91:227–229.
12. Fisher CM. Observations of the fundus oculi in transient monocular blindness. *Neurology* 1959;9:333–347. The history of the recognition and description of retinal emboli is reviewed in Graff-Radford J, Boes CJ, Brown RD. History of Hollenhorst plaques. *Stroke* 2015:46:e82–e84.
13. Fisher CM. *Memoirs of a Neurologist.* Rutland, VT: Sharp, 2006, Vol. l, p. 153.
14. Ojemann RG, Crowell RM, Roberson GH, Fisher CM. Surgical treatment of extracranial carotid occlusive disease. *Clinical Neurosurgery* 1975;22:214–263.
15. The washout hypothesis is discussed in Caplan LR, Hennerici M. Impaired clearance of emboli (washout) is an important link between hypoperfusion, embolism, and ischemic stroke. *Archives of Neurology* 1998;55:1475–1482; and Caplan LR, Wong KS, Gao S, Hennerici MG. Is hypoperfusion an important cause of strokes? If so, how? *Cerebrovascular Diseases* 2006;21:145–153.
16. Dr. Martin Reivich and colleagues called attention to patients with attacks of dizziness and vertigo, sometimes precipitated by arm exercise, who had occlusive lesions involving the subclavian artery proximal to the vertebral artery origin. Reivich M, Holling HE, Roberts B, et al. Reversal of blood flow through the vertebral artery and its effects on the cerebral circulation. *New England Journal of Medicine* 1961;265:878–885. Fisher, in an unsigned editorial in the same issue of the *New England Journal of Medicine*, coined the term "subclavian steal" to describe the radiographic findings. Fisher CM. A new vascular syndrome—"the subclavian steal." *New England Journal of Medicine* 1961;265:912.

17. The studies on the posterior circulation (vertebral and basilar artery territory) included Fisher CM, Karnes WE, Kubik CS. Lateral medullary infarction: The pattern of vascular occlusion. *Journal of Neuropathology and Experimental Neurology* 1961;20:323–379; Fisher CM. Occlusion of the Vertebral Arteries. *Archives of Neurology* 1970;22:13–19; Duncan GW, Parker SW, Fisher CM. Acute cerebellar infarction in the PICA territory. *Archives of Neurology* 1975;32:364–368; Kistler JP, Buonanno FS, DeWitt LD, Davis KR, Brady TJ, Fisher CM. Vertebral–basilar posterior cerebral territory stroke delineation by proton nuclear magnetic resonance imaging. *Stroke* 1984;15:417–426; Fisher CM. The posterior cerebral artery syndrome. *Canadian Journal of Neurological Sciences* 1986;13:232–239; Fisher CM, Tapia J. Lateral medullary infarction extending into the lower pons. *Journal of Neurology, Neurosurgery, and Psychiatry* 1987;50:620–624; and Fisher CM. The "herald hemiparesis" of basilar artery occlusion. *Archives of Neurology* 1988;45:1301–1303.
18. The studies on the intracranial carotid artery and its branches included Fisher CM, Gore I, White PD, Okabe N. Calcification of the carotid siphon. *Circulation* 1965;32:538–548; and Hinton RC, Mohr JP, Ackerman RH, Adair LB, Fisher CM. Symptomatic middle cerebral artery stenosis. *Annals of Neurology* 1979;5:152–157.
19. Fisher CM. Clinical syndromes in cerebral arterial occlusion. In W Fields (Ed.), *Proceedings of the Annual Meeting of the Houston Neurological Society*. Springfield, IL: Charles C Thomas, 1961, pp. 151–181.
20. The first edition of *Principles of Internal Medicine* [Harrison TR, Beeson PB, Resnik WH, Thorn GW, Wintrobe MM (Eds.). *Principles of Internal Medicine*. Philadelphia: Blakiston, 1950] had 1,554 pages. It did not have a section on disorders of nervous function. It contained 48 pages that briefly described various neurological conditions, among which 10 pages were devoted to diseases of the blood vessels of the brain and spinal cord. The neurological section was entirely written by Drs. Houston Merritt and Dan Sciarra from Colombia.
21. An account of the choice of Adams to become an editor of Harrison's *Internal Medical* text is found in Laureno R. *Raymond Adams: A Life in Mind and Muscle*. New York: Oxford University Press, 2009, pp. 61–62. Dr. Tinsley Harrison was a Southern gentleman, born in Alabama and educated at Vanderbilt University. How was it that Harrison came to choose a Northerner, Boston academic neurologist Adams, to edit an important section in his popular textbook? One of the editors, Dr. George Thorn, the Hersey Professor of the Theory and Practice of Physic at Harvard and Physician in Chief of the Department of Medicine at the Peter Bent Brigham Hospital, told Harrison that Adams was the person for the job. Harrison had trained at the Brigham under Thorn and highly valued his opinion. Adams' neurology section appeared in Harrison TR, Adams RD, Beeson PB, Resnik WH, Thorn GW, Wintrobe MM (Eds.). *Principles of Internal Medicine* (2nd ed.). New York: Blakiston, 1954.
22. Fisher CM, Karp HR, Adams RD. Cerebrovascular diseases. In Harrison TR, Adams RD, Bennett I Jr., Resnik WH, Thorn GW, Wintrobe MM (Eds.), *Principles of Internal Medicine* (3rd ed.). New York: McGraw-Hill, 1958, pp. 1560–1606.
23. Harrison's internal medicine textbook became one of the most widely read internal medical texts not only in the United States but also, with the availability of translated editions, throughout the world. The income from this text, Adams said, helped fund the neurology department at MGH.
24. Adams RD, Victor M. *Principles of Neurology*. New York: McGraw-Hill, 1977.

25. Ojemann RG, Fisher CM, Rich JC. Spontaneous dissecting aneurysms of the internal carotid artery. *Stroke* 1972;3:434–440.
26. The pressure within the wall of a dissected artery can break through the inner lining of the wall, the endothelium, and so introduce into the lumen of the artery fresh blood clot and other chemical factors usually contained within the wall. That blood and the swollen wall can obstruct the artery and become the source of blood clot embolizing into the brain, causing a brain infarct—a stroke.
27. Fisher CM. *Memoirs of a Neurologist*. Rutland, VT: Sharp, 2006, Vol. l, p. 157.
28. Hochberg FH, Bean CS, Fisher CM, Roberson GH. Stroke in a 15 year old girl secondary to terminal carotid dissection. *Neurology* 1975;25:725–729; Fisher CM, Ojemann RG, Roberson GH. Spontaneous dissection of cervicocerebral arteries. *Canadian Journal of Neurological Science* 1978;5:9–19.
29. In order for readers to fully understand Fisher's contribution regarding hydrocephalus, I briefly review the anatomy and function of the fluid within the skull. The brain is surrounded by liquid termed cerebrospinal fluid. Cerebrospinal fluid contains sugar and electrolytes. Cerebrospinal fluid is made by chemically active vascular structures within the ventricles of the brain—the choroid plexi. The largest ventricles are within the cerebral hemispheres on each side. The fluid then passes through a hole (the foramen of Monro) into the third ventricle, which lies in the midline in the posterior and deep portion of the cerebral hemispheres. Then, the fluid passes through a channel (the aqueduct of Sylvius) within the upper portion of the brainstem—the midbrain. It then passes into an expanded fluid-containing space, the fourth ventricle, that is located within the caudal portions of the brainstem—the pons and the medulla oblongata ventrally and the cerebellum dorsally. The fluid exits through holes within the fourth ventricle, and fluid then circulates around the cerebral hemispheres and passes down to bathe the external aspects of the spinal cord. The pressure and content of the fluid can be assessed by placing a needle in the low back (a lumbar puncture, otherwise called a spinal tap). The fluid is absorbed through chemically active tissue within the meninges that surround the brain and spinal cord. Normally, the same amount of fluid made within the ventricles is absorbed so that the water spaces remain the same size during adult life. Fluid can build up within one or more of the ventricles when the pathway is blocked (e.g., by a tumor or cyst). This is called noncommunicating hydrocephalus because the communication between the ventricles is obstructed. If too much fluid is made or too little is absorbed, then all the ventricles enlarge; this is termed communicating hydrocephalus because there is no blockage within the ventricular pathways. The fluid acts during trauma as a buffer to prevent brain tissue from hitting the craggy regions of the hard skull.
30. Adams commented on this patient in Laureno R. *Raymond Adams: A Life in Mind and Muscle*. New York: Oxford University Press, 2009, pp. 140–142; and Fisher included descriptions of the patient and the events in his memoirs: Fisher CM. *Memoirs of a Neurologist*. Rutland, VT: Sharp, 2006, Vol. 3, pp. 66–68; Vol. 2, pp. 103–104; Vol. 5, pp. 18–20. Quotation from Fisher CM. *Memoirs of a Neurologist*. Rutland, VT: Sharp, 2006, Vol. 3, p. 67.
31. Laureno R. *Raymond Adams: A Life in Mind and Muscle*. New York: Oxford University Press, 2009, p. 141.
32. Fisher CM. *Memoirs of a Neurologist*. Rutland, VT: Sharp, 2006, Vol. 2, p. 104.
33. Louis Pasteur, lecture, University of Lille (December 7, 1854).

34. Hakim, a child of Lebanese immigrants, had shown interest in science, electricity, and fluid dynamics since childhood—areas in which he continued his research during his entire career. He was educated in Bogota, Colombia, and spent time at Harvard and MGH on a grant from the Harrington Fund of Harvard Medical School. He had also acquired a PhD in neuropathology. He spent much of his later career in Colombia performing research on hydrocephalus and shunts and became one of the leading experts on shunting of fluid and the dynamics of the brain's cerebrospinal fluid circulation. He funded his extensive research from moneys earned providing clinical care.
35. Hakim S, Adams RD. The special clinical problem of symptomatic hydrocephalus with normal cerebrospinal fluid pressure: Observations on cerebrospinal fluid hydrodynamics. *Journal of Neurological Sciences* 1965;2:307–327.
36. Adams RD, Fisher CM, Hakim S, Ojemann RG, Sweet WH. Symptomatic occult hydrocephalus with "normal" cerebrospinal fluid pressure: A treatable syndrome. *New England Journal of Medicine* 1965;273:117–126.
37. Fisher CM. *Memoirs of a Neurologist*. Rutland, VT: Sharp, 2006, Vol. 1, pp. 150–151.
38. Fisher CM. *Memoirs of a Neurologist*. Rutland, VT: Sharp, 2006, Vol. 2, p. 105.
39. Ojemann RG, Fisher CM, Adams RD, Sweet WH, New PF. Further experience with the syndrome of "normal" pressure hydrocephalus. *Journal of Neurosurgery* 1969;31:279–294.
40. Fisher CM. The clinical picture in occult hydrocephalus. *Clinical Neurosurgery* 1977;24:270–284.
41. Fisher CM. Hydrocephalus as a cause of disturbances of gait in the elderly. *Neurology* 1982;32:1358–1363.
42. Fisher CM. *Memoirs of a Neurologist*. Rutland, VT: Sharp, 2006, Vol. 2, pp. 105–106.
43. Unpublished paper, Symptomatic normal pressure hydrocephalus (1984); Fisher CM. *Memoirs of a Neurologist*. Rutland, VT: Sharp, 2006, Vol. 2, pp. 103–109.

CHAPTER 12

Atrial Fibrillation, Memory, Timing and Quantity of Behavior, Randomized Therapeutic Trials and Anticoagulation of Brain Ischemia Patients, and Headache and Migraine

ATRIAL FIBRILLATION AS A COMMON CAUSE OF BRAIN EMBOLISM

During Fisher's year of training at Boston City Hospital with Raymond Adams in 1949 (for the initial discoveries, see Chapter 6), he had become interested in atrial fibrillation. One day early in his training, he examined the cerebral arteries in three patients who had large hemorrhagic brain infarcts and found them free of thrombi. All these patients had had atrial fibrillation during life. All had infarcts in the spleen and kidneys in addition to the brain. He wondered at that time if atrial fibrillation was an important cause of brain embolism.[1,2]

Fisher continued his research on brain embolism and its causes while in Montreal and finally published the work many years later.[3] While performing postmortem examinations in Boston in his neuropathology laboratory at Massachusetts General Hospital (MGH), he continued to be impressed by the frequency of atrial fibrillation in patients whose brains showed embolic infarcts. He had previously demonstrated that studies of serial sections of the left atrial appendage in patients who had had embolic brain infarcts invariably showed mural thrombi within the interstices of the trabeculae carnae of the appendage. A clinical experience further stimulated his impressions about atrial fibrillation:

> A leading Boston cardiologist had been Master of ceremonies one evening at a huge testimonial banquet. His performance was remarkable for its sparkle, wit, and polish. The following noon, I received an urgent call that while having lunch this same individual had suddenly developed a right hemiplegia and aphasia and was now in the Emergency Ward. He was in atrial fibrillation and obviously had a cerebral embolism. He was severely impaired and had in the past made it clear that should he ever become paralyzed, he wanted no measures applied that would preserve him in a deteriorated state. He died two weeks later. This unexpected tragedy caused me to ponder on the possibility of using anticoagulants to prevent such an event.[4]

Fisher tested this notion at lunch one day with colleagues. He wrote about this meeting in his memoirs:

> I voiced my proposal (about anticoagulating those with atrial fibrillation) at the luncheon table one day and in return received from my colleagues a chorus of skepticism at such an impractical idea. Dr. A said "Why I saw Mr. B in my office this morning. He has atrial fibrillation and you mean to tell me he should be on anticoagulants." I averred that that would be the correct inference. Dr. A said that he would have Mr. B seen by one of the world's foremost cardiologists, Dr. C, and get his opinion about the matter. A few days later, I was informed that in Dr. C's opinion, anticoagulants were not indicated. . . . Four months later Mr. B. a brilliant administrator was brought to the Emergency Ward having suddenly developed a receptive aphasia from which he failed to recover with the prospect that he would be left a pitiful wreck for the rest of his days. A year later Dr. C himself was admitted to the hospital because of the sudden onset of a left hemiparesis and parietal lobe deficit. He was known to have paroxysmal atrial fibrillation. One and a half years later he was admitted again because of the sudden onset of a right hemiplegia and stupor. He was in atrial fibrillation. One year later, Dr. A, who was present at the original discussion was admitted because of the sudden onset of aphasia and he too was in atrial fibrillation. Thus all three individuals involved in the original discussion had fallen victim to cerebral embolism associated with atrial fibrillation.[5]

Fisher continued to make observations about atrial fibrillation and stroke. He sent a letter to the *Lancet*, published in 1972, that stated,

> In our cerebrovascular studies, we have been struck by the number of patients in atrial fibrillation who have a severe stroke as the first manifestation of embolism. All

patients with chronic atrial fibrillation should be considered for prophylactic anticoagulant therapy . . . to avoid a fate worse than death.[6]

These initial observations about atrial fibrillation were anecdotal. With his stroke fellows and cardiology colleagues, Fisher organized a study to formally examine the heart and other organs at autopsy to clarify the role of atrial fibrillation in causing brain embolism.[7] At the time of this 1977 study, the only generally accepted role of atrial fibrillation in causing brain embolism was in patients who had rheumatic heart disease with stenosis of the mitral valve. Fisher and colleagues summarized their findings from this study as follows:

> *Atrial fibrillation is well known to increase greatly the risk of systemic arterial embolism in patients with mitral valve disease. . . . A study was made of embolic occurrences in 333 autopsy patients with atrial fibrillation associated with various kinds of heart disease. Considering only symptomatic emboli with pathologic or surgical confirmation, embolism occurred in 41% of patients with mitral valve disease, 35% of those with ischemic heart disease, 35% of those with coexisting mitral and ischemic heart disease, and 17% of those with "other" types of heart disease. Embolism was found in only 7% of a control group of 58 autopsy patients with ischemic heart disease without atrial fibrillation. These findings suggest a high risk of embolism from atrial fibrillation of any origin.*[7]

A year after this study, an epidemiological analysis of the role of atrial fibrillation in patients with stroke was published as part of the Framingham Heart Study. This report was led by Phil Wolf, a trainee of Fisher. It confirmed a high frequency of embolism in patients with atrial fibrillation who had no cardiac valve disease.[8] After 24 years of follow-up in the Framingham Heart Study, 345 strokes had occurred; 27 had occurred in individuals with chronic atrial fibrillation—7 with rheumatic heart disease and 20 with non-rheumatic atrial fibrillation. In those with atrial fibrillation and rheumatic heart disease, the incidence of stroke was increased 17.6-fold, and in those with atrial fibrillation in the absence of heart valve disease, there was a 5.6-fold increased stroke frequency.[8]

Cardiologists continued to be skeptical because they followed many elderly patients with long-term atrial fibrillation who did not have strokes. They were also wary about anticoagulation because it carried risks especially in the elderly. In 1979, Fisher published a plea for considering anticoagulation in patients with persistent or paroxysmal atrial fibrillation before brain ischemia developed.[9] He reviewed the hospital records of 100 patients who had atrial fibrillation (83 with no heart valve disease and 17 with valve disease). Of 109 episodes of stroke among the 100 patients, 71% resulted in death or in an unacceptable neurological deficit, emphasizing the severity of the initial stroke. Fisher also reviewed random records of 100 patients who were hospitalized with atrial fibrillation but not anticoagulated: 35 had embolic events (86% brain and 14% systemic). Among 48 patients who did not have strokes initially, 35% had typical embolic strokes during the 4 years of follow-up.[9]

It was not until formal randomized therapeutic trials, led by neurologists, during the 1990s that treatment of patients who had atrial fibrillation was shown definitively to prevent brain embolism. Fisher had been prescient based on his own experiences and early studies, but few non-neurologists heeded his advice until formal trials proved him right.

THE BRAIN ANATOMY OF MEMORY FUNCTION AND PERSISTENT AND TEMPORARY AMNESIA

Fisher and colleagues made important contributions to knowledge concerning the acquisition and retention of memories. The first case and publication concerned a patient of his whom he had followed for years.[10] While in his 50s, this hypertensive man began to have transient ischemic episodes and small strokes all involving the posterior, vertebrobasilar, circulation of his brain. In 1953, he developed a severe decline in vision and lost the ability to make new memories. The memory disorder persisted until his death 3 years later. His general intellectual functions were preserved. Events that occurred before 1951 were recalled accurately. Fisher et al. noted,

> *The patient's ability to recall recent events and to learn and retain new facts were both seriously affected. He would ask the same questions over and over again. He spent hours watching baseball on television, but, as soon as the set was turned off, he was unable to remember the score or any other details of the game. However, he was able to recall the highlights of games that had been played years before. . . . He would forget simple instructions given by his wife, and would neglect to read notes which had been left to reinforce his memory. During this period he was still able to play bridge adequately and actually taught his nephew the game of solitaire, but he was unable to learn new card games.*[10]

The autopsy performed in 1956 showed that both of the posterior cerebral artery territories supplying his visual cortex in the occipital lobes and the hippocampal regions in his temporal lobes had been infarcted. Fisher and colleagues reviewed the literature available at that time and Fisher attended a meeting devoted to memory function and its brain anatomy. Fisher and colleagues concluded in their report that the hippocampi—small structures that resemble seahorses located in the deep portions of the temporal lobes—were heavily involved in memory acquisition and retention.[10] In this patient and in all past reported cases of severe persistent memory loss, the hippocampi and/or their connections were severely damaged on both sides of the brain.

During the ensuing decades, Fisher was impressed that some of his patients who had strokes in the territory supplied by one of the posterior cerebral arteries had developed confusion and memory loss. In 1986, he reviewed his experience in the *Canadian Journal of Neurological Sciences* concerning the findings in his patients with posterior cerebral artery territory strokes.[11] Among 70 patients who had a stroke in the territory of the posterior cerebral arteries, 25 had important memory loss. In 24 of these 25 patients, the dominant cerebral hemisphere (nearly always the left) was involved. He also noted that some of these patients developed hyperactivity, agitation, and delirium. He concluded that involvement of the hippocampal region in the dominant cerebral hemisphere, a region supplied by the posterior cerebral artery, could cause memory impairment. He did not comment on how long the memory deficit persisted, but later reports indicated that the deficit in memory acquisition and retention was usually temporary, lasting approximately 6 months.[12] In subsequent writings, he commented on the occurrence of hyperactivity.

Stimulated by experience in patients with memory deficits that persisted, Fisher and Raymond Adams began to be consulted on patients who developed severe loss of memory that lasted less than a day. In 1964, they penned a 76-page detailed report on a syndrome that they dubbed "transient global amnesia" (TGA).[13] Fisher and Adams described 17 patients seen personally during a period of 9 years who developed sudden episodes of temporary amnesia usually lasting a few hours, after which they returned to their previous capabilities. Sixteen of the patients had one attack and the other patient had three attacks before the episode described. The onset was abrupt, and in 13 of the 17 patients, a witness to the onset could reliably describe the individual's behavior. The patient would suddenly seem bewildered and would ask repetitive queries, repeating the same questions despite being repeatedly told the answers. During the examinations by Fisher and Adams, usually hours later, the patients could not retain any information for more than a few seconds. Amnesia was patchy for events that had occurred during the previous days, weeks, months, and even years. Personal identity was always retained, and the patients could reliably relate events of their early life. Language and mathematical abilities were retained, and there were no elementary neurological abnormalities including vision, limb movements, sensation, and gait. The patients functioned normally except for their inability to make new memories. Gradually during hours, the retrograde amnesic period shrunk so that they later recalled events up to the time of onset of the amnesia. None ever regained memories of the period during which they were amnesic. Patients were middle aged or elderly. Precipitants in these patients included hot showers, sex, swimming in cold ocean water, severe pain, and a stressful interview. Fisher and Adams speculated on the possible causes of the syndrome. They concluded,

> A clinical syndrome of episodic global amnesia is herein documented for the first time. . . . The syndrome consists of the abrupt onset of disorientation due principally to a loss of immediate and recent memory. The episode has lasted usually for only a few hours, after which all psychic and other neurological functions are fully restored. . . . Clinical study has provided no clue as to the mechanism of the attacks.[13]

In 1982, Fisher reported some of his later observations on this fascinating TGA syndrome.[14] He reviewed his experience with 78 patients for whom details surrounding the onset of memory loss were known. Precipitating events were reported in 26 of the 85 spells and included highly emotional experiences (8), sexual intercourse (6), during pain (2), after a dip in the cold Atlantic Ocean (3), and while a nerve was stimulated (1). The youngest patient was aged 48 years, and the oldest was 84 years old. Fisher commented,

> TGA (transient global amnesia) illustrates with unusual purity the classic elements of acute impairment of memory: 1) inability to form new memories of anything occurring during the episode, 2) a temporary long-ranging retrograde amnesia for days, months, or years, and 3) relatively short permanent retrograde amnesia of one half to 8 hours of the most recent memories. And as the temporary amnesia resolves, returning memories follow the same rule, with older memories coming back first, followed by more recent ones. Yet during the attack the patient remains alert, attention is maintained, cortical functions are relatively intact.[14]

The brain functions differently from other body organs. In the skin, heart, lungs, liver, etc., one region looks and acts much the same as all other areas. In the brain, one region subserves a specific function. Certain regions are concerned with movements, others sensation, still others vision, hearing, memory functions, and other areas speech and language. Amnesia can be likened to the use of a tape recorder that has been loaded with dictations and malfunctions without the person who is dictating recognizing it. Because the recorder is not working, it fails to record any of the subsequent dictation. In addition, the malfunction may affect the recently dictated information acquired before the malfunction. The hippocampi and their connections must function similar to a tape recorder. They might be rendered inactive by a variety of insults.[15]

Fisher described two other amnesic syndromes—concussion amnesia and whiplash amnesia.[16,17] In 1966, he reported the remarkable case of a woman who developed amnesia after a head injury. While standing on a chair reaching for a can of coffee on a top shelf, a 41-year-old woman fell backwards, striking her head with a loud thud. She got up quickly and asked her sister-in-law, whom she had known for 28 years and who had witnessed the fall, "Who are you? What are you doing here? What happened? I can't remember a thing." She continued to repeat the same questions and remarks. Fisher examined her 3 hours later. She could not retain his name for more than 30 seconds and denied being told his name. She gave the date as 1½ years earlier and had no knowledge of the assassination of John Kennedy that had occurred during that interval period. (No normal individual living at that time could possibly forget Kennedy's murder.) After 24 hours, she recovered normally. Her first post-fall recall was the events that occurred 10 hours after the injury. Fisher commented on the disassociation of her alertness and other cognitive functions and her complete loss of memory during the episode.[16]

In 1982, Fisher described a patient who developed amnesia after a whiplash injury.[17] A 67-year-old woman was a passenger in a car that was struck by a truck. The driver saw that the patient was thrown forward and then backwards but did not strike her head. Fisher examined her 10 hours after the accident. She could not make new memories or recall events of the past 3 days. Later, her retrograde amnesia shrunk so that she was able to recall events that occurred just before the accident.[17]

Fisher, Adams, and colleagues brought to the attention of the medical community the phenomenology and anatomy of memory functions and persistent and temporary amnesia. They were reticent in defining precisely the mechanism of amnesia in these diverse situations that they encountered and reported. These observations preceded by more than a quarter of a century the current interest in sports-related concussions and blast-related brain injuries in military personnel.

THE BRAIN ANATOMY RELATED TO THE TIMING, PERSISTENCE, AND QUANTITY OF BEHAVIOR

Fisher recognized that strokes offered an opportunity to learn how various areas in the brain functioned. He became avidly interested in all aspects of cognition and behavior. The preceding paragraphs focused on a qualitative loss of one function—memory, mostly attributable to injury to the hippocampi and other adjacent structures in the medial temporal lobes. Fisher also became interested in the quantitative aspects of behavior and abnormalities in the brain that were related to both a decrease and an excessive increase in an individual's activity level and in the timing and persistence of responses. In 1968, he delivered a talk titled "Intermittent Interruption of Behavior" at the annual meeting of the American Neurological Association.[18] In the presentation, he called attention to a "neurological state in which a patient alternatively responds to questions and commands for seconds or minutes and then for an interval fails to do so."[18] During the period of not responding, the patient remains alert and may perform stereotyped movements such as rubbing the nose, flexing a leg, or looking at his or her watch. One patient described in the report alternated between a 5-minute period of responding and a 7- to 10-minute period of no activity. That patient remarked, "I had it in mind to respond but nothing happened."[18]

When he was the honored guest of the Congress of Neurological Surgeons at its annual meeting in Chicago in 1983, Fisher shared his thoughts on behavior and its brain anatomy (Figure 12.1).[19] Seeking a term for a pathological decrease in activity, he resurrected an old psychological term *abulia*, which was used to describe a lack of will or a weakness of will. Characteristically, he described what he meant by abulia in specific terms—a decrease in spontaneous speech and activity, an absence or latency in responding to queries or requests, and, when responses did occur, terse brief responses of one or two words or a single phrase. When asked a question, the patient might look at the examiner and not reply or reply only after the question was repeated once or several times. A belated but accurate response showed that the query was understood and the answer known to the patient.

Fisher described the abulic patient as speaking with a soft or faint voice, whispering. Speech was monotonous and "matter-of-fact." Motor responses were often slow and hesitant. A handshake might consist of tentative contractions. Occasional patients might not respond when confronted in

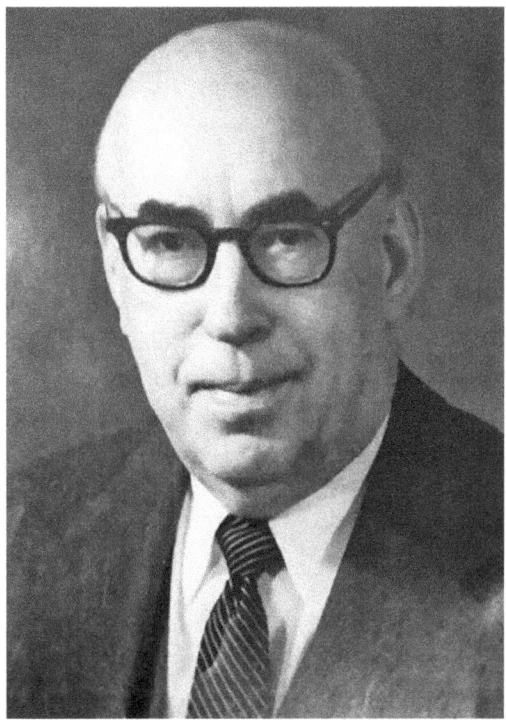

Figure 12.1 Fisher at the time of his presentation as an honored guest of the Congress of Neurological Surgeons in 1983.
Source: Reprinted with permission from Caplan LR. *Caplan's Stroke: A Clinical Approach* (4th ed.). Philadelphia: Elsevier, 2009.

person but would hold a conversation when called on the telephone (the "phone sign"):[20]

> In severe abulia the patient who is speechless when addressed in person may speak virtually normally when addressed on the telephone from out of the room. The telephone effect has been observed in anterior cerebral artery occlusion and in advanced hydrocephalus. In one instance the patient also wrote."[21]

Some of the patients whom Fisher had reported on previously who showed intermittent interruptions of behavior went on to later become persistently abulic. He considered this intermittent condition as a less advanced degree of abulia. Fisher reviewed the anatomic correlates of abulia—the reduced behavior state. The abnormalities were almost always confined to the anterior portion of the cerebrum—the frontal lobes and basal ganglia or the upper brainstem. In contrast were those patients who exhibited excess behavior. They were often described as agitated, hyperactive, restless, and talkative. These patients most often had abnormalities limited to the posterior portions of the cerebral hemispheres, especially the medial temporal lobes within the supply of the posterior cerebral arteries.[19]

Early in his career, before brain imaging became available, Fisher had described a quite different behavioral abnormality: difficulty persisting with tasks.[22] In this condition, which he called "motor impersistence," patients carried out voluntary acts quite well but they did not sustain the action. He described 10 patients, all of whom had strokes that caused some degree of paralysis of the left limbs. His attention was drawn to this syndrome when he noticed that all of the patients could not maintain eye closure. If he asked them to close their eyes, they did so quickly but did not keep the eyes closed even when urged to do so. Characteristic of his methods was to render an operational definition in practical concrete terms. He defined motor impersistence using six tests:[22]

1. Inability to maintain conjugate gaze to one side
2. Inability to keep the mouth open, especially when asked to stick out the tongue. The patient would quickly protrude their tongue but then pull it back in the mouth and close the mouth.
3. Inability to keep the eyes fixed on the examiner's nose during testing of the visual fields
4. Inability to keep the eyes closed during testing of sensation on the face or limbs. Patients could not resist opening their eyes and peeking at the area of the body touched.
5. Inability to hold a deep breath
6. Inability to exert steady pressure during hand grip or a handshake

These patients all most likely had brain damage to their frontal lobes, and Fisher opined that this brain region might relate to the ability of individuals to persist with actions. He also commented on the patients' impulsivity with quick but briefly sustained responses.

These abnormalities described by Fisher—decrease in activity, hyperactivity, and impersistence—are all quantitative rather than qualitative. Many daily activities and jobs depend on the amount of activity performed, its efficiency, and the ability to persevere with tasks. These abnormalities can explain why some individuals with normal cognition fail in their performance at home and on the job.

RANDOMIZED THERAPEUTIC TRIALS: ANTICOAGULATION TREATMENT OF PATIENTS WITH BRAIN ISCHEMIA

Fisher was a key member and proponent of the first randomized clinical trial of treatment of any neurological condition. In 1958, the Stroke Service at MGH, under his direction, began participating in the national cooperative study of anticoagulant therapy in patients who had transient ischemic attacks (TIAs) and ischemic strokes.

Dr. Irving Wright, a professor of medicine at the New York Hospital–Cornell University, had stimulated interest in cerebrovascular disease by organizing the first Princeton Conference of Cerebrovascular Disease held in January 1954.[23] Fisher attended the meeting and noted that among the 34 participants, only 5 or 6 had clinical experience in the field of stroke. This meeting stimulated the National Institute of Neurological Diseases and Blindness to appoint an ad hoc committee to develop uniform criteria to classify and diagnose cerebrovascular diseases.[24] From the deliberations of that committee came the idea to undertake an investigation of the effect of anticoagulation on the natural course of cerebrovascular disease. Anticoagulants had been used by internists to try to prevent brain and pulmonary embolism.

Fisher commented in his memoirs,

> *The study ... helped in creating one of the great turning points of all time in medical education, namely the introduction to students of the principle of valid randomization in scientific therapeutic trials. Almost overnight in the late 1950s students for the first time began to ask for the evidence concerning every claim or statement made in medical instruction. One must have experienced this period of transition to realize the magnitude of the impact. An actual anecdote will provide a striking illustration. One evening when I had concluded a randomization which seemed to have come out to the disadvantage of the patient, according to the then current wisdom, the chief of a major service got wind of it all and astonished me at the ward desk in the presence of several visitors and in loud tones, saying that I was guilty of a criminal act and should be prosecuted. Within a year or two when any point in therapeutic management arose this same individual assiduously inquired whether there had been randomization, promulgating the process as if it were his invention.*[25]

After the study was agreed upon, three organizational and planning meetings were held to discuss nomenclature, goals, clinical criteria, methods of randomization, methods of anticoagulation, and end points. The participating nine investigators were, in addition to Fisher, Harry Fang of Los Angeles; Al Heyman of Duke University; Herb Karp of Atlanta; Ellen McDevitt of Cornell University, New York; Clark Millikan of the Mayo Clinic, Rochester, Minnesota; Adolph Sahs of the University of Iowa; Peritz Scheinberg of Jackson Memorial Hospital, Miami University; and Lawrence Barrows and Jim Toole of the University of Pennsylvania. Money had to be sought to fund the study. The investigators agreed upon the wording and constituents of the grant proposal that was to be submitted to the National Institutes of Health, but because of the cooperative nature of the study, each participating center had to submit its own proposal which was to be the same in all cases. Two of the centers bowed out at the last moment and, without giving any explanation, did not apply. The study was funded and patients began to be enrolled in January 1958. The patients entered into the study were not required to give informed consent nor were they informed about randomization. To be eligible for the study, patients must have had an ischemic episode within 8 weeks; they were given a placebo capsule or anticoagulant (dicumerol with or without heparin).

Fisher was the chairman and director of the coordinating center at MGH, at which records from the other participating centers were evaluated. He wrote an interim report published in 1961.[26] At the time of this report, 384 patients had been studied. Approximately 70% had had episodes within the past 7 days. There were 37 deaths among the 182 control placebo-treated patients and 38 among the 195 patients who received anticoagulants. Fisher concluded,

> *Long-term anticoagulation therapy does not appear to reduce the mortality in occlusive cerebrovascular disease and, indeed is associated with an added risk of death due to the hemorrhagic complications. The number of transient cerebral ischemic attacks is reduced by anticoagulation.*[26]

A final report on the anticoagulation study was published in 1962 but the results had not changed since Fisher's interim report.[27]

Being the first randomized trial, there was much learned in creating the trial and defining the various subgroups and their management and the method of evaluating results. This trial was performed before brain imaging. The ischemic subgroups were small. Blood pressure was difficult to control, as was intensity of anticoagulation. There were many glitches in performing the study because the process was new to all:

> *This study was probably the first properly randomized therapeutic trial in the history of neurology. The bleeding complications of poorly regulated coumadin therapy proved*

to be an insurmountable hurdle and the study had to be halted. Nonetheless much was learned about strokes that had not been appreciated in the past. Spin-off of knowledge is an important aspect of therapeutic studies, one not fully recognized.[28]

Fisher's enthusiasm for trials waned during his later experience. As the principal investigator at MGH in a cooperative study, he was required to fill out 28 sheets of data entry in each case. He found this a time-consuming, taxing endeavor, but he strived to enter the data as accurately as possible. He commented to the director of the study how arduous the entry process was for him. The director replied, "Oh, I have the medical students do it."[29] This answer made Fisher painfully aware how much the results of studies depended on who was entering the information and the accuracy of the data.

HEADACHE AND MIGRAINE

Fisher had a career-long interest in headache, and he cared for many patients in whom headache was the predominant symptom and health problem. He was a member of the advisory board of the headache center at the Faulkner Hospital in Boston. During his career, he made important contributions with regard to migraine, one of the most common problems encountered in medical and neurological practices.

He studied and reported in the *Handbook of Clinical Neurology* the frequency, location, nature, severity, and timing of headache and neck pain in patients with various ischemic and hemorrhagic stroke syndromes and vascular lesions.[30] Figures 12.2A and 12.2B are drawings that show headache locations in patients with carotid artery occlusion and infarcts in the medulla often caused by vertebral artery occlusions.

Fisher's major contributions regarding headache were related to migraine, a condition known for centuries but poorly understood. While working in Montreal during the early 1950s, Fisher became aware of transient visual symptoms affecting one eye as a very important clue to the presence of carotid artery disease in the neck. He wrote extensively in both neurological and ophthalmological journals about the presence, nature, frequency, and timing of these transient visual attacks (for additional details, see Chapter 7).[31] After setting up practice in Boston, he maintained a major interest in visual symptoms and findings.

In 1968, he presented a report at a meeting of the American Neurological Society in which he compared the visual symptoms described by patients during migraine accompaniments with those reported by patients with

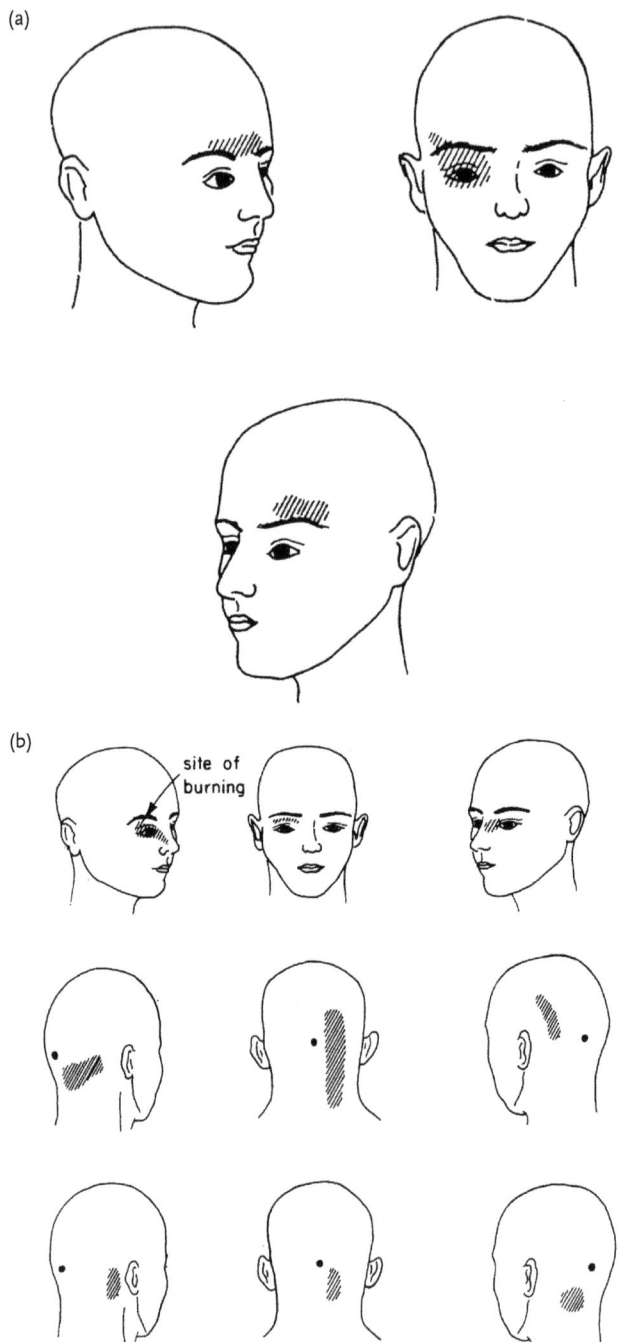

Figure 12.2 (A) Location of frontal headache in occlusion of the internal carotid artery. (B) Location of typical headache in lateral medullary syndrome.
Source: Reproduced with permission from Fisher CM. Headache in cerebrovascular disease. In Vinken PJ, Bruyn GW (Eds.), *Handbook of Clinical Neurology, Volume 5: Headaches and Cranial Neuralgias*. Amsterdam: North Holland, 1968, pp. 124–156.

brain infarctions.[32] He collected the descriptions of 68 of his patients—32 who had migraine accompaniments with headache and 36 who had migraine accompaniments without headache. He compared their descriptions with those of 57 patients who had visual symptoms because of non-migrainous occlusions of their posterior cerebral arteries. The migrainous visual symptoms were described as spots, lines, or geometric objects that flickered, moved, or scintillated. They began in one part of the visual field and moved slowly across vision, leaving in their wake an area of visual loss. Visual symptoms characteristically lasted approximately 20 minutes. The severity of the visual symptoms peaked in 3–45 minutes. Sensory symptoms often began after the visual symptoms cleared and could start in one body part and spread gradually to other parts on the same side. Headache might follow cessation of the visual and/or sensory symptoms or could be absent. In contrast to the monocular symptoms related to carotid artery disease, closing one eye did not obliterate the visual symptoms in migraineurs. Visual symptoms in patients with posterior cerebral artery occlusion did not spread gradually, and symptoms never began with visual symptoms followed by sensory abnormalities.

When he was 59 years old, Fisher began to develop transient visual attacks that were characteristic of those that migraineurs had described to him. He described his own experience in a 23-page unpublished paper that was included in his memoirs.[33] Descriptions by physicians on a topic about which they are knowledgeable serve a very useful function.[34] Recall number 13 of "Fisher's Rules" cited in Chapter 9: "Pay particular attention to the specifics of the patient with a known condition and diagnosis; it will help later when similar phenomena occur in an unknown case." A common and principal way that physicians make a diagnosis is to pattern match. In this process, the doctor matches the new patient's symptoms and findings with those of previous patients who have a known proven diagnosis. In his descriptions of migraine accompaniments and of transient visual loss, Fisher created detailed distinct patterns that could prove useful to physicians in diagnosing an unknown case; that is the major utility in reporting these observations concerning headache and migraine. The details of a particular symptom or finding can also stimulate research in better understanding and treating the cause of the condition.

Fisher had 36 attacks between ages 59 and 84 years. He had no history of these visual symptoms before but had had recurrent headaches between ages 11 and 18 years. The average duration was 15 minutes. The right visual field was involved in 20 spells, and the left was involved in 16. The only symptoms during the attacks were visual. None were followed by headache.

Spells often began with a vague feeling of visual impairment—like something was in the eye:

> After 40 seconds to 5 minutes, most commonly 2–3 minutes, a small faint flickering brightness appeared at about 5 degrees from the center of fixation intercepting the equator and lying slightly in the lower quadrant. Gradually this became a flickering line, enlarging and migrating to the periphery. The scotoma that followed in the wake of the expanding zigzag occupied only a narrow zone and lasted but a minute or two.[35]

As was his custom, Fisher reviewed the literature of other descriptions of the visual symptoms in patients with migraine, commented on similarities and differences between individuals and in different attacks, and reflected on the likely mechanism of the phenomenon. Perhaps stimulated by his own experience, he began to collect examples of visual and other migraine accompaniments that developed later in life. Most prior literature considered migraine as involving predominantly youths and young adults. He also wondered whether some transient neurological episodes labeled as TIAs were actually late-life migraine accompaniments. As such, the cause would be benign, and aggressive treatments would not be applied. He conducted a survey of patients attending a neurological clinic for reasons other than headache: One-sixth of those older than age 55 years reported the late development of migrainous visual accompaniments.

When asked to deliver the very prestigious Charcot lecture in Paris in 1979, Fisher first described late-life migrainous accompaniments as an important entity.[36] He published his early patient experience with the topic in the *Canadian Journal of Neurological Sciences* a year later:

> Occasionally patients in the stroke age-bracket over 40 have unexplained transient cerebral ischemic attacks in association with normal cerebral angiograms. From this group 120 have been collected in whom the transient episodes resembled the neurological accompaniments of migraine. According to symptoms, the patients were categorized as follows: Visual accompaniments (patients with only ordinary scintillating scotoma were excluded), 25; visual and paresthesias, 18; visual and speech disturbance, 7; visual and brain stem symptoms, 14; visual, paresthesias, and speech disturbance, 7; visual, paresthesias, speech disturbance, and paresis, 25. . . . Typical of migrainous accompaniments are the buildup and migration of visual scintillations, the march of paresthesiae, and progression from one accompaniment to another, characteristics that do not occur in thrombosis and embolism. Diagnosis facilitated when 2 or more similar episodes have occurred or migraine-like scintillations are present. Headache occurred in 50% of cases.[37]

Six years later, Fisher published his subsequent experience in the journal *Stroke* with 85 new patients who developed late-life migraine accompaniments. The results corroborated his previous experience and reports. He concluded, "The condition can justifiably be regarded as benign. Migrainous accompaniments account for some of the cases of transient ischemia with normal angiograms. Knowledge of the condition helps in the planning of rational management."[38]

Fisher also recognized that rarely a seemingly typical migrainous attack could be followed by persistent brain damage—a so-called migrainous stroke. He reported a single instance of this in the journal *Headache*. In this report, he commented on the importance of reporting single unique cases:

> *The different patterns that migraine can assume, whether a matter of headache or neurological accompaniment, seem to be countless. Unusual cases, while disconcerting to the clinician, have a special importance, for any theory of the mechanism of migraine must explain not only the commonplace but also these aberrant forms; indeed in our current state of knowledge they provide special information and may suggest additional avenues for speculation.*[39]

To Fisher, every case, every patient was important. The intricate details were important in furthering knowledge and, it was hoped, improving logical care. Some of these unique stroke cases were collected in a long and detailed report in the journal *Neurosurgery*.[40]

NOTES

1. Fisher CM. *Memoirs of a Neurologist*. Rutland, VT: Sharp, 2006, Vol. 1, pp. 48–49; Vol. 2, pp. 277–279.
2. An account of Fisher's publications and that of others on the topic of atrial fibrillation have been included in a recent report: Caplan LR. Atrial fibrillation, past and future: From a stroke non-entity to an over-targeted cause. *Cerebrovascular Diseases* 2018;45:149–153; and in Wolf PA. Awareness of the role of atrial fibrillation as a cause of ischemic stroke. *Stroke* 2014;45:e19–e21.
3. Fisher CM, Adams RD. Observations on brain embolism with special reference to hemorrhagic infarction. In Furlan AJ (Ed.), *The Heart and Stroke*. Berlin: Springer-Verlag, 1987, pp. 17–36.
4. Fisher CM. *Memoirs of a Neurologist*. Rutland, VT: Sharp, 2006, Vol. 1, pp. 153–154.
5. Fisher CM. *Memoirs of a Neurologist*. Rutland, VT: Sharp, 2006, Vol. 1, p. 154.
6. Fisher CM. The treatment of atrial fibrillation [Letter to the Editor]. *Lancet* 1972;299:1284. This letter was called to my attention by Dr. Robert Hart.

7. Hinton RC, Kistler JP, Fallon JT, Friedlich AL, Fisher CM. Influence of etiology of atrial fibrillation on incidence of systemic embolism. *American Journal of Cardiology* 1977;40:509–513.
8. Wolf PA, Dawber TR, Thomas HE Jr., Kannel WB. Epidemiologic assessment of chronic atrial fibrillation and risk of stroke: The Framingham study. *Neurology* 1978;28:973–977.
9. Fisher CM. Reducing risks of cerebral embolism. *Geriatrics* 1979;34:59–61, 65–66.
10. Victor M, Angevine JB Jr, Mancall EL, Fisher CM. Memory loss with lesions of hippocampal formation. *Archives of Neurology* 1961;5:244–263.
11. Fisher CM. The posterior cerebral artery syndrome. *Canadian Journal Neurological Sciences* 1986;13:232–239.
12. The topic of the ability to make new memories in patients with posterior cerebral artery occlusive disease is reviewed in Caplan LR, Hedley-White T. Cuing and memory dysfunction in alexia without agraphia: A case report. *Brain* 1974;97:251–262; and in Benson DF, Marsdaen CD, Meadows JC. The amnesic syndrome of posterior cerebral artery occlusion. *Acta Neurologica Scandinavica* 1974;50(2):133–145.
13. Fisher CM, Adams RD. Transient global amnesia. *Acta Neurologica Scandinavica* 1964;40(Suppl. 9):1–83.
14. Fisher CM. Transient global amnesia: Precipitating activities and other observations. *Archives of Neurology* 1982;39:605–608.
15. The entity transient global amnesia and the role that Fisher played in its initial recognition and research are reviewed in detail in Daniel BT. *Transient Global Amnesia*. Copyright 2012 Britt Talley Daniel.
16. Fisher CM. Concussion amnesia. *Neurology* 1966;826–830.
17. Fisher CM. Whiplash amnesia. *Neurology* 1982;32:667–668.
18. Fisher CM. Intermittent interruption of behavior. *Transactions of the American Neurological Association* 1968;93:209–210.
19. Fisher CM. Honored guest presentation: Abulia minor versus agitated behavior. *Clinical Neurosurgery* 1984;31:9–31.
20. One day, Fisher and I repeatedly spoke to an abulic patient in his room but got no response. While we were there, the phone rang and the patient carried on a conversation. After the phone call, we again spoke directly to him but, again, there were no responses. We stepped out of the room and called his phone and were able to converse with him.
21. Fisher CM. *Memoirs of a Neurologist*. Rutland, VT: Sharp, 2006, Vol. 6, p. 147.
22. Fisher CM. Left hemiplegia and motor impersistence. *Journal of Nervous and Mental Disease* 1956;123:201–218.
23. Wright I, Millikan CH. *Cerebrovascular Diseases: Transactions of the First Conference Held January 24–26, 1954 at Princeton, New Jersey*. New York: Grune & Stratton, 1954.
24. The committee report was published in 1958: A classification and outline of cerebrovascular diseases. *Neurology* 1958;8:188–216. It was also included as an appendix to publication of the transactions of the second conference of cerebrovascular diseases held at Princeton, New Jersey, under the auspices of the American Heart Association. Wright IS, Millikan C (Eds.). *Cerebrovascular Disease*. New York: Grune & Stratton, 1958.
25. Fisher CM. *Memoirs of a Neurologist*. Rutland, VT: Sharp, 2006, Vol. 1, pp. 141–142.

26. Fisher CM. Anticoagulant therapy in cerebral thrombosis and cerebral embolism: A National Cooperative Study, interim report. *Neurology* 1961;11:119–131.
27. Baker RN, Broward JA, Fang HC, Fisher CM, Groch SN, Heyman A. Anticoagulant therapy in cerebral infarction. *Neurology* 1962;12:823–835.
28. Fisher CM. *Memoirs of a Neurologist*. Rutland, VT: Sharp, 2006, Vol. 1, p. 141.
29. Comment made by to me by Fisher.
30. Fisher CM. Headache in cerebrovascular disease. In Vinken PJ, Bruyn GW (Eds.), *Handbook of Clinical Neurology, Volume 5: Headaches and Cranial Neuralgias*. Amsterdam: North Holland, 1968, pp. 124–156.
31. Fisher CM. Transient monocular blindness associated with hemiplegia. *American Medical Association Archives of Ophthalmology* 1952;47:167–203; Fisher CM. Occlusion of the internal carotid artery. *Archives of Neurology and Psychiatry* 1951;65:346–377; Fisher CM. Occlusion of the carotid arteries. *Archives of Neurology and Psychiatry* 1954;72:187–204; Fisher CM. Transient monocular blindness associated with hemiplegia. *Transactions of the American Neurological Association* 1951;76:154–158.
32. Fisher CM. Migraine accompaniments versus arteriosclerotic ischemia. *Transactions of the American Neurological Association* 1968;93:211–213.
33. The description is included in his memoirs: Fisher CM. Late-life migrainous scintillating scotoma without headache: One person's 26-year experience. In *Memoirs of a Neurologist*. Rutland, VT: Sharp, 2001, Vol. 3, pp. 311–334.
34. An example of medically trained individuals describing their own neurological maladies is the following book: Kapur N. (Ed.). *Injured Brains of Medical Minds: View from Within*. New York: Oxford University Press, 1997. I also began to develop visual scintillations nearly identical to those described by Fisher at approximately age 60 years.
35. Fisher CM. *Memoirs of a Neurologist*. Rutland, VT: Sharp, 2001, Vol. 3, p. 314.
36. Fisher CM. Late-life migrainous accompaniments as a cause of unexplained cerebral attacks. Charcot lecture, 1979, Hôpital de la Salpêtrière, pp. 293–324.
37. Fisher CM. Late-life migraine accompaniments as a cause of unexplained transient ischemic attacks. *Canadian Journal of Neurological Sciences* 1980;7:9–17.
38. Fisher CM. Late-life migraine accompaniments: Further experience. *Stroke* 1986;17:1033–1042.
39. Fisher CM. An unusual case of migraine accompaniments with permanent sequellae. *Headache* 1986;26:266–270.
40. Fisher CM. Cerebral ischemia—Less familiar types. *Clinical Neurosurgery* 1971;18:267–336.

CHAPTER 13

Eye Signs, Syndromes, and Reviews and Opinions

ABNORMALITIES OF VISUAL PERCEPTION, EYE APPEARANCE, AND EYE MOVEMENTS ("EYE SIGNS")

Much of human brain activity relates to visual perception and exploration of the visual environment, *looking* and *seeing*. Many of Fisher's observations during his lifetime were related to the appearance of eye structures, loss of vision, abnormal visual phenomena, and movements of the eyes, qualifying him as one of the first neuro-ophthalmologists. He began his neurological clinical practice during a period when there was no effective brain imaging. He could only use his eyes, hands, and brain to test and examine patients, some of whom had reduced consciousness and could not cooperate fully. In these patients, he discovered that careful, meticulous examination of the eyes, pupils, eyelids, eye movements, and responses to visual stimuli were available bedside tests that could yield useful information about functions of various brain regions. At Massachusetts General Hospital (MGH), he was fortunate to have outstanding ophthalmological and later neuro-ophthalmological colleagues, Drs. David Cogan, Shirley Wray, and Simmons Lessell.

Some of Fisher's contributions to abnormalities of visual function were discussed in Chapters 7, 10, and 12. These observations include the visual symptoms in patients with transient loss of vision related to carotid artery disease. The visual phenomenology of migraine accompaniments was a special interest and important contribution to medical knowledge about the differential diagnosis of migraine. He studied and described the visual perceptual symptoms in patients with posterior cerebral artery occlusive disease that involved the visual cortex and its connections. He did not limit his interest and observations about visual function to stroke patients. In 1964, Fisher reviewed the literature concerning visual functions in individuals who were blind from birth due to congenital cataracts but had these cataracts removed between ages 7 and 46 years.[1] The findings were quite different from those of individuals who had good vision and later developed obstructing lesions that were repaired. Not having previous information about how things usually appeared, the congenitally blind patients were not able to regain useful vision despite the cataract surgery. Fisher wrote,

> Seeing a thing was not innate and automatic. Every element of what is called visual perception—line, curve, angle, direction, outline, shape, shadow, and form—had to be developed through the concurrence of visual and somesthetic signals. Each element had first to be recognized and acquire "meaning."[1]

Examination of the eyelids as well as the pupils—their size, shape, and response to various stimuli—has always been an important part of the neurological examination. Fisher correlated the size of the pupils with lesions, mostly infarcts and hemorrhages, in various parts of the brainstem. The pupils were often very small, pinpoint, in lesions of the pons. Using a bright light and a magnifying lens, the very small pupils could be shown to react to light stimulation. The pupils could be widely dilated or midposition in patients whose lesions were in the midbrain. Fisher also reported unexpected changes in pupillary size in patients whose lesions were not in the brainstem. The pupil could be dilated and unreactive on the side of a carotid artery occlusion, the mechanism being ischemia to the iris of the eye.[2,3] Some patients with tuberculous meningitis had dilated pupils that were nonreactive or poorly responsive to light.[2] An oval shape of the pupils was most often a sign that accompanied severe strokes, usually indicating pressure on the midbrain.[4]

He also studied and commented on the significance of blinking, asymmetrical blinking, and the cessation of blinking. He noted the situations associated with drooping of one or both eyelids (ptosis). He reported that in some patients with strokes, especially those with left limb paralysis, the eyes were difficult to examine because of forced closure of the eyelids. He called this newly described sign "reflex blepharospasm."[5] The stimulus of lifting the eyelid to examine the eye led to strong involuntary forced closure of the eyelid on the nonparalyzed side. He posited that the most likely localization of the causative lesion was in the frontal lobe, but at the time of this observation, no brain imaging was available to prove or disprove this postulate. In stuporous and comatose patients, he showed that the reflex movement of the eyes when the head was moved horizontally and vertically had important localizing value.[2] Some patients closed one eye repeatedly without being aware that they were doing so, a sign that Fisher dubbed "unwitting closure of one eye."[2] This was a subtle indication that the patient was likely seeing double—diplopia.

Fisher analyzed unusual situations in which one or both eyes failed to move normally, and he was the first to describe the "one-and-a half syndrome."[2] In this condition, both eyes failed to move on gaze to one side. On gaze to the other side, only one eye moved. If gaze to each side was counted as one, the patient had only ½ gaze to one side so that 1½ of gaze was lost. This finding was diagnostic of a lesion in the upper, medial portion of the pons within the brainstem. In some patients, there was abnormal spontaneous movement of one or both eyes. Intermittent rhythmical up and down movement of the eyes, vertical nystagmus, indicated a lower brainstem localization.[2] He was the first to describe a different type of abnormal vertical motion of the eyes found in unresponsive patients: "In a typical case, the eyeballs intermittently dip briskly downwards through an arc of a few millimeters and then return to the primary position in a kind of bobbing action."[6] Ocular bobbing indicated a hemorrhage or infarct in the pons.

Paralysis of the movement of one eye caused by a lesion of one of the nerves to the eye (ophthalmoplegia) was known to be a common occurrence in diabetic patients, but the mechanism was not known. Fisher and colleagues showed that the cause was an infarction of the nerve related to occlusion of small arteries that fed that nonfunctioning nerve.[7] Similar ocular palsies could also occur in patients with temporal arteritis and other forms of arterial inflammation.[8]

Giant cell arteritis, an important treatable cause of blindness and other neurological disabilities in the elderly, became a focus of attention early in Fisher's career. The original name, temporal arteritis, was used because inflammation (arteritis) invariably involved the superficial temporal arteries located on the upper face. The name was later changed to giant cell arteritis because giant cells were among the inflammatory cells within biopsied arterial walls. Because the superficial temporal arteries were readily available to observe and feel, Fisher studied the diagnostic utility of feeling these and other facial and superficial arteries, such as the occipital arteries.[9] He recognized that in giant cell arteritis, the superficial temporal artery was thickened by a proliferation of connective tissue. When the inflamed thickened artery was compressed by the palpating finger, "the vessel cannot be flattened to the point of disappearance or obliteration but a firm cord persists."[9] Normal thin walled arteries can be completely compressed. Along the superficial temporal arteries, Fisher found focal firm regions that could not be easily compressed and had no pulsations. This finding was diagnostic of temporal arteritis. He later wrote about the importance of feeling the arteries of the face in the diagnosis of carotid artery occlusion.[10] The alert master clinician should use their eyes and fingers to aid in diagnosis.

CLINICAL SYNDROMES

Soon after taking up his position at the MGH, Fisher submitted a report about a particular non-stroke syndrome. The report became the lead article in the *New England Journal of Medicine*, and the syndrome has ever since been called the Miller Fisher syndrome or the Miller Fisher variant of the Guillain–Barré syndrome.[11] Two patients were seen by Fisher in Montreal, with a third examined at MGH. He admitted that he did not recognize the syndrome or its importance until the third case was studied. The three patients all had preceding respiratory infections, and their neurological abnormalities evolved gradually over days. All had complete ophthalmoplegia with no voluntary following or reflex movement of the eyes: The pupils either did not react to light or responded poorly. In addition, all the patients had severe gait ataxia, with one patient telling Fisher that "the ward was not wide enough for me to walk." Their limbs were clumsy and uncoordinated but not appreciably weak, and deep tendon reflexes were absent. Two of the patients reported that their fingers tingled, but there was no important sensory loss. All three patients made remarkable recoveries during the 3 months after leaving the hospital. Lumbar puncture to analyze the content of the fluid surrounding the spinal cord and brain was a routine procedure during the 1950s and 1960s. Fisher noted that the spinal fluid protein level was much elevated while the patient was still hospitalized. Fisher pointed out similarities to the polyneuritis described by Guillain and Barré in which the protein content of the spinal fluid was elevated. Since the original description, Miller Fisher syndrome has become quite well known, but little has changed in its description.

In 1982, Fisher described a syndrome that he called "disorientation for place."[12] One patient was described in detail, and six others were discussed briefly. The index patient was an architect who had had a recent right internal carotid artery occlusion that had caused slight weakness of his left limbs and a left visual field deficit. Computed tomography (CT) scanning showed a right parietal–occipital lobe brain infarction. Although the patient identified the MGH or a branch of the MGH as the name of the hospital, he variously located it in London, Paris, China or Japan, California, Bagdad, somewhere in New England, Arizona, etc. When his family was leaving, he asked, "Are you going upstairs now?" Fisher commented, "Disturbance of orientation for place seemed out of proportion to the rest of his behavior."[12] The other six patients all had strokes involving the right cerebral hemisphere, and four had left visual field deficits. One patient thought her house was attached to the hospital, noting that "my kitchen is down the corridor although in my mind I know it can't be." He opined that the right parieto-occipital brain region was the region especially concerned with orientation to place.[12]

In 1988, Fisher and colleagues called attention to a previously undescribed syndrome characterized by temporary narrowing of arteries within the cranium.[13] Their report described 4 patients—two women and two men aged 19, 34, 37, and 47, respectively—and reviewed 3 other cases that they had seen and the reports of 12 other patients described in the literature. Among the 19 patients, 16 were women. Six incidences occurred during the postpartum period after delivering a baby. The syndrome began with a "sudden, high-intensity headache" often accompanied by nausea, vomiting, and sensitivity to light. Seizures and multifocal neurological symptoms and signs were also common. All had focal regions of segmental vascular vasoconstriction. Narrowed arteries and dilated arteries could produce a sausage-shaped deformation of regions along the intracranial arteries. The symptoms lasted from 16 days to 6 months. Recovery was the rule. Follow-up arteriography, when performed, showed resolution of the regions of vasoconstriction. The importance of this report was to differentiate these patients who had reversible vasoconstriction from those who had inflammation of the arteries—that is, arteritis. Before this report, these patients with reversible vasoconstriction were often labeled as having cerebral arteritis and given potentially hazardous immunosuppressive treatment. Since publication of this seminal report, others have collected numerous examples, and these sudden-onset headaches have been dubbed "thunderclap headache." The syndrome has been renamed the reversible cerebral vasoconstriction syndrome (RCVS) and has become widely known among neurologists.[14]

In 1978, Fisher opined that some patients who had paralytic attacks likely had nonconvulsive seizures.[15] He described 11 patients, 4 of whom had brain tumors, 6 had old brain infarcts or hemorrhages, and 1 had a degenerative condition. The duration of the attacks was 2 minutes in 2 patients, 5–30 minutes in 5 patients, 1 hour in 1 patient, 3 hours in 1 patient, and 1 full day in 2 others. Several points argued for a seizure origin of the attacks: (1) Seizures involved the same brain functions that were abnormal between attacks, (2) electroencephalograms were abnormal, (3) there was cessation of attacks after anticonvulsants were prescribed, and (4) there was an absence of explanatory vascular lesions on cerebral angiography. Characteristically, Fisher reviewed the literature and noted that others had written about so-called inhibitory seizures and ictal paralysis.[15]

REVIEWS AND OPINIONS

Fisher considered himself a general neurologist, not just a "stroke doctor." He was fascinated by how the brain worked, and many of his observations and characterizations involved patients' cognition and behavior—so-called higher cortical functions. Chapter 12 provided descriptions of his writings concerning abulia, a name that he coined for decreased behavior, initiative, and persistence. Patients with temporary spells of abulia he dubbed as having "intermittent interruption of behavior." A very different condition, motor impersistence, described rapid following of requests or orders to perform a motor task such as closing the eyes, shaking hands, protruding the tongue yet an inability to persevere with the tasks. He also wrote extensively about amnesia and disorders of memory.

After Fisher stopped consulting regularly on patients, he wrote reviews of topics he had worked on or thought about during his more active career. Looking back on his experience with lacunar infarcts and information from magnetic resonance imaging (MRI), he summarized information about the more than 20 lacunar infarct syndromes and the pathology underlying the condition.[16] He also summarized information about the white matter abnormalities that had been recognized in patients with chronic hypertension and penetrating artery disease, Binswanger encephalopathy.[17] In this review, he commented on the historical background, CT findings, MRI results, epidemiology, pathology, clinical picture, laboratory findings, differential diagnosis, and treatment of the condition with some original thoughts. He noted that the penetrating arteries in the condition were hyalinized and thickened, but the lumens were usually open. His two cases of Binswanger encephalopathy studied with serial sections failed to show an occluded or severely narrowed penetrating artery.[17]

He delved into more complex topics, such as emotions, thoughts, and behaviors. He often included in his reviews verbatim patient notes that he had collected. He shared his large and long experience, his observations, and his thought about various topics.

He opined that "neurologists experienced in the interpretation of disease in terms of disordered action of the nervous system should be well suited to extend their field of interest to the more complex disorders of human behavior."[18]

After describing unusual behaviors in a review titled "The Reach of Neurology," he wrote in conclusion,

> *The neural organization of human behavior is complex beyond imagination. Action is determined by inherited neurophysiological tendencies, maturation, training, experience and the ideational–emotional circumstances of the moment. . . . The challenge is to improve our current analysis and explanation of behavior. . . . Inquiry into complex disorders of behavior is inseparable from the broad subject of normal mental activity, the neural organization subserving all human thought, emotion, and action.*[19]

NAMING OF SYMPTOMS OR PHENOMENA

Fisher tried to choose a word, a bon mot, or a short phrase that would characterize a symptom, finding, or behavior. Characterizations that defined and described helped introduce uniform language to describe complex behaviors to aid comparisons and collections of phenomena. He described and named behaviors in demented patients.[18] *Insistence* was a term that he coined to describe the tendency of patients to stubbornly insist on continuing whatever they were saying or doing despite dissuasion, explanation, appeals, and counterproposals. *Balking* described refusing to cooperate in routine tasks—for example, bathing, dressing, and going to bed. When cajoled or coerced, the patients often became hostile. *Insertions of inobvious origin* was a term Fisher used to describe irrelevant responses and comments that often harked back to previous conversations. *Ambient echoalia* described patients' outpourings during incoherent mumblings to continue to repeat words or phrases heard from nearby conversations or the radio or television. *Substitution for the first-person pronoun* was used to described demented patients who often used "he" or "she" or "him" or "her" instead of "I" or "me" when referring to themselves. *Lability of temper* was a descriptor that he coined to connote patients' tendency to switch moods back and forth from hostile to pleasant demeanors without obvious reason. *Amphigory* was a word coined to characterize fluent, nonsensical nonaphasic speech unrelated to the topic of discussion and unresponsive to queries or distractions.[20] An individual would continue to ramble from topic to topic even when no one was listening. *Reaching out and holding and handling* described a tendency of demented individuals to reach for a person or object and to continue to hold and manipulate objects. *Constancy of errors* described the tendency to repeat the same mistakes—for example, in counting backwards from 100 by 7's or 3's.[18]

Fisher also commented on other common terms used often in neurological practice.[18] *Anosognosia* was a term introduced originally by Babinski to describe a patient's unawareness that he or she was paralyzed on one side. Others had used the term to denote denial or unawareness of other tangible deficits, such as deafness, blindness, and inability to read. Fisher broadened the term to include unawareness or lack of insight into any deficit. *Confabulation* (inadvertent replacement of memories from the past into the present) occurred only when individuals were unaware of their loss of the ability to make new memories. Fisher also shared his opinions about perseveration, memory and amnesia, restlessness and agitation, failure of gesture in aphasics, pain localization, and selective localization of functions in the brain.

SELF-OBSERVATION

Fisher urged neurologists to engage in self-observation:

> *I think there is a place for the scrutiny of personal experience and for self-experimentation. Physicians, particularly neurologists, are in an advantageous position to utilize the analysis of personal events for insights they may provide into the biology of the nervous system—migraine, pain, referred pain, malaise, emotion, depression, mood, worry, headache, discovery, ideas, thinking, diagnosis, and so on.*[18]

In his memoirs, Fisher included detailed descriptions of his own experiences with myocardial infarction,[21] migraine,[22] and back pain.[23]

NOTES

1. Fisher CM. The late acquisition of vision by persons born blind as the result of bilateral congenital cataracts. *Transactions of the American Neurological Association* 1964;89:195–197.
2. Fisher CM. Some neuro-ophthalmological observations. *Journal of Neurology Neurosurgery and Psychiatry* 1967;30:383–392.
3. Fisher CM. Dilated pupil in carotid occlusion. *Transactions of the American Neurological Association* 1966;91:230–231.
4. Fisher CM. Oval pupils. *Archives of Neurology* 1980;37:502–503.
5. Fisher CM. Reflex blepharospasm. *Neurology* 1963;13:77–78.
6. Fisher CM. Ocular bobbing. *Archives of Neurology* 1964;11:543–546.

7. Asbury A, Fisher CM, Aldredge H, Hershberg R. Diabetic ophthalmoplegia: A clinico-pathologic investigation. *Transactions of the American Neurological Association* 1969;94:64–68; Asbury A, Aldredge H, Hershberg R, Fisher CM. Ocular palsy in diabetes mellitus: A clinico-pathologic study. *Brain* 1970;93:555–566.
8. Fisher CM. Ocular palsy in temporal arteritis. *Minnesota Medicine* 1959;42:1258–1268, 1430–1437, 1617–1630.
9. Fisher CM. Palpation of arteries in temporal arteritis: Reemphasis of the value of careful palpation. *Journal of the American Medical Association* 1961;175:325.
10. Fisher CM. Facial pulses in internal carotid artery occlusion. *Neurology* 1970;20:476–478.
11. Fisher M. An unusual variant of acute idiopathic polyneuritis (syndrome of ophthalmoplegia, ataxia, and areflexia). *New England Journal of Medicine* 1956;255:57–65.
12. Fisher CM. Disorientation for place. *Archives of Neurology* 1982;39:33–36.
13. Call GK, Fleming MC, Scalfon S, Levine H, Kistler JP, Fisher CM. Reversible cerebral segmental vasoconstriction. *Stroke* 1988;19:1159–1170.
14. RCVS has been widely studied and further characterized: Ducros A, Boukobza M, Porcher R, et al. The clinical and radiological spectrum of reversible cerebral vasoconstriction syndrome: A prospective series of 67 patients. *Brain* 2007;130:3091–3101; Ducros A. Reversible cerebral vasoconstriction syndrome. *Lancet Neurology* 2012;11:906–917; Singhal AB, Haij-Ali RA, Topcuoglu MA, et al. Reversible cerebral vasoconstriction syndromes: Analysis of 139 cases. *Archives of Neurology* 2011;68:1005–1012.
15. Fisher CM. Transient paralytic attacks of obscure nature: The question of non-convulsive seizure paralysis. *Canadian Journal of Neurological Sciences* 1978;5:267–273.
16. Fisher CM. Lacunar strokes and infarcts: A review. *Neurology* 1982;32: 871–876; Fisher CM. Lacunar infarcts: A review. *Cerebrovascular Diseases* 1991;1:311–320.
17. Fisher CM. Binswanger's encephalopathy: A review. *Journal of Neurology* 1989;236:65–79.
18. Fisher CM. Neurologic fragments I: Clinical observations in demented patients. *Neurology* 1988;38:1868–1873; Fisher CM. Neurologic fragments II: Remarks on anosognosia, confabulation, memory, and other topics; and an appendix on self-observation. *Neurology* 1989;39:127–132.
19. Fisher CM. The reach of neurology. *Archives of Neurology* 20013;60:173–177.
20. Fisher CM. Nonsense speech–amphigory. *Transactions of the American Neurological Association* 1970;95:238–240.
21. Fisher CM. A personal account of an MI (1988). In *Memoirs of a Neurologist*. Rutland, VT: Sharp, 2006, Vol. 1, pp. 229–230.
22. Fisher CM. Late-life migrainous scintillating scotoma without headache: One person's 26-year experience. In *Memoirs of a Neurologist*. Rutland, VT: Sharp, 2001, Vol. 3, pp. 311–334.
23. Fisher CM. Personal diary: Notes on low backache. In *Memoirs of a Neurologist*. Rutland, VT: Sharp, 2006, Vol. 5, pp. 142–147.

PART VI
The Last Decades of Fisher's Life

Although he formally retired in 1980, Fisher continued to make important observations even during the early years of the 21st century. His last years were fraught with health issues.

CHAPTER 14

Retirement and Beyond

Fisher's Last Decades

In September 1980, Dr. C. Miller Fisher officially "retired." Drs. E. P. Richardson, Raymond Adams, and J. Philip Kistler sent out the following letter inviting current and former fellows, colleagues, and friends to attend a program in his honor:

> This year Miller Fisher is retiring as Professor of Neurology and as Neurologist at the Massachusetts General Hospital. This marks the 26th year of his service to the Massachusetts General Hospital and of his devoted tutorship of the Neurology residents. He will, of course, continue here as a Senior Consultant and as Emeritus Professor at Harvard Medical School, working "the night shift" as usual with future generations of residents and students in the Emergency Room and the wards. And, of course, he still has thousands of boxes of slides to study.[1]

His retirement was celebrated with a full-day scientific program—C. Miller Fisher Day—held at the Ether Dome at Massachusetts General Hospital (MGH) on September 7, 1980. I opened the presentations with "Fisher's Rules," a summary of some of his guiding principles. These rules were described and annotated in Chapter 9. Fellows and colleagues made 30 presentations during the day. In the evening, there was a celebratory dinner in his honor at a local Boston hotel.

ACTIVE "RETIREMENT," 1980–2003

Of course, Fisher had no intention at all to really retire. He continued to be quite active during the next 25 years. After breakfasting together, Doris continued to drive him to work each morning. She would usually make lunch for him to eat in his office. He stopped taking a regular turn as attending physician on the neurology ward service at MGH. The neurology department set aside an hour each week for Fisher Rounds, which was held in a conference room on White 12, the floor that housed the neurology ward patients. Residents would choose a case from the wards, and Fisher would discuss the case with the residents, fellows, and staff attendees. The discussions would be in great depth, with Fisher leading by using his inimical Socratic technique. Fisher would sit at the head of the table facing the patient. The patient would often gaze at the portrait of Fisher on the wall above. Often, the rounds would last for hours. Fisher continued to regularly attend the weekly brain cutting sessions and to comment on each brain studied. He also attended grand rounds and sometimes was asked to be the discussant. He regularly attended the meetings of the Boston Stroke Society, a city-wide Boston organization of physicians interested in stroke and cerebrovascular disease. The first meeting was in October 1984 at MGH. Years later, the name of the organization was changed to the Miller Fisher Society.

Much of Fisher's time was spent in his office examining slides, thinking, and writing. He was always available to residents and colleagues who came to his office to discuss a case, an idea, an event, or to just schmooze. He continued to see consults on patients housed in the private sections of the hospital when requested by the patients' physicians. He made himself available to the residents and fellows who would ask him to see a patient with them or discuss aspects of a case they had seen. He continued to see private patients in his office on Kennedy 9. He kept his own schedule with the help of department secretaries. Doris did the billing and always chided him on his very low fees, which he refused to raise. His office and the tables in it were packed with boxes of pathology slides, books, and papers. Lantern slides for presentations were piled on his desk. He would see and examine the patients amid this disarray. Invariably he would stay late each night. When finished, he would call Doris to come pick him up in their car.

He continued to publish important papers and observations in medical journals. These consisted of his clinical observations gained from a single patient or group of patients—for example, "An Unusual Case of Migraine Accompaniments"[2]; "Late-Life Migraine Accompaniments: Further

Experiences"[3]; "The 'Herald Hemiparesis' of Basilar Artery Occlusion"[4]; "Clinical Observations in Demented Patients"[5]; "Visual Hallucinations and Racing Thoughts on Eye Closure After Minor Surgery"[6]; "Unexplained Sudden Amnesia"[7]; and "Disorientation for Place."[8]

Some contributions reflected anatomical or pathological observations Fisher made from examining specimens and slides—for example, bilateral distribution of end branches of pontine arteries,[9] demonstration of the source of bleeding in a patient with hypertensive brain hemorrhage,[10] and bilateral eye signs from occlusion of a single branch artery.[11] Other contributions represented reviews and comments on topics that he had written on previously—for example, lacunes, small deep infarcts[12]; transient ischemic attacks[13]; a review of Binswanger's encephalopathy[14]; and a review of the alien hand phenomenon with six personal cases.[15]

During his later years, Fisher published some of his thoughts and musings about his own career and on general topics of philosophy and behavior—for example, "If There Were No Free Will"[16]; "A Career in Cerebral Vascular Disease"[17]; "The Reach of Neurology:[18]; and remarks on anosognosia (lack of awareness of a deficit), confabulation (fabricated, distorted, or misinterpreted memories), all aspects of memory and other topics; and self-observation.[19]

In 1986, Fisher began to work on his memoirs, which were first published in 1992 by a small publishing house in Vermont under the aegis of Montreal General Hospital and Massachusetts General Hospital. He continued to add to the memoirs, publishing additional volumes in 1999, 2001, 2004, 2006, 2007, and 2008. The memoirs consisted of autobiographical information; remarks made on various occasions; published and unpublished papers and lectures; stories; limericks and verses; and many thoughts, observations, and teachings. His daughter in-law Susan would help type material for the manuscripts of his memoirs. She was a frequent visitor and a strong and able supporter of Fisher. A short paperback autobiography was created and Susan Fisher, Alex (Fisher's grandson), and Phil Kistler handed out 500 copies to attendees at the annual American Academy of Neurology meeting in Boston in 2007. Drs. Natalia Rost and Aneesh Singhal handed out the remaining volumes of a portion of Fisher's autobiographical memoirs at the annual meeting of the American Academy of Neurology in Honolulu, Hawaii, in 2011.

In 1988, Fisher had his first serious medical illness, a myocardial infarction. At the time, he was seriously overweight; performed little, if any, exercise; and paid little attention to the contents of his diet or to his health in general. The manner in which he handled his symptoms conveys much about his personality and behavioral tendencies. He included a description of the events of that day in his memoirs. He became ill on a Sunday, a day that he almost always spent in his office working:

> *While in the surgery [his office] tidying up on a Sunday afternoon, moderately severe pain came on in the thoracic spine. After 10 minutes, it persisted and precluded sitting quietly. Concentrating on desk work was impossible due to pain and a distinct malaise. Lying or sitting in various positions, standing, walking, and stretching in the back by hanging from a doorjamb did not affect the pain; nor did abundant antacid. After 30 minutes the back pain was more authoritative, and aching had begun in both cheeks.... The soft part of the nose was ice-cold, whereas the lips and ears were warm.... After an hour of restlessly moving about, it was decided to carry out what I call a pain-o-gram, a methodical detailed analysis of all aspects of the pain. It was an ache of 6/10 intensity, constant, not cramping or throbbing. It was deep, posterior, in the spine or close to it in the midline, 8½ inches below the vertebra prominens. Bending, tilting, twisting, and jarring did not aggravate the pain.... On and off deep aching appeared in both upper arms and in the right forearm.*[20]

Fisher approached his own symptoms as if he were the physician attempting to diagnose the illness. He used a very methodical approach. He characterized the symptoms qualitatively and quantitatively. He made hypotheses as he tested himself. Was it an aortic dissection? He felt his limb and carotid pulses and found them normal—evidence against a dissection. Was it a myocardial infarction? There was no chest pain save for occasional brief aching in both axillae. There was no angor animi, shortness of breath or cough. The pain was not related to exercise, breathing, or coughing."[21] He checked his blood pressure and pulse. He also wondered about an ulcer or other gastrointestinal cause.

Finally, Fisher called his wife and asked her to come and bring him home because he could not continue working. Doris responded, "Miller, you must be very sick. You have never done this before. Go immediately to the emergency room and have them check you out."[22] Fortunately, he did follow her advice. He had had an inferior myocardial infarction that was complicated by hypotension and bradycardia. He made a very good recovery, and within weeks he was back to work as before. While in the hospital, he noted that he had an uncharacteristic lack of energy—"no get up and go." This stimulated him to think about and explore inertia and motivation in neurological phenomenology.

AWARDS

Honors and awards began to accrue. In 1982, he had been awarded the Jacoby Award of the American Neurological Association at its annual meeting in Washington, DC. This award was given every 3 years "to a member of the American Neurological Association who has conducted especially meritorious experimental work on any neurological or psychiatric subject during the preceding 3 years." The Congress of Neurological Surgeons honored Fisher by inviting him to be the honored guest at their annual meeting in Chicago in 1983. This selection was a rarity. Almost all of the previous honored guests were neurosurgeons. It was very unusual for a neurologist to be chosen. Fisher presented two major lectures at the meeting—one concerning the neurological basis of inactivity and overactivity, agitation, and another on painful states. He also delivered advise to neurosurgical residents.[23]

As a testimony to his continued interaction with neurology residents, he was awarded the Teacher of the Year Prize and plaque in 1990 by the neurology service at MGH, 10 years after his official "retirement." Fisher was very proud of this award because he considered himself primarily a learner and a teacher. In 1993, he received the Mihara Memorial Research Grant awarded by a Cerebrovascular Disorders Committee in Japan. In 1994, the American Association of Neurological Surgeons (the senior neurosurgical society in the United States—formerly the Harvey Cushing Society) decided to fund and collect interviews of a small group of honored neurologists, neuroscientists, and neurosurgeons in the archives of their society. I was chosen to interview Fisher. Approximately 3 hours of discussion was later condensed to one long audiotape recording.[24] In 1997, the New England chapter of the American Heart Association inaugurated the C. Miller Fisher Award to be given annually to individuals who had made important contributions to knowledge in the field of stroke and cerebrovascular diseases. Fisher delivered comments honoring the awardees at annual meetings at which the awards were presented. The first physicians honored (Drs. Nicholas Zervas, myself, Robert Ojemann, J. Philip Kistler, Robert Ackerman, Phillip Wolf, and Carlos Kase) were colleagues or mentees of Fisher. The honor that he cherished above the others came to Fisher in 1998 when he was chosen to enter the Canadian Medical Hall of Fame. Despite leaving Canada nearly a half century before, Fisher always considered himself a proud Canadian and was mindful of his Canadian heritage.

LATER YEARS, 2003–2012

After the turn of the century, health and mobility issues began to plague Fisher and his wife. He and Doris were in their late 80s. His gait began to deteriorate, and he became rather unsteady when he walked, especially on uneven terrain and on stairs and inclines. He developed glaucoma and cataracts, and his vision gradually failed. Beginning in approximately 2003, Doris began to develop physical and mental symptoms. She broke her hips twice and finally completely stopped driving in 2005. She began to show memory and behavioral signs that gradually worsened so that by 2006 she required a nursing home placement and had severe dementia. Doris died in November 2008. Figure 14.1 is a photograph of Doris with Fisher taken in 1995 before her decline. Figure 14.2 is a photograph of Doris and Fisher at a dinner arranged by Ackerman.

When Doris could not drive and finally stopped driving, Fisher had no way to regularly come to the hospital from his home in Winchester. His poor vision prevented him from driving. At home, there was a flight of stairs from the pavement to the front porch that was not easy for him to navigate. His poor vision also made it a challenge to get about in the house and up and down the stairs. Winter snow and ice made entering

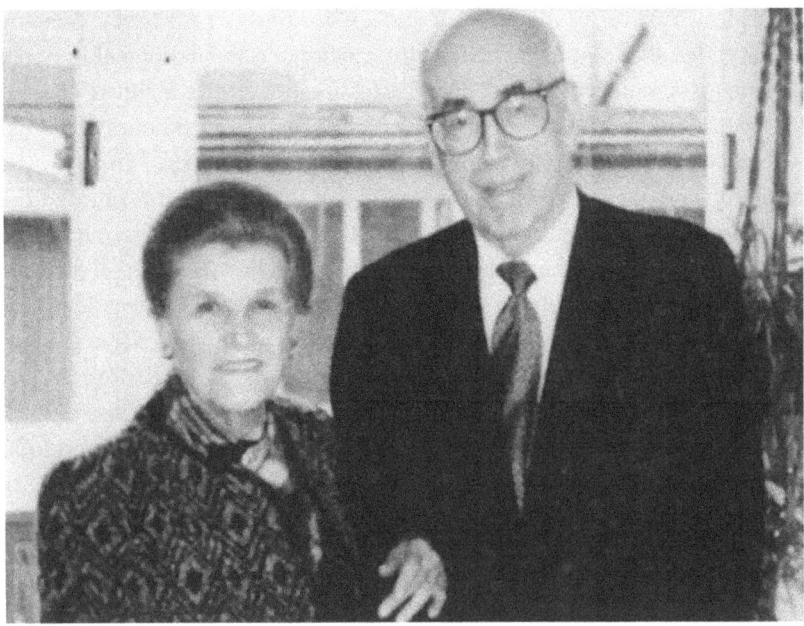

Figure 14.1 Fisher with his wife, Doris, in 1995.

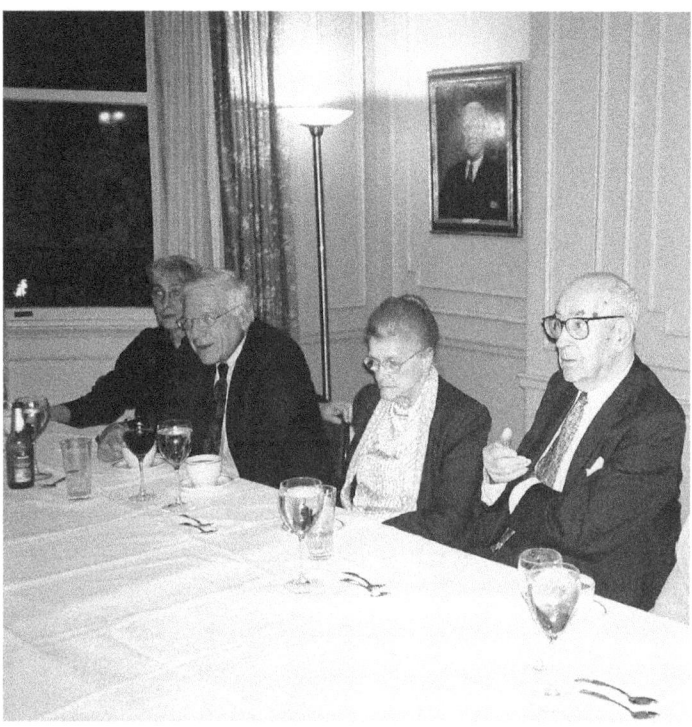

Figure 14.2 (From left to right) Brenda Caplan, Louis Caplan, Doris Fisher, and Fisher at a dinner at St. Botolph Club in Boston arranged by Dr. Robert Ackerman.

and leaving the house virtually non-navigable for him. When Doris was in the nursing home, he would find a way to visit her often. Kistler would drive Fisher to the nursing home, wait for him in the car, and then drive Fisher back to his home. In addition, Kistler would drive him to doctor visits. Colleagues, family, and friends would occasionally visit the Fisher home. Dr. Joe Hanaway would visit the Winchester home whenever he was in Boston. Visitors would often bring a sandwich or other food that Fisher liked. Fisher's son Hugh and his wife Susan would keep close tabs on him and would visit from Albany periodically. MGH neurologists would on occasion be brought to visit Fisher in his home. Kistler, Ackerman, and occasionally others would drive him on special occasions to MGH (e.g., for a meeting of the Boston Stroke Society). Figures 14.3A and 14.3B are photographs of various physicians visiting Fisher in and near his home.

The regular Fisher's rounds ended in 2004. His oldest child, Elizabeth, now a retired attorney living in New Mexico, would order regular food deliveries, and a friend who lived nearby would visit once or twice a week and bring a home-cooked dinner. Fisher remained alert and inquisitive, becoming

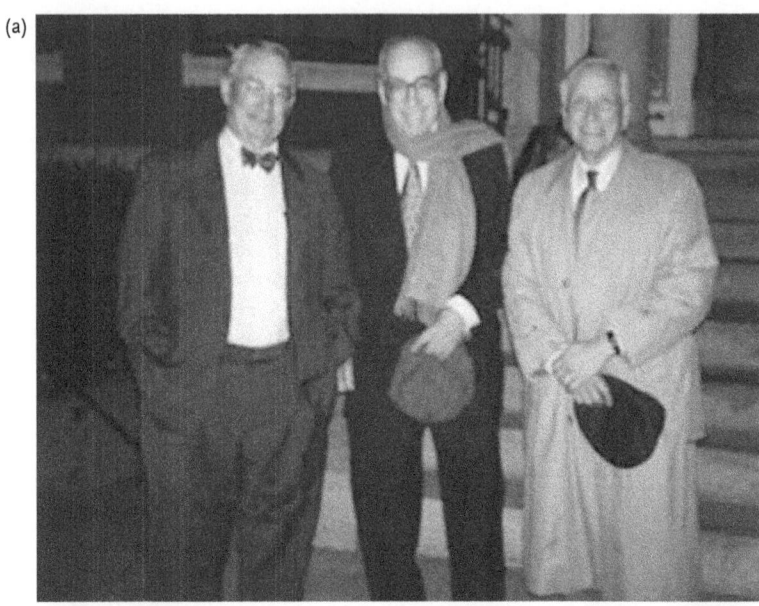

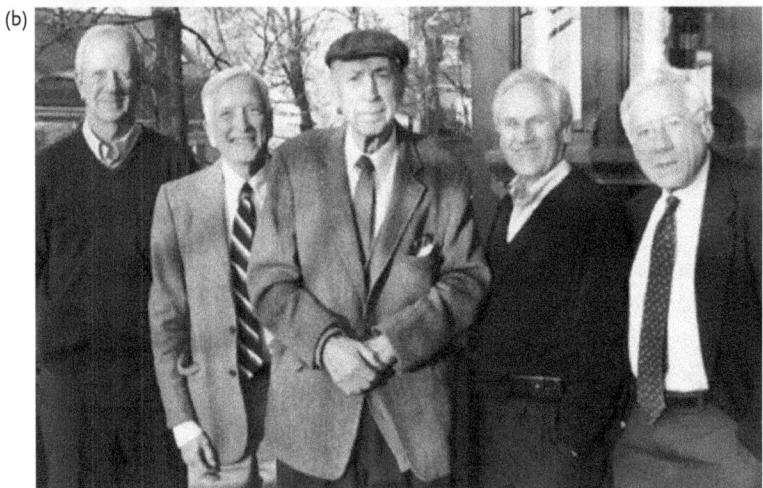

Figure 14.3 (A) Drs. Mohr, Fisher, and Ackerman on one of the in-town trips. (B) From left to right: Drs. Kase, Ackerman, Fisher, Wolf, and Caplan outside the Fisher residence.
Source: A, reproduced with permission from Caplan LR. *Caplan's Stroke* (5th ed.). Cambridge, UK: Cambridge University Press, 2016.

fascinated by genetics, a topic in which he had had no formal education or training; in fact, he bought and studied a textbook of genetics. But the lonely isolated existence became boring and depressing, especially in winter.

Fisher continued to read in his home using a magnifying glass to methodically and slowly navigate the enlarged print on each page. He continued to dictate his memoirs. A typing service and later his daughter Elizabeth and his daughter-in-law Susan would type up his dictations. In 2007, Fisher agreed to undergo cataract surgery. This helped his vision slightly. He carefully studied and noted fluctuations in his visual abilities and the related circumstances. After eye surgery, he developed some visual allusions and visual hallucinations. Miller became despondent, and it was clearly unsafe for him to live in the large Winchester home by himself.

Dr. Hugh Fisher, Fisher's youngest son and a urologist, insisted that his father move to Albany in 2008, where Hugh lived and practiced. Fisher was first housed at the Atria Senior Living facility in Albany. A number of other retired physicians also lived in this one-story facility, including a retired ophthalmologist with whom Fisher shared stories and information about changes in medicine. Fisher had a relatively large living and sleeping room and a bathroom. He continued to work on his memoirs there. He had his microscope and could also look at pathological slides. He had a magnifying glass with which he laboriously read the piles of papers that were strewn around the room. He regularly visited the home of Hugh and Susan and delighted in playing with his grandchildren. On one of these visits, Hugh was surprised at how avidly his father played the role of conductor of a train and entered gleefully in managing a train trip with the grandchildren. Fisher was always an accomplished actor. He often played possum with patients and trainees by pretending not to understand. He had often played the naive, bumbling speaker and other roles. This persona was part of his teaching technique throughout the years. It was no surprise that he could avidly assume a new acting role with his grandchildren.

Fisher developed more difficulty swallowing and navigating, requiring a walker for safe travel on foot. He developed a cough and became ill with pneumonia. He refused treatment, and Atria Senior Living told him that he could no longer stay and needed to be moved to another facility. He moved to St. Peter's and had a much smaller living space—essentially one room. He continued to try to keep up with reading and the neurological literature and continued to write. He ate sparingly, became more asthenic, had more difficulty breathing, and finally, at age 98 years, breathed his last breath.

He was 98 years old and had witnessed remarkable changes during his near century of life. Much of the change in the care of patients with stroke and cerebrovascular disease could be directly attributable to his research, writings, and teachings and to the physicians he had mentored lovingly during his long and fruitful career. Obituaries published after his death celebrated his life and his accomplishments.[25]

NOTES

1. Letter from Dr. E. P. Richardson to Louis R. Caplan, MD, February 26, 1980.
2. Fisher CM. An unusual case of migraine accompaniments with permanent sequelae. *Headache* 1986;26:266–270.
3. Fisher CM. Late-life migraine accompaniments: Further experience. *Stroke* 1986;17:1033–1042.
4. Fisher CM. The "herald hemiparesis" of basilar artery occlusion. *Archives of Neurology* 1988;19:1159–1170.
5. Fisher CM. Neurological fragments I: Clinical observations in demented patients. *Neurology* 1988;38:1868–1873.
6. Fisher CM. Visual hallucinations and racing thoughts on eye closure after minor surgery. *Archives of Neurology* 1991;48:1091–1092.
7. Fisher CM. Unexplained sudden amnesia. *Archives of Neurology* 2002;59:1310–1313.
8. Fisher CM. Disorientation for place. *Archives of Neurology* 1982;39:33–36.
9. Fisher CM. Bilateral distribution of the end branches of the pontine paramedian branches of the basilar artery. *Journal of Neuro-Ophthalmology* 2003;23:181.
10. Fisher CM. Hypertensive cerebral hemorrhage: Demonstration of the source of bleeding. *Journal of Neuropathology and Experimental Neurology* 2003;62:104–107.
11. Fisher CM. Neuroanatomic evidence to explain why bilateral internuclear ophthalmoplegia may result from occlusion of a unilateral pontine branch artery. *Journal of Neuro-Ophthalmology* 2004; 24:39–41.
12. Fisher CM. Lacunes: Small deep cerebral infarcts. *Neurology* 2011;77:2104.
13. Fisher CM. Transient ischemic attacks. *New England Journal of Medicine* 2002;347:141–142.
14. Fisher CM. Binswanger's encephalopathy: A review. *Journal of Neurology* 1989;236:65–79.
15. Fisher CM. Alien hand phenomena: A review with the addition of six personal cases. *Canadian Journal of Neurological Sciences* 2000;27:192–203.
16. Fisher CM. If there were no free will. *Medical Hypotheses* 2001;56:364–366.
17. Fisher CM. A career in cerebrovascular disease: A personal account. *Stroke* 2001;32:2719–2724.
18. Fisher CM. The reach of neurology. *Archives of Neurology* 2003; 60:173–177.
19. Fisher CM. Neurological fragments II: Remarks on anosognosia, confabulation, memory, and other topics; and an appendix on self-observation. *Neurology* 1989;39:127–132.
20. Fisher CM. *Memoirs of a Neurologist*. Rutland, VT: Sharp, 2006, Vol. 1, p. 229.
21. Fisher CM. *Memoirs of a Neurologist*. Rutland, VT: Sharp, 2006, Vol. 1, p. 229–230.
22. Personal communication from Doris Fisher.
23. The three lectures presented to the Congress of Neurological Surgeons were later published in a volume that contained the proceedings of the meeting: Fisher CM. Abulia minor versus agitated behavior. *Clinical Neurosurgery* 1984;31:9–31; Fisher CM. Painful states: A neurological commentary. *Clinical Neurosurgery* 1984;31:32–53; Fisher CM. Remarks to neurosurgical residents. *Clinical Neurosurgery* 1984;31:54–57.

24. The interview is available on YouTube: "C. Miller Fisher, MD Interviewed by Louis R. Caplan MD," October 7, 2016.
25. Mohr JP, Caplan LR, Kistler JP. C. Miller Fisher: An appreciation. *Stroke* 2012;43:1739–1740; Caplan LR, Mohr JP, Ackerman RH. In memoriam: Charles Miller Fisher (1913–2012). *Archives of Neurology* 2012;69:1208–1209; Koroshetz WJ, Mohr JP, Caplan LR. C. Miller Fisher MD (1913–2012). *Neurology* 2012;79(10).

NAME INDEX

Figures are indicated by *f* following the page number

For the benefit of digital users, indexed terms that span two pages (e.g., 52–53) may, on occasion, appear on only one of those pages.

Ackerman, Robert, 157, 197, 247, 250*f*
Adams, Raymond, 83, 88, 90, 93–95, 94*f*, 95*f*, 96–99, 98*f*, 101, 104n14, 115, 122, 124, 126, 133, 136–38, 137*f*, 139*f*, 139–40, 157–58, 158*f*, 159*f*, 161, 198–200, 202–5, 208, 210n21, 213, 217–18, 219, 243
Angevine, Jay, 136
Arnason, Barry, 136
Ayer, James B, 97

Babinski, Joseph, 77–78n5
Baker, A. B., 208n2
Banting, Frederick, 13
Barrows, Lawrence, 223–24
Best, Charles, 13, 14–15
Blackburn, J. A., 36, 37–38
Brownlees, Peter, 59

Caplan, Brenda, 249*f*
Caplan, L. R., 161, 164, 199–200, 211n29, 230n20, 247, 249*f*, 250*f*
Carroll, Margaret, 140
Castle, William, 133–34
Caviness, Verne, 157–58, 159*f*
Charcot, Jean Martin, 77–78n5
Chiari, Hans, 115–16
Churchill, Winston, 87
Cobb, Stanley, 85–86, 97, 126, 136
Cogan, David, 136, 232
Cole, Edwin, 136
Conant, James, 87

Cone, William, 70
Cooley, Denton, 129n28
Cramer, Steve, 162–63
Cushing, Harvey, 73–75, 78n6

Dandy, Walter, 73–75
Davidson, Wilburt, 96
DeBakey, Michael, 129n28
Denny-Brown, Derek, 83–84, 86–95, 88*f*, 93*f*, 97–98, 99, 104n11, 133–34, 135–36, 140–41
DeSanctis, Roman, 156
Dodge, Phillip, 136
Duff, Lyman, 106–7
Durand-Fardel, xxx, 120–21

Eastcott, Felix, 120
Elliot, Harold, 106–7
Elsberg, Charles, 71–72
Evelyn, Kenneth, 26, 72–73, 106–7

Fang, Harry, 223–24
Ferrand, xxx, 120–21
Fields, William, 19, 21n21, 181, 182*f*
Fisher, Doris (neé Stiefelmeyer), 19, 27–28, 34, 42, 67, 76, 108*f*, 138–39, 141–42, 147–48, 160, 244, 246, 248*f*, 248–49, 249*f*
Fisher, Elizabeth (child of Miller), 67, 76, 108*f*, 249–50
Fisher, Elizabeth (neé England), 5
Fisher, Ella (neé Knechtel), 9

Fisher, Frieda (neé Kaufman), 5, 6, 8–9
Fisher, George Middleton, 5, 6f, 6–8
Fisher, Hugh (child of Miller), 76, 108f, 163, 248–49, 251
Fisher, Mirabeau M., 5
Fisher, Peter (child of Miller), 76, 108f
Fitzgerald, R. R., 117
Foix, Charles, xiv–xv, xvi–xviin6
Foley, Joseph, 90
Freemont-Smith, xxx, 86
Freud, Sigmond, 77–78n5
Friedlich, Allan, 156
Fulton, John, 86–87

George V (King of England), 4
Gibbs, Frederick/Erna, 86
Gowers, William, 77–78n5
Greenfield, Godwin, 78n6
Gregg, Allan, 70–71, 84–85, 86
Gress, Daryl, 158–59

Hakim, Salomon, 164, 202–5, 208, 212n34
Ham, Arthur, 14–15
Hanaway, Joe, 248–49
Hanes, xxx, 96–97
Harris, Wilfred, 75–76
Harrison, Tinsley, 198–99, 210n21, 210n23
Hebb, Harvey, 32–33
Heyman, Al, 223–24
Hitler, Adolf, 25, 48, 60
Holmes, Gordon, 77–78n5, 78n6
Hortop, William, 4

Jackson, Hughlings, 77–78n5

Karp, Herb, 190n33, 199, 223–24
Kase, Carlos, 247, 250f
Kistler, J. Phillip, 157, 158–59, 187–88, 199–200, 243, 247, 248–49
Kitchener, Horatio Herbert, 4
Knight, Gavin, 51
Koroshetz, Walter, 158–59
Kubik, Charles, 97, 139–40

Lennox, William, 86
Lessell, Simmons, 232
Long, Crawford, 154n4

MacLeod, Wendell, 67
Mancall, Elliott, 136
Mandela, Nelson, 62n18
Marie, Pierre, 77–78n5, 120–21
Martin, Joseph, 140–41, 157–58, 158f, 159f
McDevitt, Ellen, 223–24
McDougall, David, 100
McKay, Fred, 72
McKay, Grace, 89–90
McKissock, Wylie, 185
McNaughton, Francis, 106–7, 127
Meakins, Jonathan, 25–26
Means, James Howard, 133–34
Merritt, Houston, 86, 97–98, 198–99, 210n20
Michelsen, Jost, 137
Millikan, Clark, 191n40, 223–24
Mills, Edward, 126
Minot, George, 133–34
Mohr, J. P., 156–57, 158–59, 199–200, 250f
Molins, Mahels, 119–20
Moniz, Egaz, 114, 127–28n9
Morton, William T. G., 154n4
Munro, Donald, 85–86
Myerson, Abraham, 85–86

Nelson, Horatio, 32

Oertel, Horst, 68–69
Ojemann, Robert, 156, 158–59, 187–88, 198, 200–1, 206, 208, 247
Osler, William, 13, 20n6, 68–69, 78n6, 116–17

Pasteur, Louis, 204–5
Penfield, Wilder, 69–72, 73–75, 74f, 78n6, 83, 84–85, 126
Peterson, Norman, 72, 107–9
Pickering, George White, 120
Prince, Morton, 84, 103n7
Putnam, Tracy, 85–86

Rabinovitch, Reuben, 54–55, 75. *See also* Vosic, Harry
Ramon y Cajal, Santiago, 70, 77–78n5
Reivich, Martin, 209n16
Richards, Norma, 89–90

Richardson, E. P., 139*f*, 139–40, 156, 158*f*, 159*f*, 243
Rio-Hortega, Pio del, 70
Robb, Charles, 120
Robb, Preston, 73–75, 127
Roberson, Glenn, 187–88
Romanul, Flaviau, 90
Romberg, Moritz, 77–78n5
Roosevelt, Franklin, 87
Ropper, Alan, 158–59, 199–200
Russel, Colin, 70, 72

Sahs, Adolph, 223–24
Samuels, Martin, 174, 189n13, 199–200
Scheinberg, Peritz, 223–24
Sciarra, Dan, 210n20
Seagram, Joseph E., 4
Sherrington, Charles, 78n6, 86–87, 89
Shirras, David, 72
Smith, Donald, 69
Sperber, Mihil, 52–53
Stalin, Joseph, 48
Stauffenberg, Claus von, 60
Stephen, George, 69
Swank, Roy, 83, 103n3
Swearingen, Brooke, 158–59
Sweet, William, 202–4
Symonds, Charles, 99, 119–20, 186–87

Tagrin, Edith, 176–77, 193–94
Thorn, George, 210n21
Toole, Jim, 223–24
Tyler, H. Richard, 133–34

Victor, Maurice, 139*f*, 139–40, 199–200
Victoria (Queen), 69
Vincent, Clovis, 54–55
Virchow, Rudolph, 62n19
Vosic, Harry, 54–55. *See also* Rabinovitch, Reuben

Waksman, Byron, 136
Webber, Samuel Gilbert, 84
Webster, Donald, 26–27
Wernicke, Carl, 77–78n5
Whipple, Allen, 70
White, Paul Dudley, 156, 193
Willis, Thomas, 116–17
Wilson, Kinnier, 77–78n5
Wolf, Phillip, 247, 250*f*
Wray, Shirley, 136, 232
Wright, Irving, 223

Yakovlev, Paul, 97, 136
Young, Arthur, 72

Zervas, Nicholas, 247

SUBJECT INDEX

Figures are indicated by *f* following the page number

For the benefit of digital users, indexed terms that span two pages (e.g., 52–53) may, on occasion, appear on only one of those pages.

ABC (facial) pulses, 195–96, 196*f*
abulia, 220–22, 230n20, 237
air bombings (WWII), 29–30, 57–58
Alcantara, HMS, 35, 37–38
Alexandria Hospital for Infectious Diseases, 25–26
Alzheimer disease, 147
ambient echoalia, 238–39
American Association of Neurological Surgeons, 247
amnesia, 216–19, 230n20
amphigory, 238–39
aneurysms, 177, 186–88, 191n36
angiography, 114, 127–28n9, 144, 187–88, 202
Annaburg, Germany, 59–60
anosognosia, 239
anticoagulation therapy, 215–16, 223–25
"An Unusual Case of Migraine Accompaniments," 244–45
appendicitis, 55
Aquavit, 39
arterial dissection, 200–2, 211n26
arterial pulse examination, 173
arteries, narrowing studies, 125–26, 176–77, 234–35
atheromatous branch disease, 179*f*, 179–80
atherosclerosis, 192–95, 194*f*, 208n2
atrial fibrillation, 101–2, 125, 213–16
Atria Senior Living facility, 251
awards, 247

bacterial endocarditis, 102
balking, 238–39
balloon catheter, 129n28
basilar branch infarcts, 179–80
Battle of Dunkirk, 27–28
Bedford Basin (Halifax, Canada), 28
Best and Taylor's Textbook of Physiology, 14–15
Binswanger encephalopathy, 237
blinking, examination of, 233–34
body fluids measurement, 72–73
Boston City Hospital
  background, 84–88, 85*f*
  conferences, 92–95
  described, 133–35
  Fisher's fellowship, 83–84, 89–95, 99–103
  grand rounds, 90–91, 92*f*
  living conditions, 99
  Mallory Building, 83, 93–95, 94*f*
  necropsy/autopsy, 100
  nervous system disease care, 84–85
  Neurological Research Unit, 88–95, 97–98, 136
  Neuropathology Department, 96–103
  sensory charts, 91, 92*f*, 93
  Thorndike Memorial Laboratory, 133–34
Boston University, 133–34
brain
  anatomy in memory function, 216–19
  cognition/behavior studies, 220–22

brain (*cont.*)
　damage studies, of Fisher, 101–3, 115–17, 118, 139–40
　embolism, 102, 121–24, 123*f*, 124*f*, 196, 197*f*, 213–16, 223
　ischemia, anticoagulation therapy, 215–16, 223–25
　ischemia/infarction, 192–95, 194*f*
British Broadcasting Corporation, 53
Bullfinch, Charles, 134–35

C. Miller Fisher Award, 247
C. Miller Fisher Day, 243
Canadian Medical Hall of Fame, 247
Carnavon Castle, HMS, 35, 37–38
carotid artery disease, 109–20, 111*f*, 129n28, 192–200, 194*f*, 225–27, 226*f*
cataract surgery, 250–51
cerebellar hemorrhage, 101–2, 181–88, 183*f*, 187*f*, 190n33
Charcot lecture, 228
Charles Mueller Cooperage, 5
China, stroke prevalence, xiii–xiv
cholera epidemic, 84
chronic diseases, 84
circle of Willis anomalies, 193–94, 194*f*
clinical observation rule, 164
"Clinical Observations in Demented Patients," 244–45
cognition/behavior studies, 220–22
community life (of Miller), 4–5
computed tomography (CT), 143, 155n13, 162, 171, 180, 187–88
concussion amnesia, 219
confabulation, 239
congestive heart failure, 73
Congress of Neurological Surgeons presentations, 220, 221*f*, 247
consciousness, physiology of, 171
constancy of errors, 238–39
Countway Medical Library, 62n19

D-Day (Operation Overlord), 58–59
delayed ischemic deficit (DID), 187–88
dementia, 238–39
diabetes, 25–26
diagnosis, Fisher's rules of, 164–66, 167–68, 227
didactic talks, Fisher's rule of, 167

dieners, 125, 192–93
diphtheria, 25–26, 55, 101
disorientation for place, 235–36
"Disorientation for Place," 244–45
dizziness/vertigo, 209n16
Donnaconda, HMS, 26–27
Duke University, 96–98

education (of Fisher). *See also* Boston City Hospital; Montreal Neurological Institute; Toronto Medical School
　early years, 9–11, 10*f*
　German medical literature, 56, 62n19
　Henry Ford Hospital internship, 18–19
　languages, in Marlag/Milag, 56–57, 62n18
　psychology, Fisher's studies of, 47–48
　Royal Victoria Hospital, 72–75
　tropical medicine, 35
　vascular pathology, 142
EEG, 136, 171
empathy, Fisher's rules of, 168
endarterectomy, 120, 129n28
episodic global amnesia, 216–19, 230n20
Erb Street home, 6, 7*f*
ether anesthesia, 154n4
eye signs
　cerebral hemorrhage, 172–73, 186, 190n33
　Fisher's examination of, 232–35
　migraine, 227–29

Faulkner Hospital, 225
Festschrift celebration, 164
findings, Fisher's rules of presentation, 166
First United Church of Waterloo, 7
Fisher, C. Miller
　background generally, xv, 1
　birth, 3
　children, 42, 76, 108*f*
　daily routine, post-retirement, 244–46
　death, 251
　early years, 9–11
　family genealogy, 5*f*, 5–6
　health decline, 248–51
　marriage, 19, 27–28
　retirement, 243
Framingham Heart Study, 215
French Underground, 54–55

gait abnormalities, 202–8, 203f, 208f
Geneva Convention, 48, 52
giant cell arteritis, 234–35
gonorrhea, 15–16
Gripsholm, 60, 61f
Guillain-Barré syndrome, Fisher variant, 125, 235

Halifax Harbour, 28, 33–34
Hamburg, air strikes on, 58
Harrison's Principles of Internal Medicine, 198–200, 201f
Harvard Medical School, 85–86, 89, 133–34, 157–58
Harvey Cushing Society, 247
headache, 225–29, 226f, 236
hematomas, 183f, 183–85
hemorrhagic infarction, 101–2, 181–88, 183f, 187f, 190n33
Henry Ford Hospital, 18–19, 181
HMCS Stadaconna, Halifax, 67
hurricanes (plane), 31
hydrocephalus, 146, 162, 202–8, 203f, 208f, 211n29
hypertension, 178, 183–84, 189n16, 193
hypertensive encephalopathy, 77
hypothesis generation/sequential testing, 150–52, 164–65

imaging studies, 124, 143, 162, 171, 180
inhibitory seizures/ictal paralysis, 236–37
insertions of inobvious origin, 238–39
insistence, 238–39
insulin, 13, 14–15
"Intermittent Interruption of Behavior," 220
internal carotid artery occlusion. *See* carotid artery disease

Jacoby Award, American Neurological Association, 247
Japan, in WWII, 48

Kitchener, Ontario, Canada, 3–4

lability of temper, 238–39
lacunes, lacunar infarction, 120–21, 174–82, 175f, 176f, 177f, 178f, 237

late-life migraine, Fisher's experience of, 227–29
"Late-Life Migraine Accompaniments: Further Experiences," 244–45
lateral medullary syndrome, 225, 226f
Lazarett, 52–53
learning, Fisher's rule of, 167
Leopoldville, 28–30, 33
Letitia, HMS, 32–34
lipohyalinosis, 176–77, 178f, 180
listening, Fisher's rules of, 167
Lord Nelson Hotel, 28
low-sodium diets, 73

Marlag/Milag
    activities, 54–57, 62n18
    anti-Nazi Germans in, 54, 58
    camp economy, 51, 58
    cigarettes in camp economy, 51
    described, 42, 43f, 49–51
    educational activities, 56–57, 62n18
    ex-prisoners annual meetings, 60
    Fisher's transfer to, 49–51
    Jews/other prisoners, treatment of, 52–53
    living conditions, 51–52
    medical facilities, 51–52
    orchestra, 56
    radio/outside information access, 53–54
    Red Cross parcels, 56–57
    repatriation, 57–61
    sports, 54–55
    theater activity, 55–56
    work detail/thefts of items, 52
Mary Imogene Bassett Hospital, 157
Massachusetts General Hospital
    Baker Building, 134–35, 142
    brain cutting conferences, 142f, 142, 143f, 174
    Bullfinch Building, 133–34, 135f
    described, 133–35
    Ether Dome, 134–35, 135f, 154n4, 243
    Fisher Rounds, 244, 249–50
    Fisher's activities/methodology, 137–44
    Fisher's invitation to directorship, 126–27, 133
    George Robert White building, 134–35
    ICU, 158–59

Massachusetts General Hospital (*cont.*)
   neurology residency program/stroke fellows, 97, 143–44, 156–59
   neuromedical service, 84, 135–37
   neuropathology laboratory, under Fisher, 139–40
   pediatric neurology program, 157–58
   Phillips House, 134–35, 142
   residency training grants, 140–41
   stroke patient management, 143–44, 150–52
   Vincent Burnham Building, 157–58
McGill, James, 68
McGill Medical School, 13, 26–27, 68, 70, 72, 106–7, 113, 126
memoirs, Fisher's work on, 245, 251
memory function, 216–19
Mennonites, 3
Methodist Victoria University, 12
microaneurysms, 177
migraine, 225–29
Mihara Memorial Research Grant, 247
military service (of Fisher). *See also* POW (Miller as)
   casualty stations duty, 32
   entrance into, via Montreal, 25–26
   Leopoldville, 28–30, 33
   Letitia, HMS, 32–34
   London, landing in, 30–31
   Portsmouth, 31–32
   Royal Canadian Navy, 26–34, 27f, 29f
   tropical gear, 35
   Voltaire, HMS, 34f, 34–38, 42
Miller Fisher syndrome, 125, 235
Montreal Neurological Institute
   background, 68–69, 70–72, 71f, 84–85
   carotid arteries, postmortem studies of, 112–13
   Fisher as Neurology Registrar, 73–77
   Fisher's education in, 25–26, 73
   as Fisher's grant time choice, 67–68
   Fisher's return to, 106, 107f, 108f
   medical projects involvement, 76–77
   nervous system diseases, 69, 70–71, 77–78n5
   Penfield, 69–72, 78n6
   stroke, Fisher's study of, 106–7
Mosquito (plane), 57–58
motor impersistence, 222, 237
movement disorders, 136

MRI, 155n13, 162, 171, 180, 237
multiple sclerosis, 136
muscle disorders, 136
Mutual Life Insurance Company, 6–7
myasthenia gravis, 136
myocardial infarction, 147–48
myocardial infarction, Fisher's, 245–46

naming of symptoms/phenomena, 238–39
National Hospital for Neurology and Neurosurgery, 71–72, 78n6
National Institute of Neurological Diseases and Blindness, 223
National Institutes of Health (NIH), 140–41, 161, 223–24
Nazi atrocities, 40, 46, 52–53
nerve disorders, 136
Neuro, the. *See* Montreal Neurological Institute
Neurological Institute of New York, 71–72
neurology training programs, 133–34, 140–41, 150–54
New York Hospital–Cornell University, 223
nicknames, 160

"Occlusion of the Carotid Arteries: Further Experiences.," 118
"Occlusion of the Internal Carotid Artery," 113
one-and-a half syndrome, 233–34
ophthalmoplegia, 234
opinions/reviews, 237–38

Parkinson's disease, 136
Pasteur, Louis, 101, 109
patients as people, Fisher's rules of, 168
pattern matching, 227
Pearl Harbor attack, 48
personal computers, 146
personality traits
   acting, 162–63
   as author, 153–54
   as colleague, 156–59
   as collector, 125, 146, 161–62, 166, 192–93, 209n6, 228
   compulsiveness, 161–62
   customary daily routine, 141–42

forward looking/flexibility, 162
hypothesis generation/sequential
  testing, 150–52
as learner-student, 75–76,
  143, 145–48
metrics, love of, 26
money/practical matters, lack of
  concern for, 160–61
note-taking/documentation, 10f, 11,
  116, 159–60, 161–62, 167, 198,
  199, 201f
parenting style, 7–8
patriotism, 163–64
as people watcher, 146–48
perseverance, 206
as physician, 148–49
as speaker, 152
as teacher/mentor, 149f, 150–54
time, lack of concern for, 159–60
work ethic, 84, 107–9, 138
Peter Bent Brigham Hospital, 83, 133–34
photographs of Fisher
  as child, 8f
  Congress of Neurological
    Surgeons, 221f
  in high school, 16f, 17f
  later years, 248f, 249f, 250f
  in medical school, 18f
  at MGH, 135f, 137f, 138f, 139f, 142f,
    143f, 149f, 158f, 159f
  at MNI, 74f
  as POW, 34f, 50f, 61f
  as Surgeon Lieutenant, 27f, 29f
pneumoencephalogram, 202–4
postpartum illness, 84
post-stenotic dilatations, 177
postural hypotension, 77
POW (Miller as). See also military service
  (of Fisher)
  camp, trip to, 39–40
  cigarettes in camp market, 45–46
  eastern front maps, 47
  escape attempt, by other
    prisoners, 48–49
  German food ration, 44–45
  letters of notification to Doris, 42
    44f–46f
  Marlag (see Marlag/Milag)
  medical facilities, 47
  Nazi atrocities, 40, 46

poker club, 48
propagandists, 48
psychology, Fisher's studies of, 47–48
Red Cross parcels, 43–44
sanitary facilities, 47
Stalag XB, Sandbostel, 40–49, 41f, 55
Princeton Conference of Cerebrovascular
  Disease, 223
Principles of Internal Medicine,
  198–99, 210n20
propaganda leaflets, 58
psychogenic disorders, 163
publications by Fisher, 112–13, 118, 171–
  72, 220, 244–45
pulmonary embolism, 223
pupils, examination of, 233

Queen Mary/Queen Elizabeth, 28–29
Queen Mary Veterans' Hospital, 107–9
Queen Square, 71–72, 78n6

ramollissements, xiv–xv, xvin5
reaching out and holding and
  handling, 238–39
reductio ad absurdum, 165
reflex blepharospasm, 233–34
Reich Labour Service, 40–41
reversible cerebral vasoconstriction
  syndrome (RCVS), 236
reviews/opinions, 237–38
rheumatic heart disease, 215
rheumatoid arthritis, 73
Rockefeller Foundation, 70–71,
  84–87, 97
rounders (game), 59
Royal Victoria Hospital, 25–26, 69,
  72–75, 127
Rules (of Fisher), 164–68, 227
Russia, German invasion of, 48

salaries, of doctors/residents, 85–86,
  97–98, 109, 137–38, 161
Seagram Distillery, 4, 5–6
Seagram's VO, 4
segmental arterial disorganization,
  176–77, 178f
self-observation, 239
small branch artery disease, 174–81,
  175f, 176f, 177f, 178f, 179f
spitfires (plane), 31

Subject Index [263]

St. Anne's Hospital, 107–9
Stalag XB, Sandbostel, 40–49, 41f, 55
stroke
    characterization, xiii
    Fisher's brain damage studies, 101–3, 115–17, 118, 174
    Fisher's presentations of research, 117–18, 119–20, 153–54, 198, 205, 206–7, 215, 225–27, 228
    historically, xiv–xv
    lesion localization, 125–26, 150–51, 172–73, 174, 180, 233–34
    pathology, Fisher's emphasis on, 15
    patient management, 143–44, 150–52
    posterior cerebral artery, 216–17
    prevalence, xiii–xiv
    pure motor/pure sensory, 181
    sensory charts, 91, 92f
    symptoms, Fisher's research on, 109–13, 119
    as targeted medical condition, xiv
    TIAs, 109–20
stupor/coma, 170–73
subarachnoid hemorrhages, 186–88
subclavian steal syndrome, 198
submarine warfare (German), 29–30, 33, 87
substitution for the first-person pronoun, 238–39
sulfonamides, 15–16, 47
surgical exploration, 73–75
sympathectomy, in treating hypertension, 76–77
syringomyelia, 77

Teacher of the Year Prize, 247
temporal arteritis, 234–35
temporal lobe tumors, 73–75
"The 'Herald Hemiparesis' of Basilar Artery Occlusion," 244–45
"The Neurological Examination of the Comatose Patient," 171–72
Thor, sinking of *Voltaire* by, 35–38, 39
thorium dioxide, 127–28n9
thunderclap headache, 236
Toronto Medical School
    Anatomy curriculum, 14–15
    background, 12–13

Biology and Medicine (B&M) curriculum, 13–15
    Burwash Hall/student housing, 17
    clinical teaching, 15–16
    Fisher's education in, 13–16
    pathology/neuropathology, 15
    pharmaceutical agents, 15–16
    physics studies, 14
    scholarship award, 11
    sports, 17f, 17
    Straight Medicine curriculum, 13–14
Toronto University. *See* Toronto Medical School
Trans Canada Airlines, 27–28
transient global amnesia (TGA), 216–19, 230n20
transient ischemic attacks (TIAs), 109–20, 195–200, 196f, 197f, 223–25, 228
"Transient Monocular Blindness Associated with Hemiplegia," 112–13
tributes to Fisher, 243
Trinity College, 12
tuberculosis, 25–26, 51, 84, 96
Tufts Medical School, 85–86, 89, 133–34

"Unexplained Sudden Amnesia," 244–45
United States, stroke prevalence, xiv

vascular anatomy, xiv–xv, xvin5
ventricular span measurements, 207, 208f
verification, Fisher's rule of, 166
vertebral artery occlusion, 225
Victory, HMS, 32
"Visual Hallucinations and Racing Thoughts on Eye Closure After Minor Surgery," 244–45
Voltaire, HMS, 34f, 34–38, 42

washout hypothesis, 209n15
Waterloo, Ontario, Canada, 4–5, 9–11
whiplash amnesia, 219
Wilhelmshaven, air strikes on, 57–58
Wimpies, 47
Winchester Hospital, 141
World War II, 87. *See also* military service (of Fisher)

www.ingramcontent.com/pod-product-compliance
Ingram Content Group UK Ltd.
Pitfield, Milton Keynes, MK11 3LW, UK
UKHW021250180426
11946UKWH00003B/63